Excimer Lasers in Corneal Diseases and Refractive Disorders

Excimer Lasers in Corneal Diseases and Refractive Disorders

MANEESH KHOBA MD

Chief Medical Officer
Department of Ophthalmology
Vardhman Mahavir Medical College and
Safdarjang Hospital
New Delhi

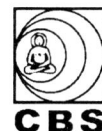

CBS PUBLISHERS & DISTRIBUTORS
NEW DELHI • BANGALORE

Excimer Lasers in Corneal Diseases and Refractive Disorders

First Edition : 2003

Copyright © Author & Publisher

ISBN : 81-239-0958-6

All rights reserved. No part of this book may be reproduced or transmitted in any form or by any means, electronic or mechanical, including photocopying, recording, or any information storage and retrieval system without permission, in writing, from the publisher.

Production Director : Vinod K. Jain

Published by :
Satish Kumar Jain for CBS Publishers & Distributors,
4596/1-A, 11 Darya Ganj, New Delhi - 110 002 (India)
E-mail : cbspubs@del3.vsnl.net.in
Website : http://www.cbspd.com

Branch Office :
Seema House, 2975, 17th Cross, K.R. Road,
Bansankari 2nd Stage, Bangalore - 560070
Fax : 080-6771680 • E-mail : cbsbng@vsnl.net

Printed at :
Asia Printograph, Shahdara, Delhi - 110032 (India)

to

all my patients, who have provided a constant stimulus for learning and challenge to seek new vistas in the horizon of medical sciences

and

my family, which has stood by me throughout the struggle for excelling in the medical field and my continuous endeavor for seeking the latest in the field of ophthalmology

Foreword

It gives me an immense pleasure to write the foreword of the book *Excimer Lasers in Corneal Diseases and Refractive Disorders* authored by Dr. Maneesh Khoba working in the department of ophthalmology of Vardhman Mahavir Medical College and Safdarjang Hospital, New Delhi. Dr. Khoba is a dedicated academician, keeping abreast with every development in subject of ophthalmology.

Subject of laser is fascinating to every one, scientists or laymen. Excimer lasers in ophthalmology have materialized as a big boon for ones who want to get rid of glasses and the ones who suffer from corneal blindness that can be possibly treated with excimer lasers.

This book covers different lasers. It gives an excellent account of lasers used in ophthalmology, in particular, excimer lasers and deals with their different applications in ophthalmology.

I commend the work of the author, which would be a tremendous help to practising as well as budding ophthalmologists.

Dr. K.P.S. Malik DOMS, MS, MNAMS, FICS
Consultant and Head, Department of Ophthalmology
Vardhman Mahavir Medical College and Safdarjang Hospital
New Delhi

Preface

The role of lasers in ophthalmology is tremendous and their applications in ophthalmological practice are well established. Lasers have now become indispensable treatment modalities in almost every field of ophthalmology, be it vitreoretinal diseases, glaucoma, ocular tumors, oculoplasty or corneal diseases and refractive disorders. Laser technologies have taken a quantum leap during the last two decades with the advent of excimer lasers and erbium: YAG laser. These lasers have completely changed the concepts of corneal, vitreoretinal and cataract surgeries; and opened new vistas, hitherto unimaginable, in these fields. Erbium: YAG laser has proved to be an excellent surgical tool for cataract and vitreoretinal surgeries.

The excimer laser corneal surgeries (refractive and phototherapeutic) are a great technological advancement. The excimer laser corneal surgeries for refractive corrections are common subject matter for the medical fraternity as well as for general public. But its application for treatment of corneal diseases is not a very familiar topic, even for many ophthalmologists. Phototherapeutic keratectomy (PTK) is a newer technique. It utilizes ArF excimer laser for treating a wide range of superficial corneal diseases. PTK is an effective and safe method in comparison to superficial keratectomy and penetrating keratoplasty, yet it is still to become popular among the excimer laser surgeons. The reasons are lack of familiarity and experience about this treatment modality. Growing commercialism is another impediment for this technique as majority of excimer laser corneal surgeries are performed for refractive corrections. PTK-induced refractive changes, mainly hyperopic shift, are common excuses offered by some surgeons. Proper strategies, improved techniques and good postoperative care can reduce the postrefractive changes and achieve very good visual results, as has been obtained by the author. This issue has been discussed in great details in this book.

Excimer laser refractive procedures have almost completely replaced other refractive surgeries. They have proved to be superior in terms of efficacy, predictability and safety in comparison to other conventional surgeries in this field. Like any other procedure, the excimer laser surgeries also have taken some time to come out from the gestation period, evolve, mature and get established. The development and refinement is still continuing due to a natural quest for achieving the best possible results. As a result of this ongoing development, we have witnessed in recent times newer technologies like customized-LASIK and LASEK to attain the maximum possible efficacy with least complications. The latest technological advancements in excimer laser refractive procedure have offered excellent results with maximum safety. Customized LASIK has been able to provide uncorrected visual acuity greater than 6/6 in may patients. It has converted the dream of having super-vision into reality.

The role of excimer laser refractive surgeries has been considered to be a cosmetic one by the medical fraternity and even by many ophthalmologists. This misconception would change if one realizes the plight of an ammetrope, whose refractive error is a handicap even in locating the spectacles. Dependence on the corrective lenses may become an impediment for routine activities. The other misconceptions are about the safety and complications of excimer laser refractive surgeries. Complications are bound to occur with any surgery. Even use of high power spectacles has many disadvantages of different magnitude. Contact lenses have their own limitations and complications. The complication rate with excimer laser refractive procedures, using the latest know-how and technology along with appropriate case selection is low in skillful hands. In fact, these procedures are the safest among all other conventional refractive surgeries. This book analyses these issues in depth. This would be appreciated as the reader goes through the relevant chapters.

Maneesh Khoba MD
January 2003

Acknowledgement

I am indebted to all my teachers, who have been a constant guiding force throughout my learning at AIIMS.

I express my special gratitude to Professor HK Tiwari, who had not only taught retina but also helped me on occasions of great distress, which no one else than myself would know. I am thankful to Professor VK Dada and Professor Rasik B. Vajpayee, who had been excellent teachers, able guides and above all good human beings throughout the period of my learning of ophthalmology and in particular excimer laser surgeries and cornea at Dr. Rajender Prasad Center for Ophthalmic Sciences, All India Institute of Medical Sciences, New Delhi. It had been a great privilege and my luck to work under their guidance.

I am thankful to my elder son Siddhartha, who had been a great moral support and younger son Nitin, who has provided excellent technical support for computer graphics, writing and giving shape to this book.

Words would not suffice to express my feelings towards Dr. K.P.S. Malik. He has been more of a friend and well-wisher than a senior and Head of the Department for me, throughout my stay in the Department of Ophthalmology at Safdarjang Hospital. He is a great person and academician. He is a big source of inspiration for all of us in the department. He provides all support and encouragement for any one striving to improve the academics in the department.

Maneesh Khoba

Contents

Foreword vii
Preface ix

Introduction 1

SECTION I

1. **Laser Terms, Definitions and Laser System** 7
   Laser terms, definitions 7
   Laser system 9
   Modes of laser delivery 11

2. **Frequency Conversion: Solid State Excimer Lasers** 13
   What is frequency conversion? 13
   How it works? 13
   Clinical applications of frequency conversion 15

3. **Effect of Different Lasers on the Ocular Tissues** 16
   Photothermal effects 16
   Photocoagulation 16
   Delivery system for laser photocoagulation 17
   Photothermal tissue shrinkage 17
   Photodisruption/optical breakdown 18
   Photovaporization/photothermal ablation 19
   Photochemical effe 19
   Natural occurring photochemical reactions 19
   Ablative photodecomposition 20
   Photodynamic effect 20
   Transpupillary thermotherapy 20

SECTION II

4. **Excimer Lasers: History** 27
   Excimer laser parameters and definitions 29

5. **Response of the Ablated Cornea to Excimer Laser** 32
   Collateral damage and thermal effect 32
   Formation of pseudomembrane 32
   Epithelial response 33
   Factors governing the epithelial healing response 33
   Adherence of newly formed epithelium to the stroma 33
   Bowman's layer response 33
   Stromal response and corneal haze 33
   Descemet's membrane response 34
   Endothelial response 34
   Corneal sensitivity 35

6. **Hazards of the Excimer Laser Radiations** 37
   Risk to the lens and phototoxicity 37
   Absorption vs. transmission of laser 37
   Scattering of the laser into the tissue 37
   Secondary fluorescence 38
   Integrity of the cornea 38
   Susceptibility to traumatic rupture 38
   Corneal ectasia 38
   Causes of corneal ectasia and forward shift of corneal curvature 40
   Predisposition to develop corneal ectasia 40
   Evaluation of central corneal thickness 40
   Methods of evaluating central corneal thickness: Optical vs. ultrasonic 40
   Variables affecting corneal thickness measurements 40
   Retinal detachment 41
   Damage to cornea by free-radicals 42
   Photokeratitis 42
   Mutagenesis 42
   Shock waves and surface waves 42

Acoustic shock waves 42
Surface waves 42
Surface heating 42

7. Excimer Laser Delivery Systems 45
Excimer laser system 45
Maintenance of the lasing medium 47
Calibration of laser energy 47
Excimer laser beam characteristics 47
Large/wide beam laser system 47
Disadvantages of large beam laser systems 49
Advantages of large beam laser systems 49
Homogenization/smoothening of large beam 49
Scanning laser systems 50
Advantages of large beam laser systems 51
Disadvantages of large beam laser systems 51

SECTION III

8. Corneal Anatomy and Physiology 55
Corneal curvature 55
Regular astigmatism 55
Irregular astigmatism 56
Apical/corneal cap or apical zone 56
Radius of curvature of the apical zone 56
Structure of the cornea 56
Functions of the epithelium 56
Regeneration of epithelial cells 57
Corneal stroma 57
Transparency of the cornea 58
Endothelium 59
Endothelial pump 59
Corneal physiology 59
Corneal metabolism 59
Corneal hypoxia 59
Maintenance of corneal thickness 60
Forces causing stromal turgescence 60
Forces causing stromal deturgescence 60

9. Corneal Degenerations and Dystrophies 62
Introduction 62
Corneal degenerations 62
Age-related degenerations 63
Corneal degenerations not caused by aging 65

Corneal dystrophies 69
Epithelial and Bowman's layer dystrophies 70
Anterior stromal dystrophies 71
Mid-stromal dystrophy 71
Posterior stromal dystrophy 73
Panstromal dystrophy 73
Endothelial dystrophy 73
Drawbacks of present treatment modalities for corneal diseases 76

SECTION IV

10. Refractive Surgical Procedures 81
Emmetropia 81
Ammetropia 81
Factors that decide the future of a refractive surgery 83
Thermokeratoplasty 83
The thermomechanical behaviour of cornea 83
Radial thermokeratoplasty (TKP) 83
Laser thermokeratoplasty (LTK) 84
LTK for hyperopic astigmatism 85
Lamellar corneal surgeries 86
Mechanical keratomileusis 85
Automated lamellar keratoplasty (ALK) 87
Epikeratophakia 88
Keratophakia 88
Synthetic implants 89
Intrastromal corneal ring segments (ICRS)/ INTACS 90
Incisional surgeries 91
Radial keratotomy (RK) 91
Factors influencing the outcome and predictability of RK 92
Astigmatic keratotomy 96
Combined radial and astigmatic keratotomy 96
Post-surgical astigmatism correction 96
Hexagonal keratotomy for hypermetropia 98
Holmium: YAG laser LTK for hyperopic astigmatism 98
Intraocular procedures 99
Clear lens extraction 99
Phakic intraocular lenses 99
Keratorefractive procedures with excimer and other lasers 101

SECTION V

11. Phototherapeutic Keratectomy: Advantages and Indications — 107

Introduction 107
Advantages of excimer laser surgeries 107
Limitations of excimer laser surgeries 108
Review of PTK literature 108

12. PTK: Preoperative Evaluation — 114

Assessment of the corneal pathology 114
  Depth of lesion: vertical distribution 113
  Horizontal distribution of the lesion 115
  Type of pathology 115
  Corneal sensation 115
  Corneal vascularization 116
  Corneal thinning 116
Recognition of absolute and relative contraindications 116
Understanding the functional needs and expectations of patients 116
Preoperative refractive error of the patient 117
Evaluation of risks and benefits to the patient 117
Preoperative intraocular pressure 117

13. PTK and PRK: Pretreatment of the Surface — 118

Pretreatment for PRK procedures 118
Pretreatment for PTK procedures 119

14. PTK: Treatment Strategies — 121

Treatment of irregular surface 121
  Masking agents/wetting agents/coupling fluids 122
  Comparison of different masking agents 122
PTK: Ablation techniques 123
  Large area photoablation 124
  Point and shoot technique 124
  Standard taper technique 124
  Modified taper technique 124
  Smoothening technique 124
  Overlapping zone vs. single zone ablation 124
  Polishing technique 125
Manual superficial keratectomy combined with large area PTK 125
Focal laser smoothening 125
Basement membrane ablation 125
Pancorneal ablation 126

15. PTK: The Operative Procedure — 128

Preoperative considerations 128
Intraoperative considerations 128

16. Corneal Surface Ablation: Postoperative Managemet — 132

Postoperative pain 132
Epitelization of the ablative surface 133
Postoperative inflammation and corneal haze 134
Prophylaxis against infectious keratitis 135
Minimizing the undesirable refractive changes 135
Topical anaesthetics 135

17. Results of PTK Studies — 137

18. Non-surgical Methods of Refractive Corrections — 151

Use of spectacle lenses 151
  General problems with spectacles 151
  Problems with the use of high-power glasses 152
  Problems in cases of astigmatism 152
  Problems in cases of anisometropia 152
Use of contact lenses 153
  Limitation of contact lenses 153
  Complications of contact lenses 153

19. Photorefractive Surgeries: Indications and Patient Evaluation — 158

Why photorefractive surgery? 158
Advantages of photorefractive procedures 159
Aim of the photorefractive surgery 159
Range of refractive corrections 160
Preoperative evaluation for photorefractive surgeries 161
  Education of the patient and informed consent 162
Patient's history 162
  Assessment of parameters concerning or affecting refractive ablation 163
  Computerized videokeratography (CVK) 166

Contraindications vs. patient's suitability:
    The final decision   171

20. Photorefractive Keratectomy: PRK — 174

History of photorefractive keratectomy   174
PRK: Definition   175
PRK: Ablation techniques   175
   Mechanical iris diaphragm   175
   *Rotating wheel with different
      apertures*   175
   A moving slit   176
   *Combination of "parallel blade shutter"
      with an expanding aperture*   176
   An ablatable mask (PMMA)   176
PRK: Techniques for myopia   176
   Single zone/transition zone ablation   176
   Multipass ablation   177
   Multizone technique   177
   Tapered transition zone ablation   179
Ablation techniques for astigmatism   179
   *"Parallel blade shutter" with an expanding
      iris aperture*   180
   Hourglass shaped rotating mask   180
Ablation techniques for hyperopia   180
   An ablatable mask   181
   Ablatable mask with an Axicon lens   181
   Non-ablatable mask   181
   A rotating small circular beam   182

21. Laser in-situ Keratomileusis: LASIK — 184

What is laser in-situ keratomileusis
   (LASIK)   184
History of laser in-situ keratomileusis   184
Advantages of LASIK   185
Limitations of LASIK surgery   185
LASIK instrumentation   185
Microkeratomes   185
   Mechanical microkeratomes   186
   *The hydrokeratomes/water-jet
      microkeratomes*   188
   Laser microkeratomes   189

22. Customized LASIK/C-LASIK and Wavefront-guided LASIK — 190

Introduction   190
Optical defects of the eye   190
Natural mechanisms to decrease optical
   aberrations   191

Customised LASIK or C-LASIK   192
Wavefront-guided LASIK   192
   *Methods of measuring optical
      aberrations*   194
   Laser ablation   194
   *Limitations of wavefront-guided
      LASIK*   195

23. Photorefractive Surgeries: The Operative Procedure — 196

Preoperative preparations   196
PRK: Surgical procedure   197
PRK: Postoperative instructions   198
LASIK: Surgical procedure   198
Postoperative management following
   LASIK   202

24. Laser-Assisted Subepithelial Keratectomy: LASEK — 205

Definition and history   205
LASEK vs. PRK   205
LASEK vs. LASIK   206
LASEK: The operative procedure   207
Postoperative care   208
Intraoperative and postoperative
   complications   208

25. Excimer Laser Surgeries: Results — 212

Results of PTK   212
Results of PRK   213
Results of LASIK   216
PRK vs. LASIK   216
Astigmatic correction with LASIK   217
Hyperopic correction with LASIK   219
Results of customized ablation and LASEK   219
   Customized LASIK   220
   Customized PRK   220
   LASEK   220

26. Complications of Excimer Laser Surgeries — 225

Excimer laser ablation: Intraoperative
   complications   227
   Intraoperative laser failure   227
   Decentration of ablation zone   227
   Inappropriate ablation   229
   *Inadequate/irregular removal of the
      epithelium*   229

Excimer laser ablation: Transient
    complications   229
    Lid swelling and ptosis   229
    Complication of topical medications   229
Excimer laser ablation: Immediate postoperative
    complications   230
    Pain   230
    Delayed epithelial healing   230
    Sterile corneal infiltrates   231
    Microbial keratitis   232
    *Reactivation of herpes simplex
        keratitis*   233
Excimer Laser ablation: Intermediate to long
    term complications   233
    Corneal haze   233
    *Steroid induced rise of intraocular
        pressure*   234
    Corneal hypoesthesia   235
    Corneal scarring   235
Complications after PTK   235
    Corneal haze   235
    *Reactivation of herpes simplex
        keratitis*   235
    PTK induced refractive changes   236
    *Recurrence of corneal dystrophies and
        degenerations*   237
Intermediate to long term complications after
    photorefractive surgeries   238
    Overcorrection and undercorrection   238
    Induced/residual astigmatism   239
    Central steep islands   240
    Decrease in visual functions   241
    *Glare, halos with or without starburst and
        ghost images*   243
    Regression   243
    *Recurrent corneal erosion/microerosions and
        dry eye*   246
Intraoperative complications of LASIK   246
    Inadequate exposure   246

Inadequate suction   247
Incomplete pass/incomplete flap   247
*Thin flaps/irregular flaps and
    buttonholes*   248
Free cap   249
Corneal perforation   249
*Intraoperatively shifted/wrinkled
    flaps*   250
*Shifted/wrinkled flaps during initial
    days*   250
Interface debris   251
Diffuse lamellar keratitis   251
Epithelial implantation and ingrowth   253
LASIK- induced optic neuropathy   255
Stromal melts   256
*LASIK- induced corneal ectasia/
    keratectasia*   256

27. Management of Refractive Complications: Conservative and Reoperations   265

Medical Management   265
Other Modalities   266
    Contact lenses   266
    Epithelial Debridement   266
Reoperations   266
    Simple reoperations   266
    Mixed reoperations   266
    Enhancements   266
    Retreatments   266
Planning reoperations   266
Choice of surgical procedure   268
Reoperations following PRK   269
Reoperations following LASIK   269
Retreatment of central steep islands   270
Retreatment of corneal haze   270
Retreatment for decentration   271
Special problems for retreatment of decentered
    ablation following LASIK   271

Index   273

COLOUR PLATE 1

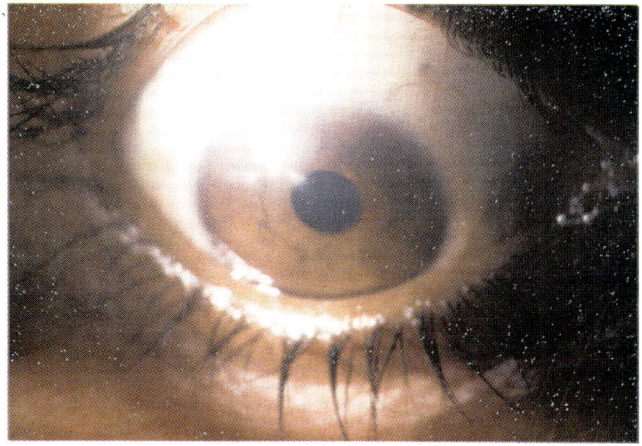

Photograph 1: Salzmann's nodules coming up to the pupillary margin

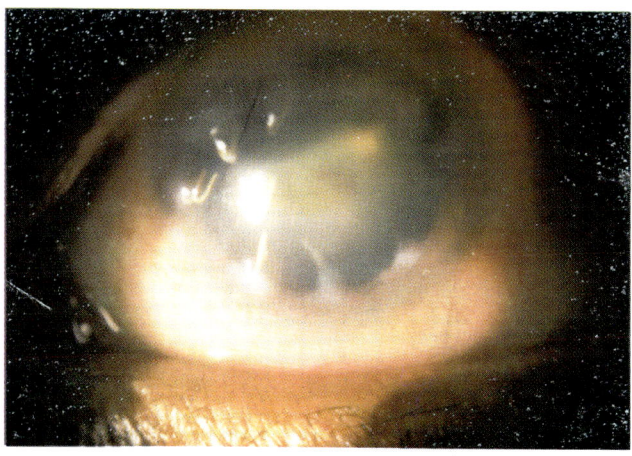

Photograph 2: Extensive Salzmann's nodules in mid periphery

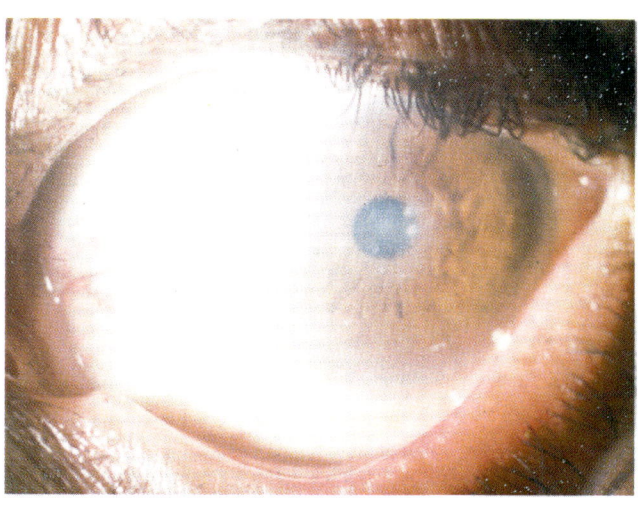

Photograph 3: Three small Salzmann's nodules within the pupillary area

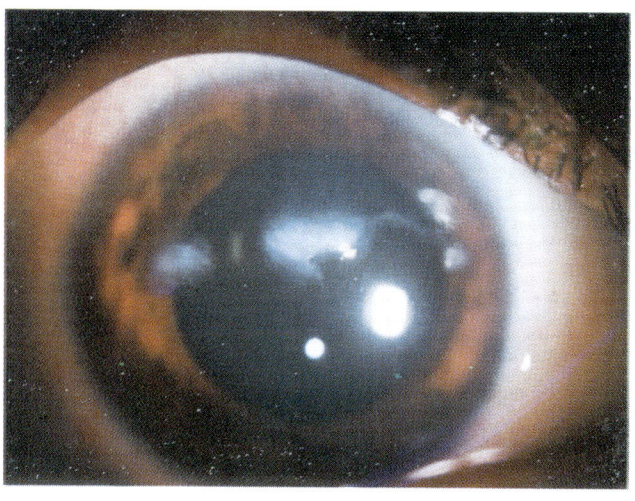

Photograph 4: Big Salzmann's nodules coming into the visual axis

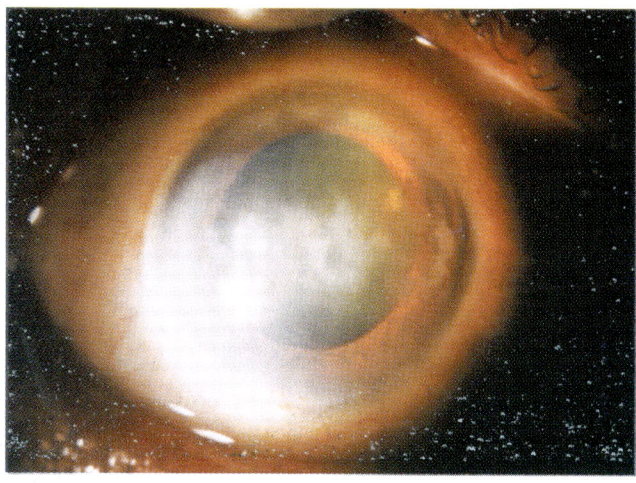

Photograph 5: Band-shaped keratopathy: Rough band

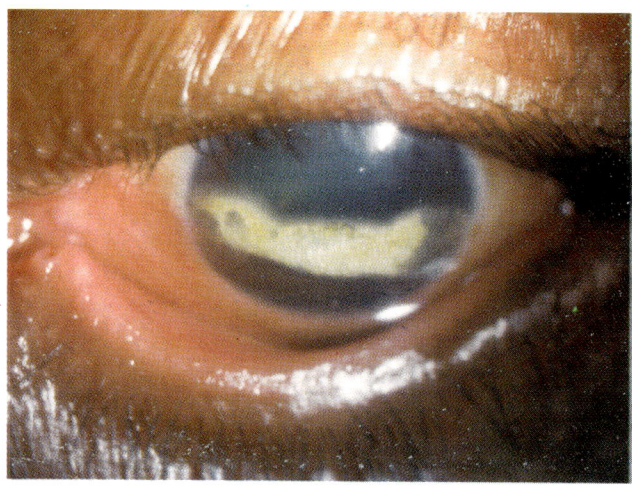

Photograph 6: Band-shaped keratopathy: Thick rough band

COLOUR PLATE 2

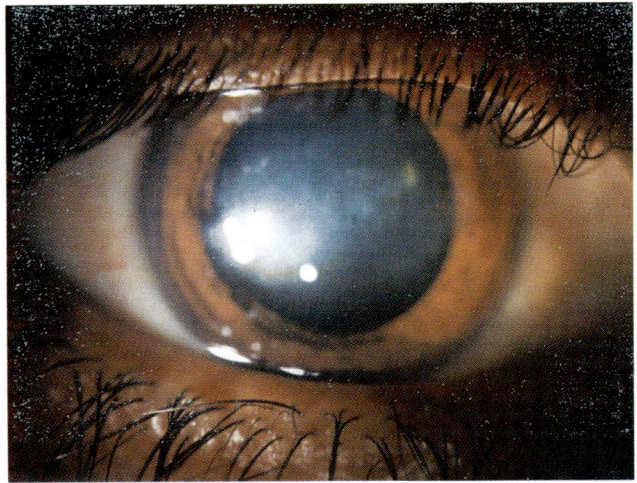

Photograph 7: Band-shaped keratopathy: Smooth band

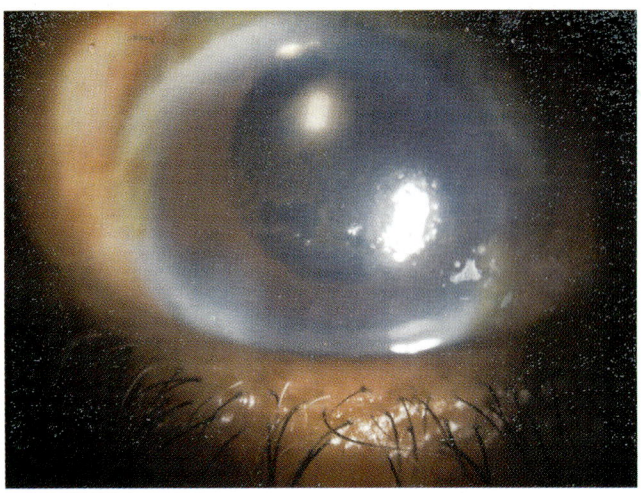

Photograph 8: Spheroidal degeneration grade III

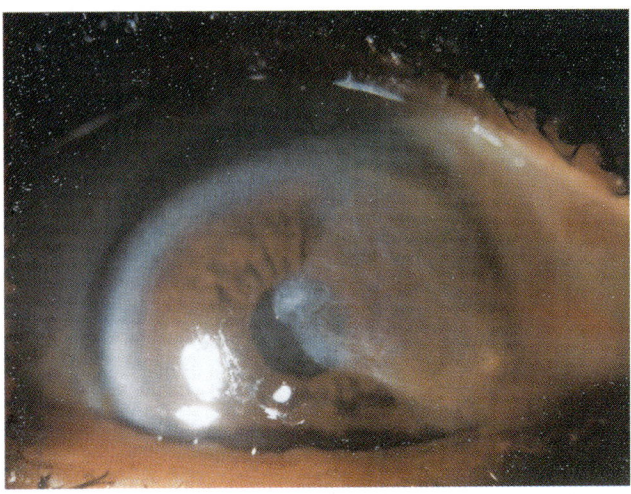

Photograph 9: Pterygium encroaching upon the visual axis

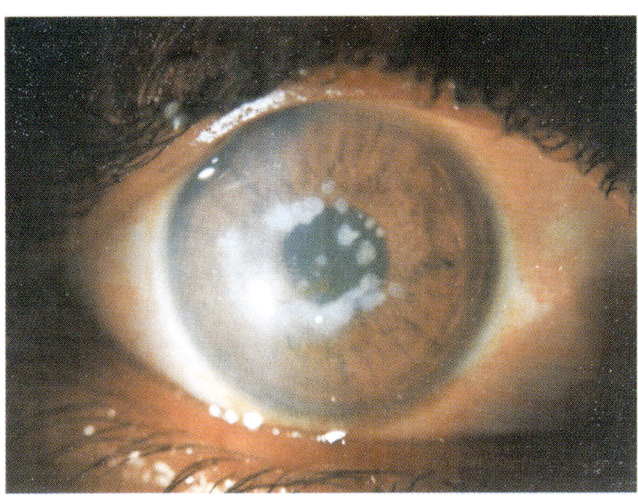

Photograph 10: Granular dystrophy type II: Disk-like opacities with clear cornea between the lesions

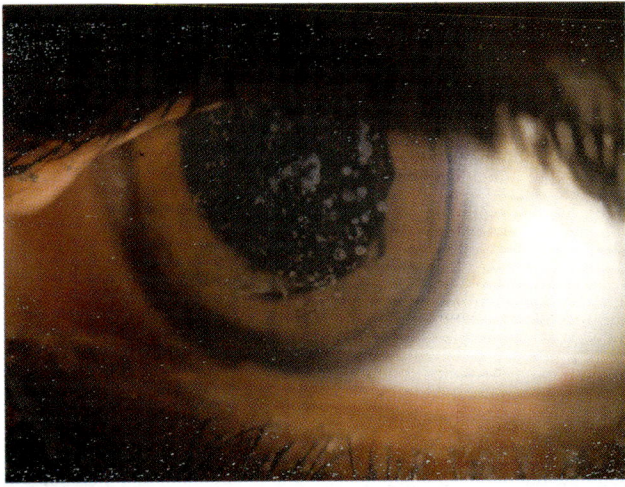

Photograph 11: Granular dystrophy type I: Small crumb-like lesions with ground-glass haze appearing between them

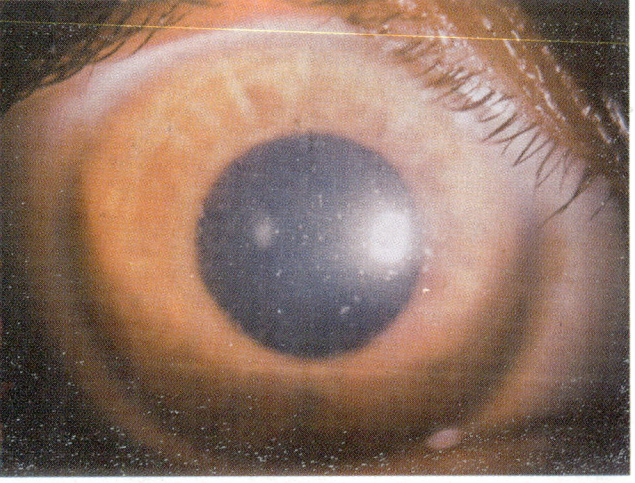

Photograph 12: Epithelial basement membrane dystrophy with dot-like opacities and recurrent corneal erosion syndrome

COLOUR PLATE 3

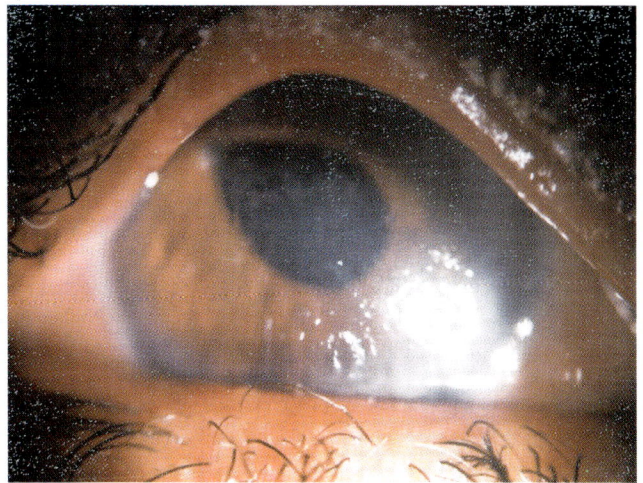

Photograph 13: Post-traumatic recurrent corneal erosions with nebular opacities after cataract surgery

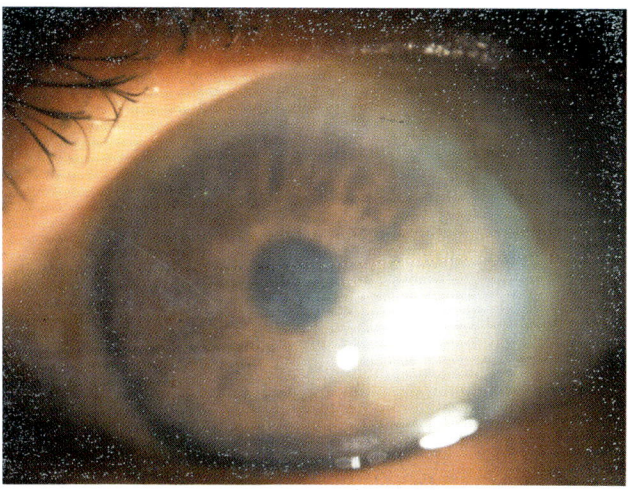

Photograph 14: Reis-Bucklers' dystrophy with recurrent corneal erosion syndrome

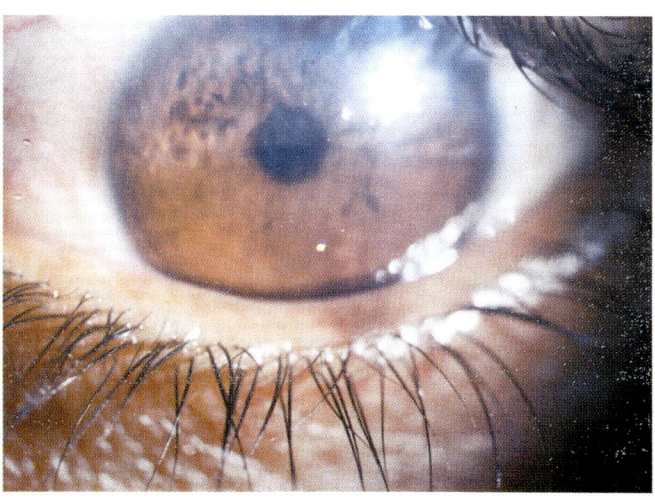

Photograph 15: Another case of post-traumatic recurrent corneal erosions with opacities in the pupillary area

COLOUR PLATE 4

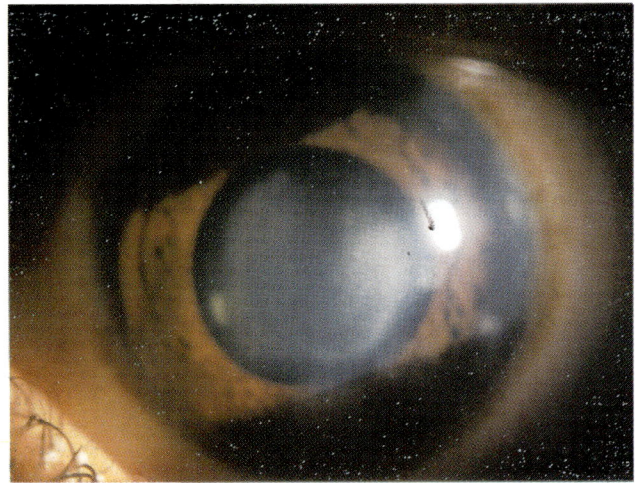

Photograph 16: Corneal opacity in a 26-year old patient

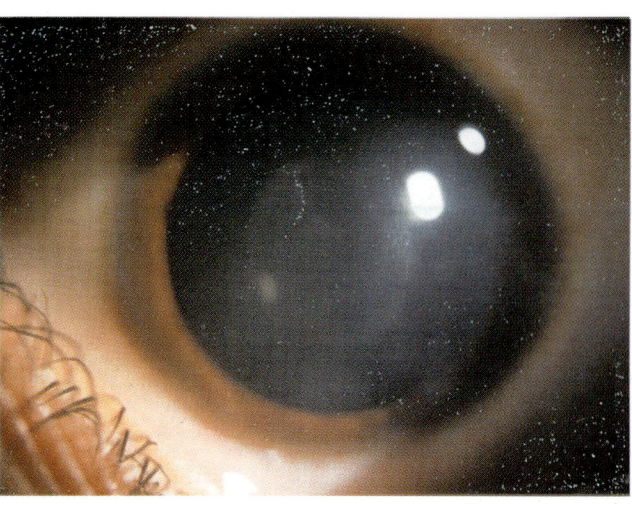

Photograph 17: Same eye as in photograph 16, one month after PTK

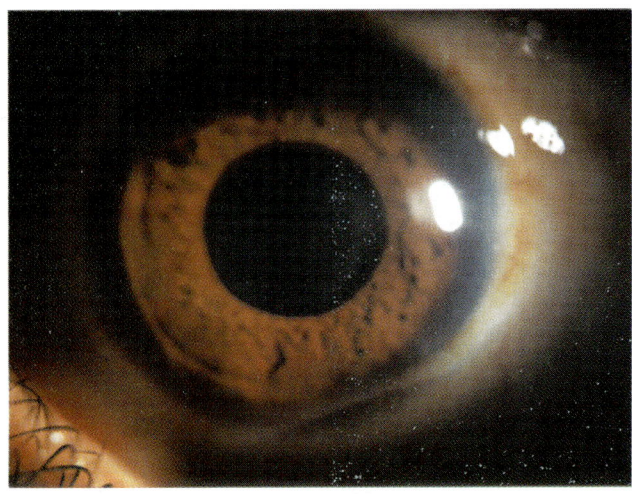

Photograph 18: Same eye as in photograph 16, six months after PTK

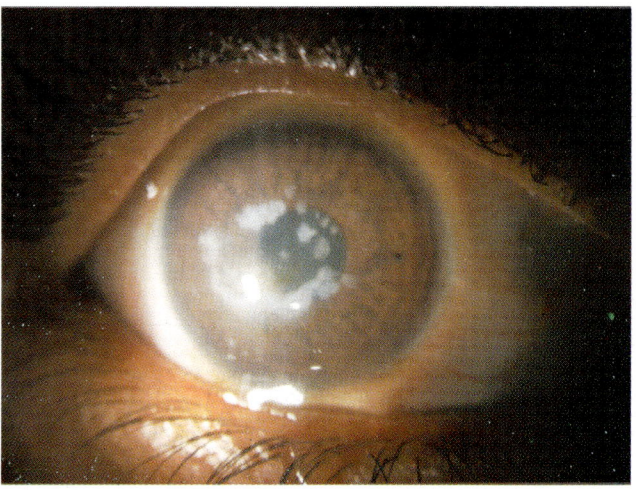

Photograph 19: A case of granular dystrophy with recurrent corneal erosions

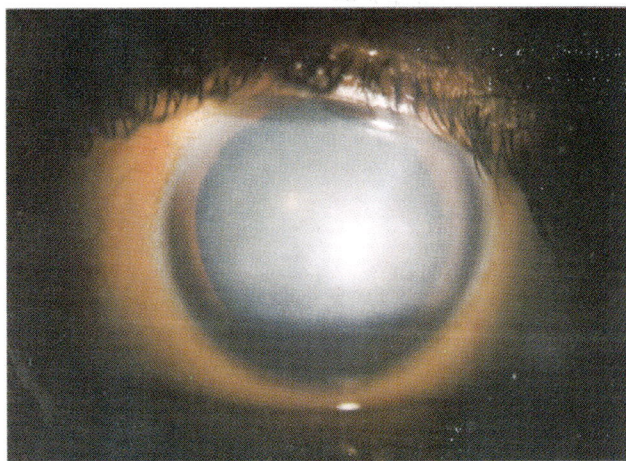

Photograph 20: Same eye as in photograph 19 after 1 month of PTK: Note the corneal haze

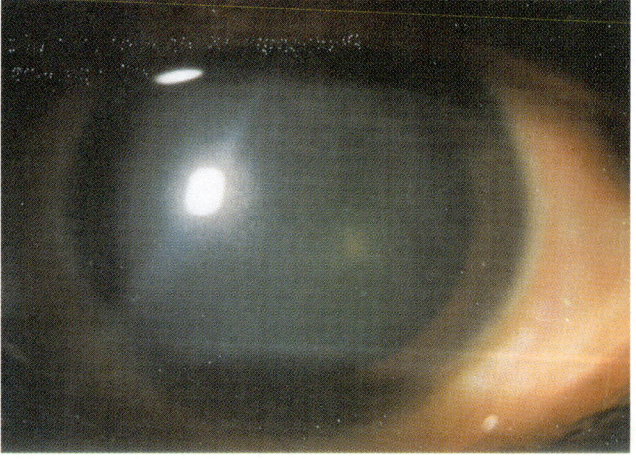

Photograph 21: Six months after PTK the corneal haze has cleared sufficiently to allow good visual acuity

COLOUR PLATE 5

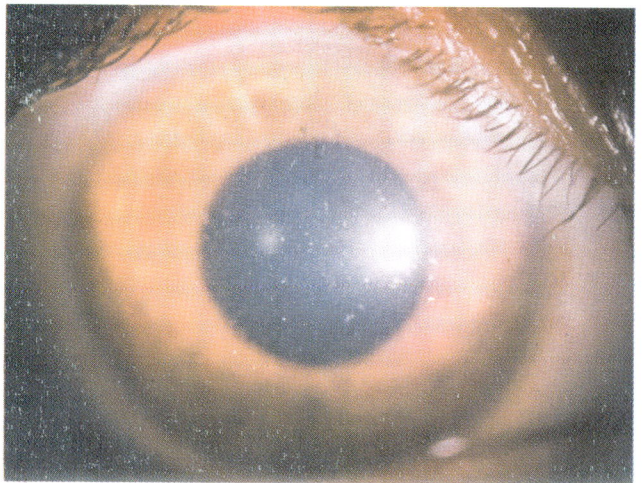

Photograph 22: Case of bilateral recurrent corneal erosion syndrome secondary to epithelial basement membrane dystrophy

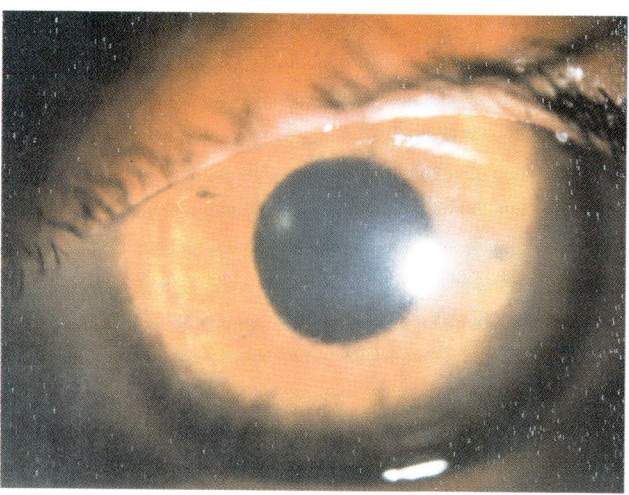

Photograph 23: Same eye six months after PTK

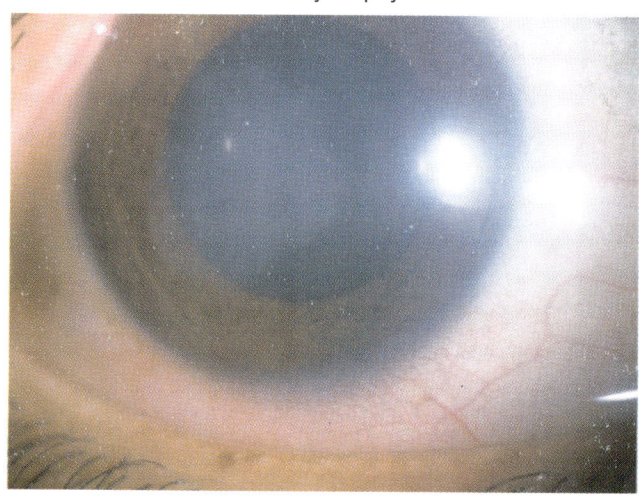

Photograph 24: Case of corneal opacity in an 18-year old boy

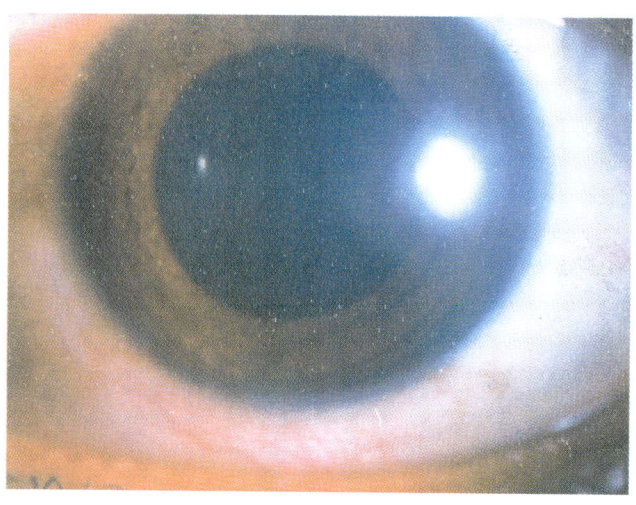

Photograph 25: Same eye three months after PTK

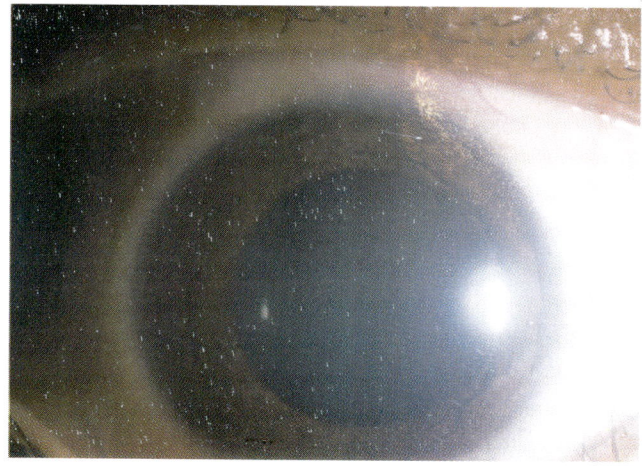

Photograph 26: Same eye as show in photograph 24 six months after PTK

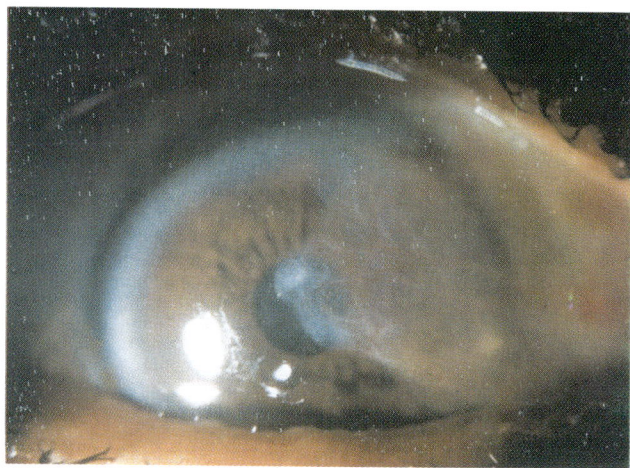

Photograph 27: A case of pterygium in 55-year old patient

COLOUR PLATE 6

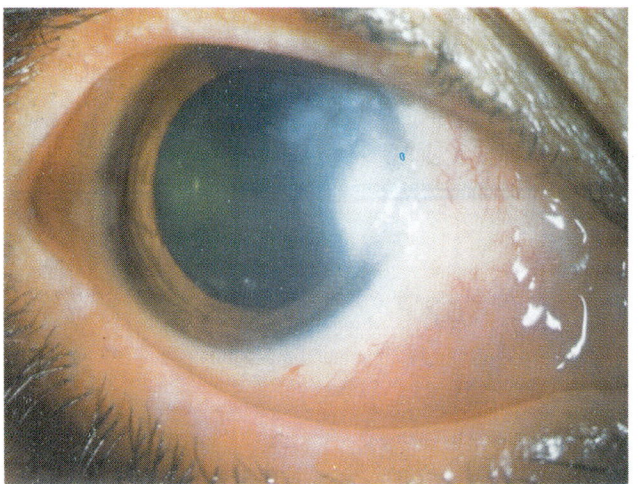
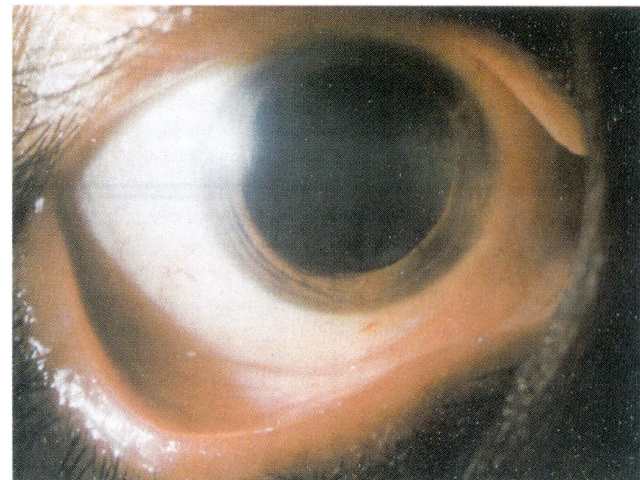

Photographs 28 and 29: Show the same eye as in photograph 27 after 1 week and 6 months of PTK

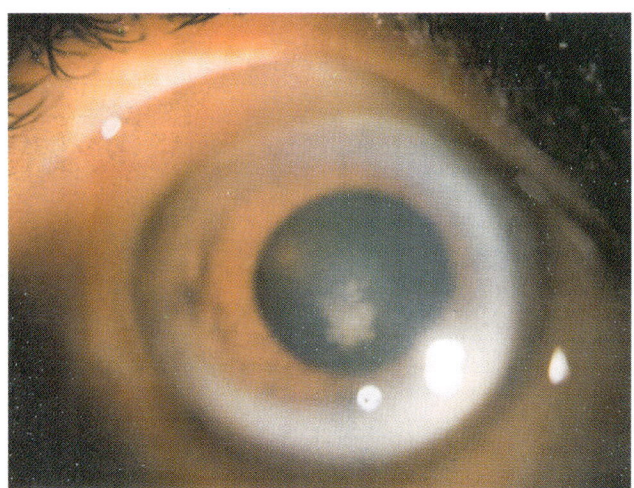

Photograph 30: Case of corneal opacity in the pupillary

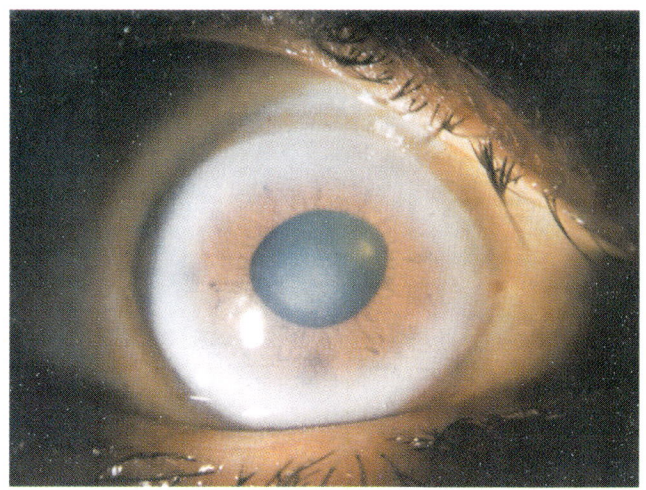

Photograph 31: Same eye as shown in photograph 30 one month after PTK

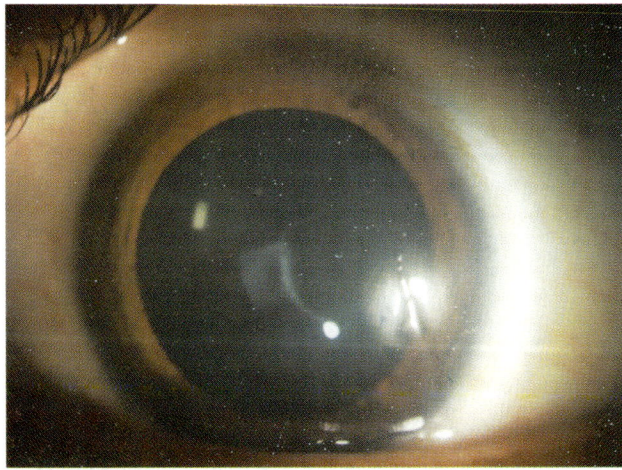

Photograph 32: Another case of corneal opacity in the pupillary area

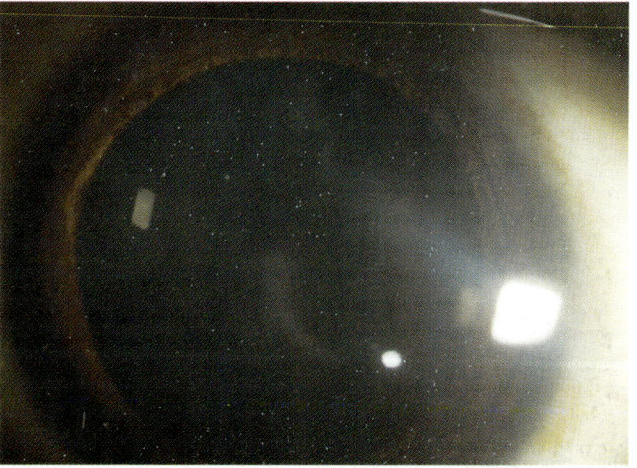

Photograph 33: Same eye three month after PTK. Note the residual opacity

COLOUR PLATE 7

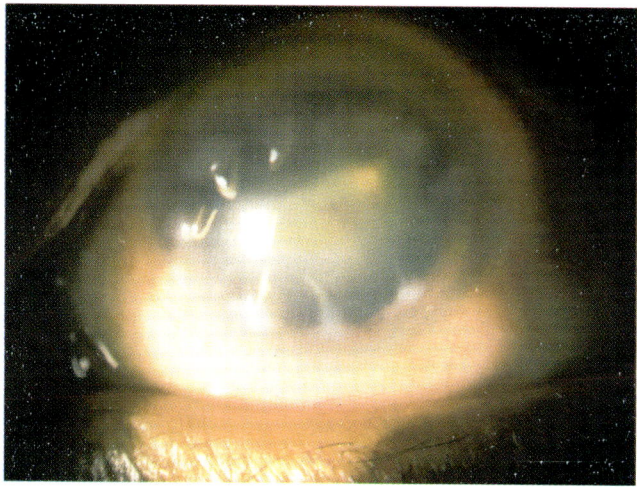
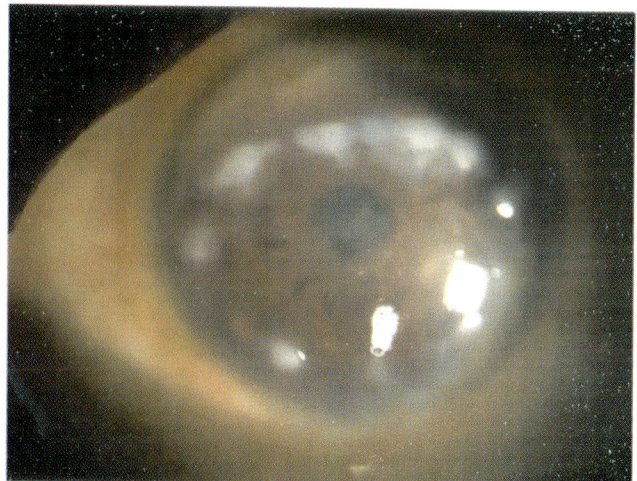

Photographs 34 and 35: Case of Salzmann's nodular degeneration with bad ocular surface

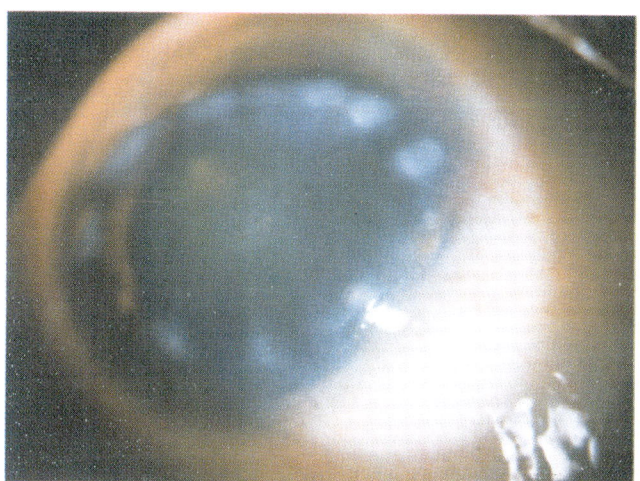

Photograph 36: Same eye as in photographs 34 and 35 three month after PTK.

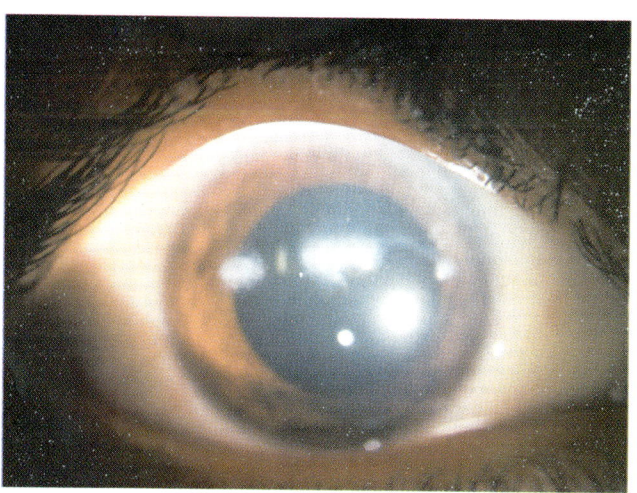

Photograph 37: Another case of Salzmann's nodular degeneration. Note that only the central, optical zone has been treated

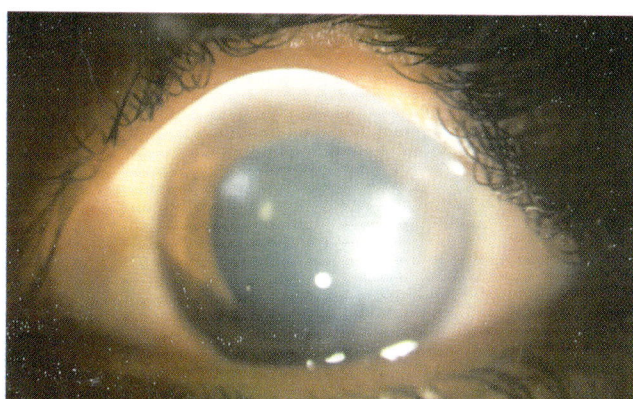

Photograph 38: Same eye as in photograph 37 three month after PTK showing corneal haze. Only the central six mm optical zone has been treated leaving lesion in the mid periphery

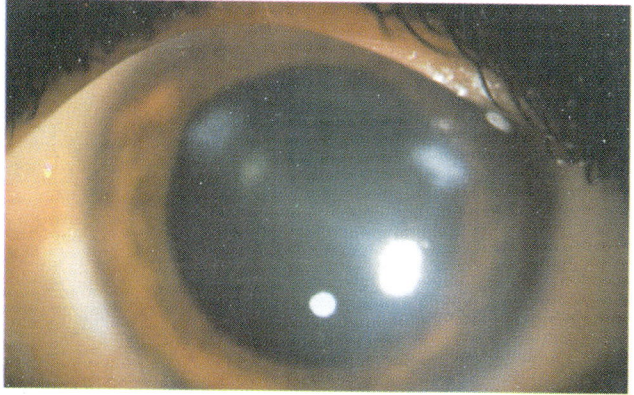

Photograph 39: Same eye as in photograph 38 showing clearing of the haze at six month

COLOUR PLATE 8

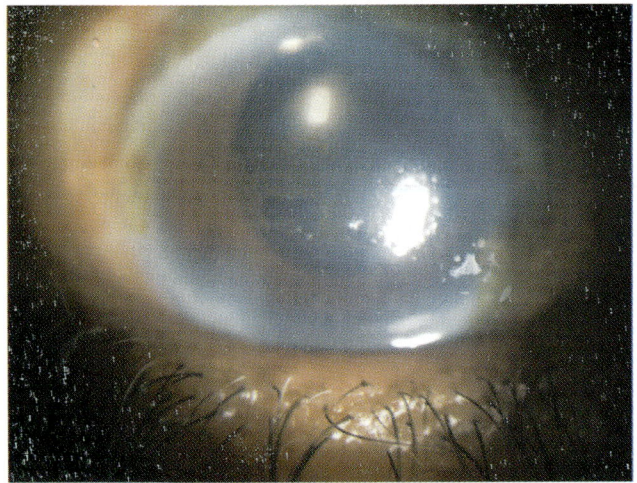

Photograph 40: Case of spheroidal degeneration with bad ocular surface

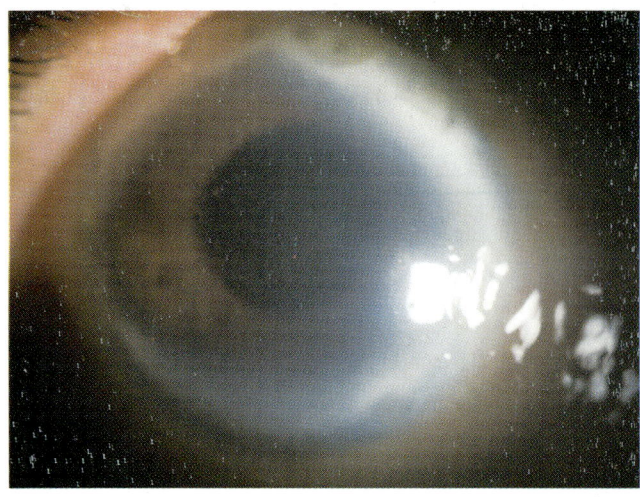

Photograph 41: Same eye as in photograph 40 showing one month after PTK

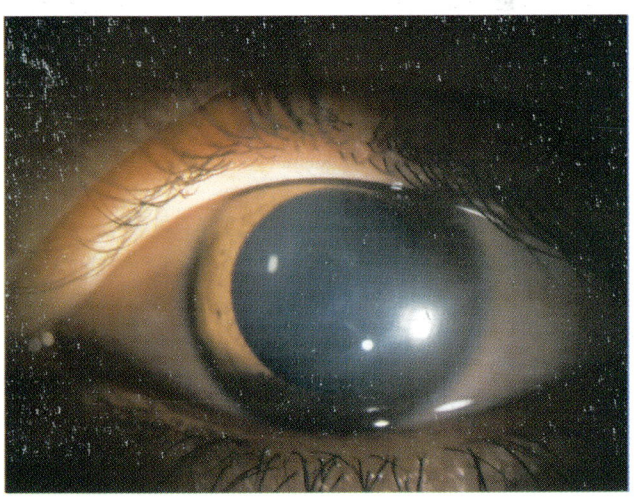

Photograph 42: Case of superficial corneal opacity post-herpetic keratitis

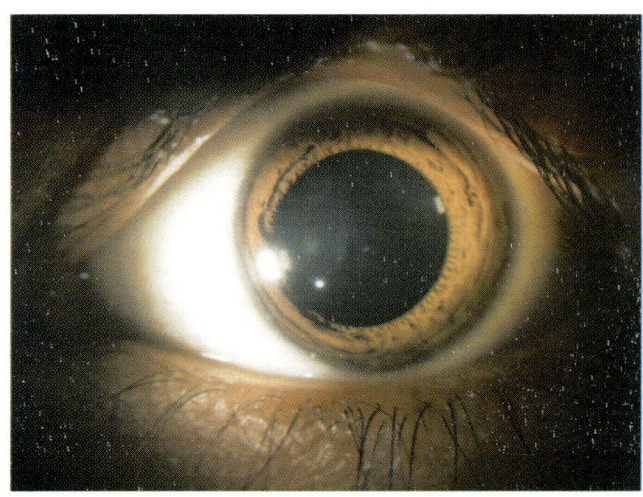

Photograph 43: Same eye as in photograph 43 six months after PTK

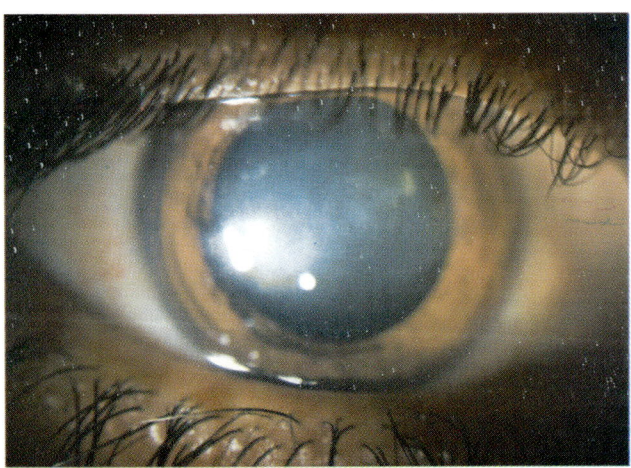

Photograph 44: Case of smooth band keratopathy

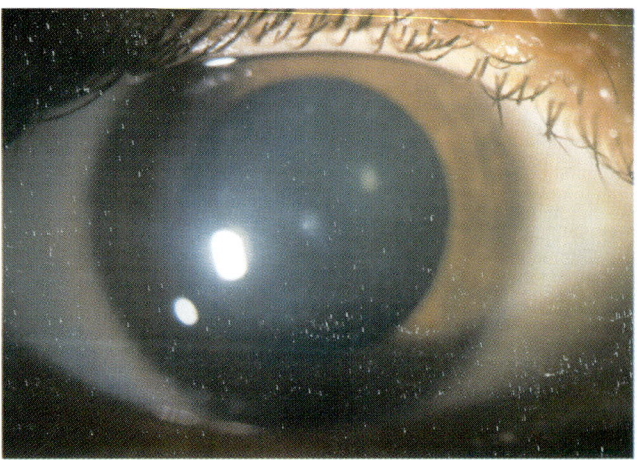

Photograph 45: Same eye as in photograph 44 three months after PTK

COLOUR PLATE 9

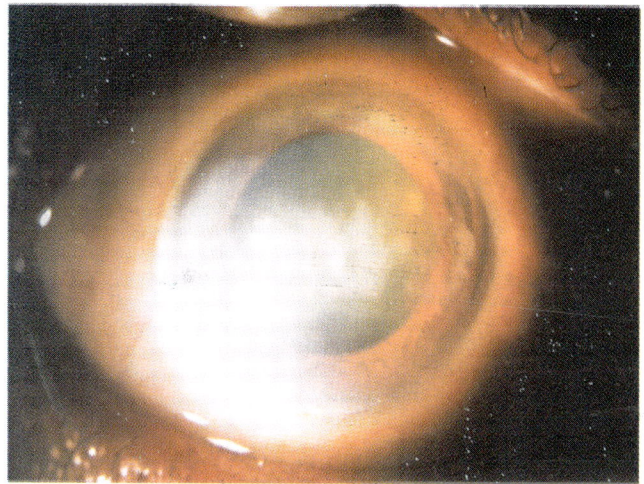

Photograph 46: Case of rough band-shaped keratopathy

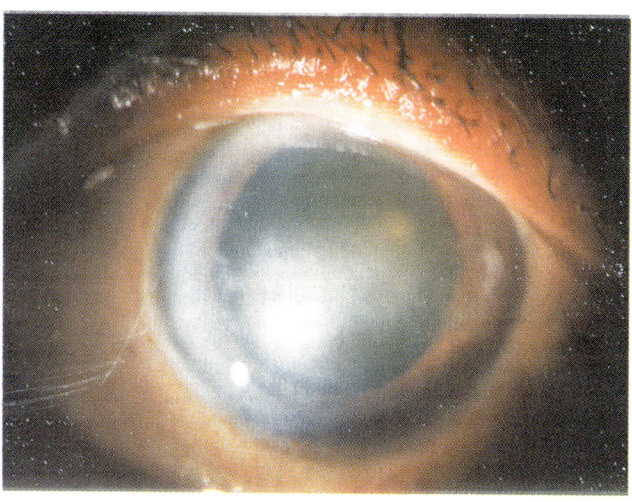

Photograph 47: Same eye as in photograph 46, one month after PTK

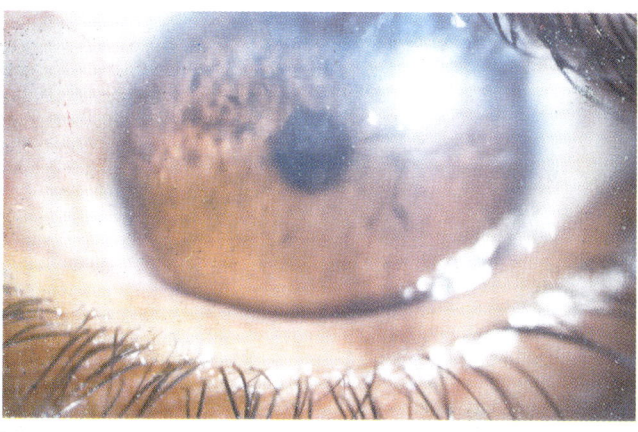

Photograph 48: Case post-traumatic recurrent corneal erosions with superficial opacity in the optical zone

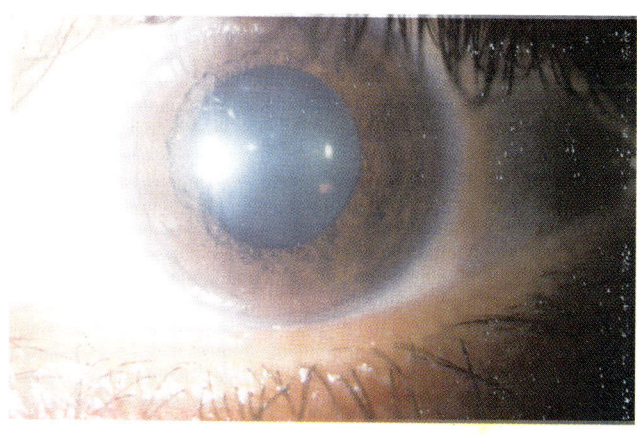

Photograph 49: Same eye six months after PTK

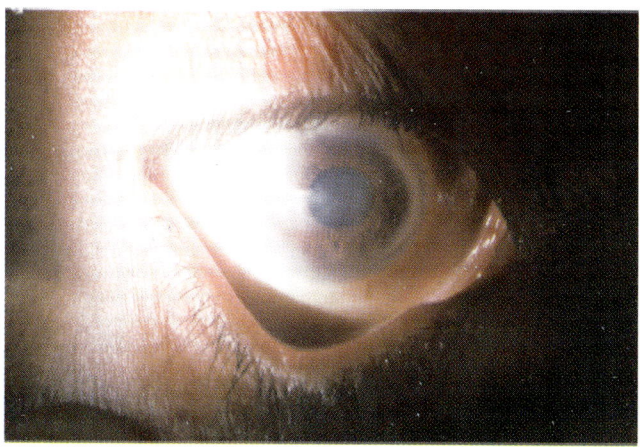

Photograph 50: Case of corneal opacity involving the pupillary area

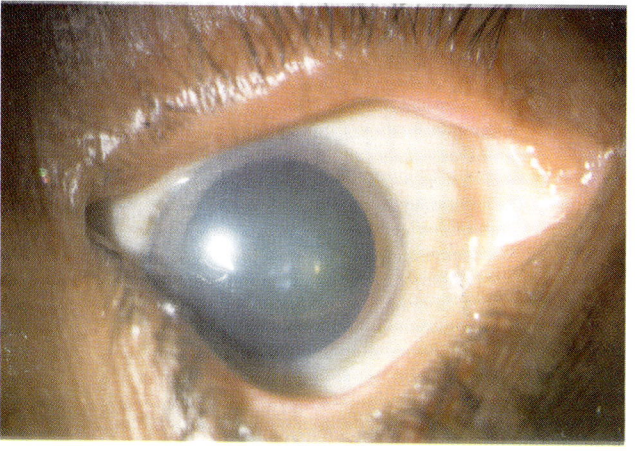

Photograph 51: Same eye three months after PTK

COLOUR PLATE 10

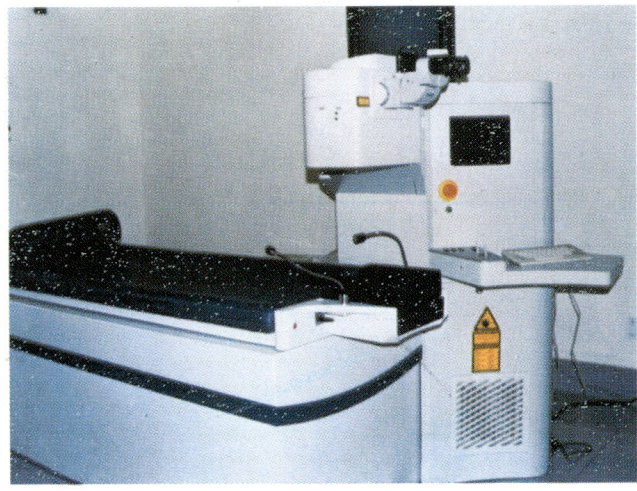

Photograph 52: The Chiron Technolas Keracor 217 C-LASIK excimer laser machine

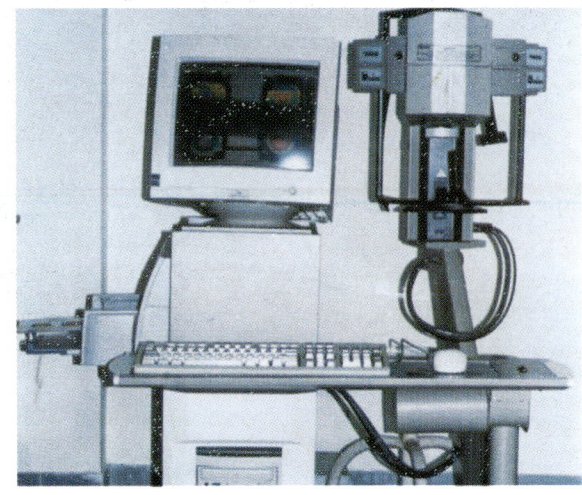

Photograph 53: The Orbscan I computerized corneal topography system

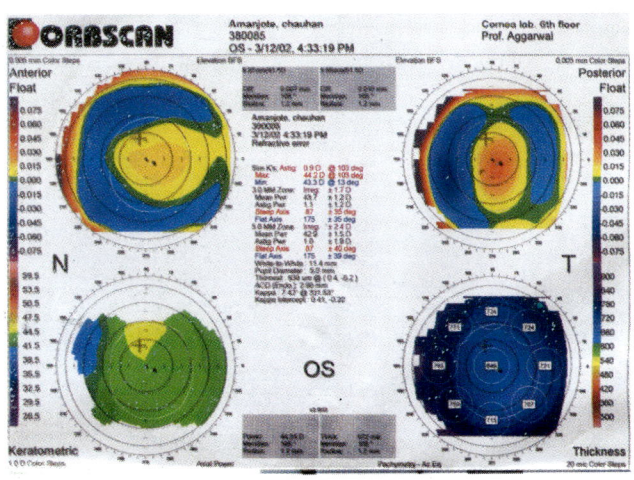

Photograph 54: An Orbscan topography map showing the corneal power, anterior and posterior surface elevation and corneal thickness at different locations

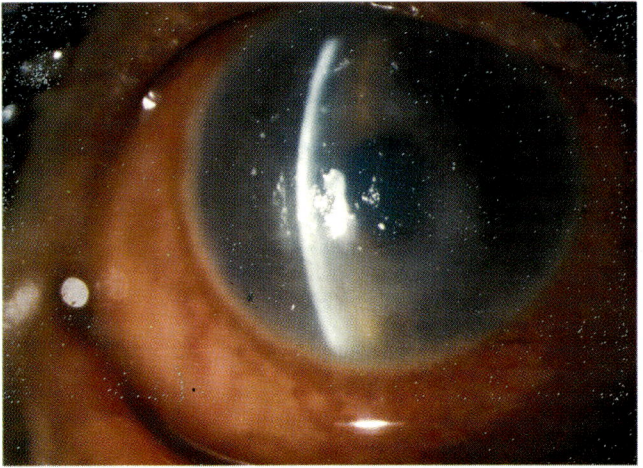

Photograph 55: Eye of the patient, who developed keratitis 2 weeks after PTK

COLOUR PLATE 11

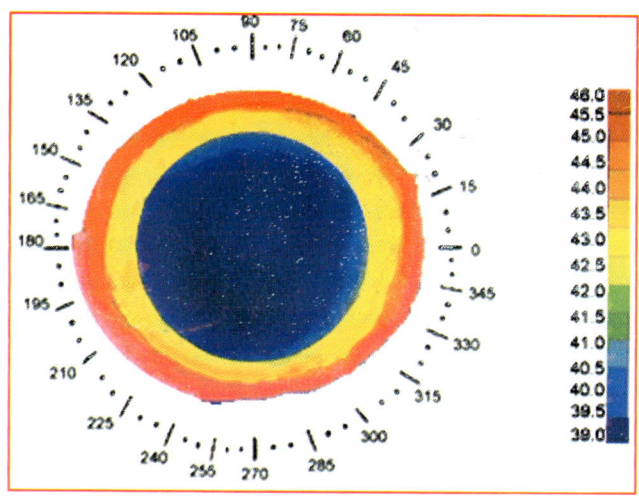

Photograph 56: CVK map of cornea after myopic photorefractive ablation showing flattening of central cornea and a well centred ablation zone

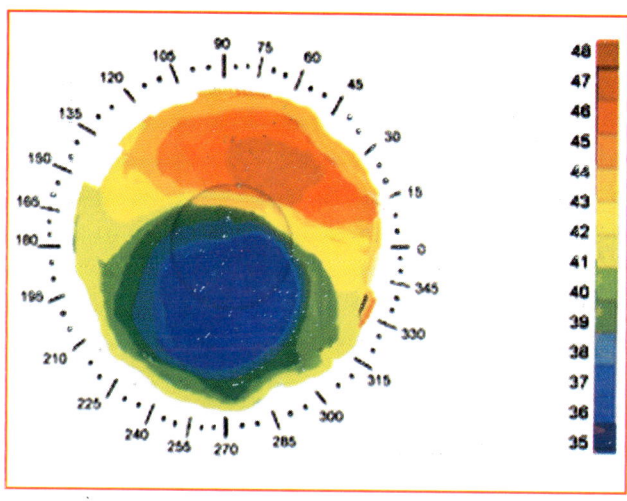

Photograph 57: CVK map of cornea after myopic photorefractive ablation showing inferior decentration of the ablation zone, the edge coming into the pupillary area

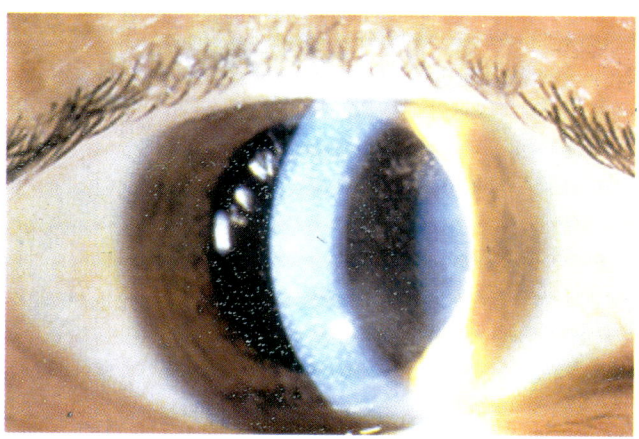

Photograph 58: Eye showing sterile peripheral corneal infiltrates

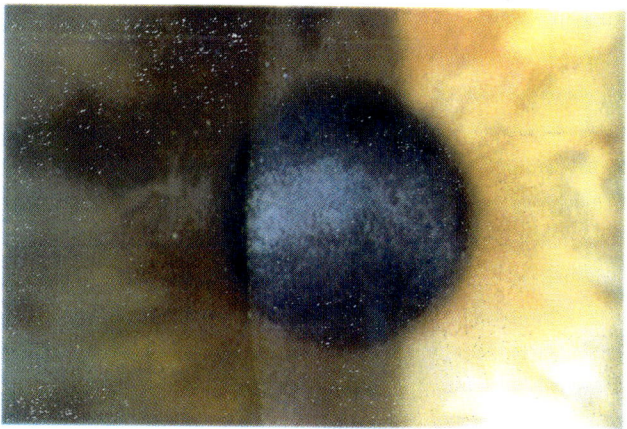

Photograph 59: Subepithelial corneal scarring following PRK

COLOUR PLATE 12

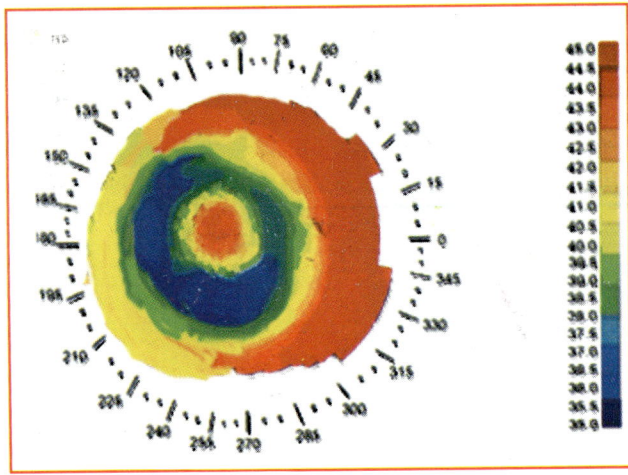

Photograph 60: Central steep island following photorefractive surgery

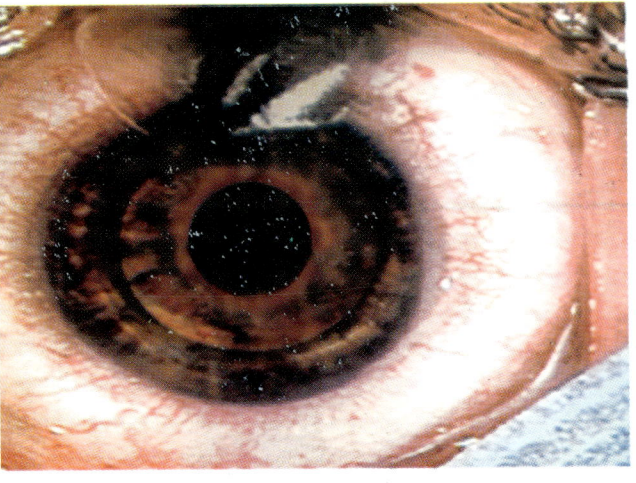

Photograph 61: Superiorly hinged corneal flap

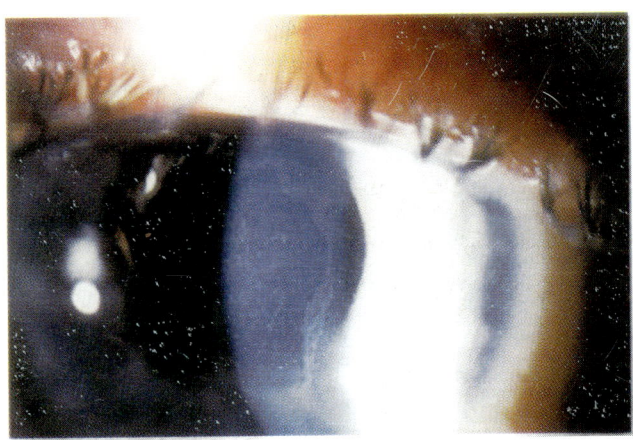

Photograph 62: Buttonhole following flap creation during LASIK

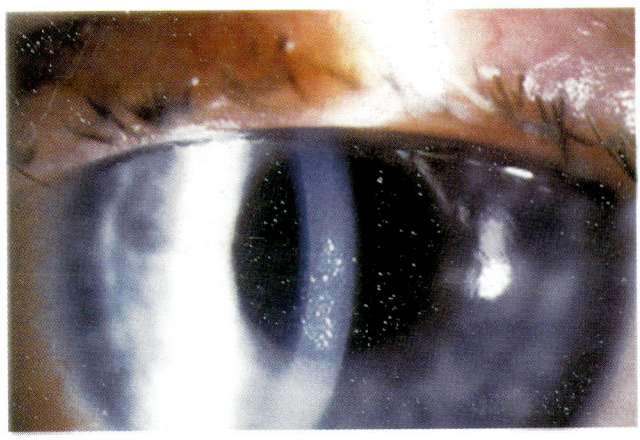

Photograph 63: Interface debris following LASIK

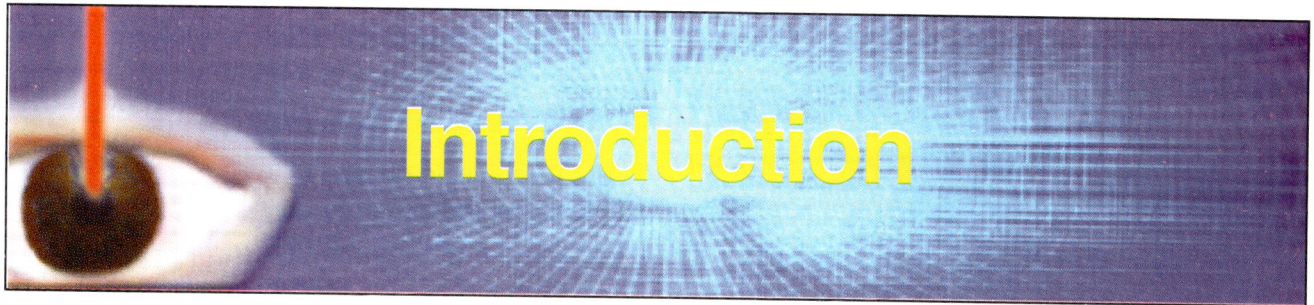

Introduction

REFRACTIVE AND CORNEAL DISORDERS

Refractive Disorders

Refractive disorders are the most common causes of ocular morbidity. They constitute the second most common cause of blindness and are the leading cause of low vision. Refractive errors account for 7.35% and aphakia for 4.69% cases of blindness in India according to the last national survey.

India was the first country to recognize that refractive disorders should be included in the list of causes of blindness. It was the absence or inaccessibility of refractive services to the masses, particularly the rural one; poverty and recurring cost of glasses which kept the common man blind or visually handicapped; and lack of awareness, which lead the National Program for Control of Blindness to perceive that the refractive disorders should be tackled on priority to control blindness.

This concept has been accepted worldover to include this problem as one of the five priority areas of the WHO program called **Vision 2020—The Right to Sight: A Global Initiative for the Elimination of Avoidable Blindness.** This program includes cataract, refractive errors, trachoma (causing corneal blindness), childhood blindness and onchocerciasis, as the five major blinding eye conditions to be tackled on priority.

Corneal Disorders

Corneal disorders are the third most common cause for blindness and low vision, after cataract and refractive errors, accounting for almost 3.3% cases of blindness in India and other developing countries. Approximately 3 million patients are waiting for corneal transplantation in India.

In addition to trachomatous opacity, human eye is affected by many other corneal disorders which give rise to corneal opacities and scars. They may be responsible for significant visual impairment in addition to being the cause of ocular discomfort and pain. These disorders of anterior cornea include various dystrophies, degenerations and surface irregularities, causing interference with vision. Recurrent corneal erosion syndrome is a notoriously disabling condition in terms of recurrent pain and ocular morbidity. Medical and surgical modes of management currently available for these conditions are unsatisfactory in terms of visual outcome and for relief of symptoms.

Corneal Blindness

Corneal blindness is avoidable, i.e. preventable and curable. Cases of corneal blindness require penetrating keratoplasty as a definitive measure. This procedure suffers from a large number of problems and constraints. Scarcity of the donor corneal buttons is the biggest limitation and there is a huge backlog of cases. Patients have to wait for years for their turn, thus losing their earning potential and leading to precious manpower and economic loss for the nation as well.

Penetrating Keratoplasty (PKP)

Penetrating keratoplasty is more invasive and demanding surgery associated with many intraoperative and postoperative complications. Graft failure and unsatisfactory visual outcome due to high irregular astigmatism and/or poor corneal clarity are its major drawbacks. Recurrence of the dystrophy or the degenerative process also demands regrafting.

Argon Fluoride Excimer Laser

After the discovery of their effects on cornea by Taboada et al in 1981, excimer lasers have been extensively studied for their interaction with cornea and safety to other ocular structures.

The physical qualities of 193 nm ArF excimer laser interaction with corneal tissue have endowed it with a magical surgical action capable of controlled removal of corneal tissue with submicron precision and of desired shapes and patterns without significant collateral damage; and predictability in terms of intended depth, length and reproducibility of cuts.

It has been suitably termed as laser scalpel that can be used to create a new corneal curvature or to reconstruct the surface of the cornea, thereby successfully replacing keratectomy, keratotomy and keratoplasty.

It is an easier to perform, non-invasive surgery. There is not much waiting time and visual rehabilitation is good and quick. Moreover, repeat surgery can be performed as long as the corneal thickness remains more than 325 microns, without endangering the corneal integrity.

Excimer laser has been utilized for the following procedures.
1. Phototherapeutic keratectomy
2. Photorefractive surgeries

PHOTOTHERAPEUTIC KERATECTOMY (PTK)

PTK is a new technique that offers an effective alternative mode for treatment of the corneal conditions mentioned before. It treats corneal disorders by removing the diseased corneal tissue and smoothening the corneal irregularities with 193 nm ArF excimer laser. It also treats iatrogenically induced refractive problems.

PHOTOREFRACTIVE SURGERIES

1. Refractive Keratotomy (RK)
   Laser keratotomy can be used for giving precise corneal incisions to alter the corneal curvature.
2. Photorefractive Keratectomy (PRK)
   This is used for changing corneal curvature by removing tissue from corneal surface.
3. Excimer Laser Intrastromal Keratomileusis (ELISK)
   In this procedure laser is used for removing stroma from the back surface of a corneal flap to bring a change in refractive power of the cornea.
4. Laser in-situ Keratomileusis (LASIK)
   LASIK is a technique of changing the refractive power of the eye through change in corneal curvature by removing tissue from the stromal bed after creation of an anterior stromal flap (along with the epithelium).
5. Customized LASIK/ wavefront-guided LASIK
   The higher-order optical aberrations suffered by an individual's eye are taken care of by a complicated software algorithm to achieve 'super visual acuity' better than 6/5. In this technique, a device called an aberrometer analyzes and constructs the deformation map suffered by the eye by using highly collimated rays incident on an individual's eye. There are three types of aberrometers in use, utilizing the Hartman-Shack method, the ray tracing technique and the Tsherning aberroscope. The data is then used for assisting the tissue removal with excimer laser.
6. Laser Subepithelial Keratomileusis (LASEK)
   This technique changes the corneal curvature by removing tissue from the corneal surface after creation of an epithelial flap with a microtrephine. Creation of epithelial flap is assisted by use of 18–20% ethanol. Then excimer laser is used to alter the corneal curvature.

Preservation of the Bowman's layer during corneal surgeries has been proven to be a myth. This layer can be violated by excimer laser without producing any opacity or irregularity. At the same time, quick and adequate re-epithelization with normal adherence of the epithelium to the underlying stroma occurs, leading to the formation of a surface which is not only smooth and clear to optical standards but also free from epithelial loss.

Many experimental and clinical studies have shown that ArF excimer laser keratectomy is safe regarding the risks of cataractogenesis, mutagenesis, photokeratitis and compromising the corneal integrity.

Gartry et al were the first to perform PTK on sighted human eyes in 1988 in UK. The Food and Drugs Administration (FDA) in USA gave conditional approval for PTK in March 1994.

McDonald and Kaufman introduced PRK in 1988 for correction of refractive errors. LASIK was introduced by Pallikaris in 1990 and wavefront-guided LASIK by Mrochen and Seiler in 1999.

Till today, innumerable clinical studies have been undertaken by different groups which have reported successful results of excimer laser surgeries in treating various refractive disorders and corneal diseases.

Over the years, surgeons have become more prudent and have acquired better understanding as to which of the corneal pathologies are more amenable to and which are poor candidates for PTK. Rapuano et al suggested that the best candidates for PTK are the eyes with superficial smooth anterior corneal opacities confined to less than 33% of corneal thickness. The second category of good candidates for PTK are eyes with elevated lesions, nodules or scars in the central cornea, which are not treatable with the blade. The last category of good candidates for PTK are eyes with recurrent corneal erosion syndrome not responding to conventional treatment. The success of PTK has been reported in 77% of eyes with painful bullous keratopathy also.

Similarily, millions of patients have undergone excimer laser surgeries for various types and different degrees of refractive errors. The results of these procedures have been critically analyzed to reach some vital and practical conclusions about the indications, efficacy, predictability and safety of various excimer laser refractive surgeries in different situations.

Suggested readings

1. Govt. of India (1992): Present Status of National Program for Control of Blindness (NPCB), 1992, Ophthalmology section, DGHS, New Delhi.
2. Govt. of India (1986), Health Information of India 1986, DGHS, New Delhi.
3. WHO (1996), Regional Health Report 1996, South-East Asia Region, New Delhi.
4. WHO (1997), The World Health Report 1997, Report of the Director-General WHO.
5. Taboada J, Archibald CJ: An extreme sensitivity in the corneal epithelium to far UV ArF excimer laser pulses: In proceedings of the 52nd annual meeting of Aerospace Medical Association, Washington DC, 1981; pp 89.
6. Trokel SL, Srinivasan R, Braren B : Excimer laser surgery of the cornea. Am J Ophthalmol 1983; 96: 710-715.
7. Marshall J, Trokel S, Rothery S, Kruger R: An ultrastructural study of corneal incisions induced by an excimer laser at 193 nm. Ophthalmol 1985; 92: 749-758.
8. Marshall J, Trokel SL, Rothery S et al : A comparative study of corneal incisions induced by diamond and steel knives and two UV radiations from excimer laser. BJO 1986; 70: 482-501.
9. KerrMuir MG, Trokel SL, Marshall J et al: Ultrastructural comparison of conventional surgical and ArF excimer laser keratectomy. Am J Ophthalmol 1987; 103 (part II) 448-453.
10. Marshall J, Trokel SL, Rothery S et al: Long term healing of the central cornea after PRK using an excimer laser. Ophthalmol 1988; (95): 1401-1421.
11. Tuft SJ, Zabble RW, Marshall J: Corneal repair following keratectomy: A comparison between conventional surgery and laser ablation. Invest Ophthalmol Vis Sci 1989; 30: 1769-1777.
12. Seiler and Bende et al: Side effects in excimer corneal surgery. Graefe's Arch Clin Exp Ophthalmology 1988; 226: 273-276.
13. Green H, Bold J, Parrish JA et al: Cyto-toxicity and mutagenicity of low intensity 248 nm and 193 nm excimer laser radiations in mammalian cells. Cancer Research 1987; 47: 410-413.
14. Nuss RC, Puliafito GA et al: Unscheduled DNA synthesis following excimer laser ablation of cornea in vivo. Investi Ophthalmol Vis Sci 1987; 28: 287-29.
15. Kochever IE, Walsh AN, Green HA et al: DNA damage induced by 193nm radiations in mammalian cells. Cancer Research 1991; 51: 288-293.
16. Sliney DH, Kruger RR, Trokel SL, Rappaport KD: Photokeratitis from 193nm ArF. Laser radiations: Photochemistry and Photobiology 1991; 53: 739-744.
17. Pitts DG, Cullen AP et al: Ocular effects of UV radiations from 295 nm to 365 nm. Invest Ophthalmol Vis Sci 1977; 16: 932-939.
18. Muller Stolzenberg NW, Muller CZ et al: UV exposure of lens during 193nm excimer laser corneal surgery. Arch Ophthalmol 1990; 108): 915-916.
19. Dehm EJ, Puliafito CA, Adller CM et al: Corneal endothelial injury in rabbits following excimer laser ablation at 193 nm and 248 nm. Arch Ophthalmol 1986; 104: 1364-1368.
20. McDonald M, Kaufman HE: Excimer laser ablation in human eye. Arch Ophthalmol 1989; 107: 641-2.
21. Pallikaris IG, Paptazanaki ME et al: Laser in situ keratomileusis. Laser surgery Med 1990; 10: 463-468
22. Gartry D, Muir MK, Marshall J: Excimer laser treatment of corneal surface pathology: a laboratory and clinical study. BJO 1991; 75: 258-269.
23. Sher NA, Bowers RA, Zebel RW et al: Clinical use of 193 nm excimer laser in treatment of corneal scars. Arch Ophthalmol 1991; 109: 491-498.
24. Stark WJ, Chamon W, Kamp MT et al: Clinical follow up of 193 nm ArF excimer laser PTK. Ophthalmology 1992; 99: 805-811.
25. Mrochen M, Kaemmerer M, Seiler T: Wavefront-guided laser in situ keratomileusis: early results in three eyes. J Refract Surg 2000 Mar-Apr;16(2):116-21.
26. Mrochen M, Kaemmerer M, Seiler T: Clinical results of Wavefront-guided laser in-situ keratomileusis 3 months after surgery. J Cataract Refract Surg 2001 Feb; 27 (2): 201-7.

27. Panagopolou SI, Pallikaris IG: Wavefront customized ablations with the WASCA Asclepion workstation. J Refract Surg 2001 Sep-Oct; 17(5):S 608-12.
28. Vonthongsri A, Phusitphoyakai N, Naripthapan P: Comparison of Wavefront-guided customized ablation vs conventional ablation in laser in situ keratomileusis. J Refract Surg 2002 May-Jun; 18(3 Suppl): S332-5
29. Dastjerdi MH, Soong HK: LASEK (laser subepithelial keratomileusis). Curr Opin Ophthalmol 2002 Aug; 13(4): 261-3.
30. Shahinian L: Laser-assisted subepithelial keratectomy for low to high myopia and astigmatism. J Cataract Refract Surg 2002 Aug; 28(8): 1334.

Section I

Basics of Various Lasers

Chapter 1
Laser Terms, Definitions and Laser System

LASER TERMS AND DEFINITIONS

The emission of radiant energy from substances may take place in two different ways:

1. Spontaneous emission
2. Stimulated emission

SPONTANEOUS EMISSIONS

The release of radiant energy from the excited atoms of a substance on its own, as they return to the more stable ground state, is termed as spontaneous emission. *No triggering mechanism is required for the emission of the energy to occur.*

Spontaneous energy emission from the molecules can be understood with the help of **Boltzmann's energy distribution theory.** It says that the atoms in the molecules of the matter are at different energy states depending on the temperature. At higher temperature they are in higher energy or the 'excited state' and at low temperature in low energy stable state or the 'ground state'. But in nature less molecules are in higher energy state as compared to those in the lower energy or ground state, i.e. *there is a natural tendency to fall to the ground state until and unless the molecules are kept in an excited state by an external energy source.* Energy is released when the molecules fall to the 'ground state'.

Fluorescence

It is an example of spontaneous emission. Fluorescence is a phenomenon in which a chemical molecule *emits photons spontaneously* after absorbing energy from photons of *a different wavelength*. Here the incident photons (from a monochromatic light of a particular wavelength) raise the electrons surrounding the nucleus of an atom to a higher energy orbit. The excited atom thus formed is unstable and falls to the ground (unexcited) state spontaneously as the energized electrons decay back to lower energy orbit by emitting photons of a different wavelength (Fig. 1.1). The whole process of light absorption, emission and fluorescence takes place in approximately 10^{-8} second.

The *property* of fluorescence *is limited* to only certain substances. The wavelength absorbed is specific for that substance and is a function of energy level characteristics of its molecules.

Examples
Sodium Fluorescein ($C_{20}H_{10}O_5Na_2$)
Excitation   490 nm (480 to 510 nm)   Blue
Emission   530 nm (peak)   Green

Indocyanin Green (ICG)
Excitation   750 nm to 810 nm
Emission   835 nm (peak)

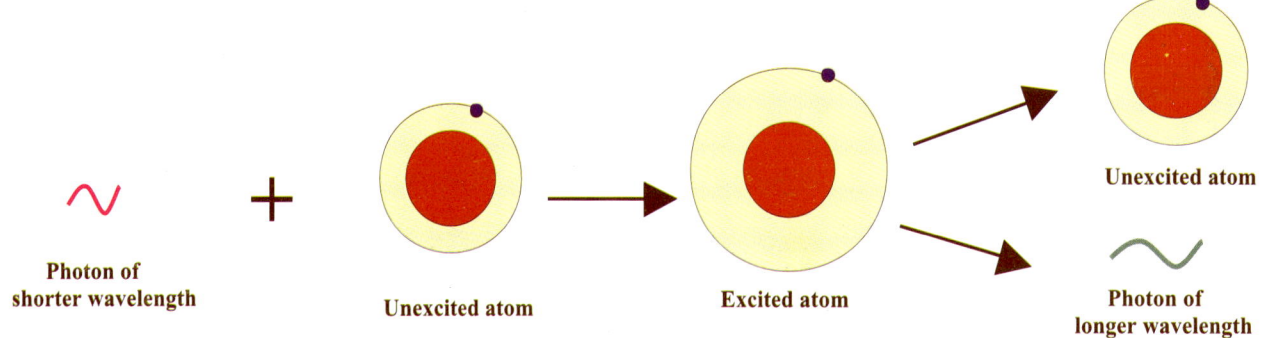

Fig. 1.1: Spontaneous emission

Stokes Law

The emitted light in all but rare instances is of a longer wavelength. Therefore the energy level of the emitted light is always lower than that of the absorbed light because the energy is inversely proportional to the wavelength as shown by the following equation:

$$\text{Energy} \propto \frac{1}{\text{wavelength}}$$

The energy is expressed in joules and the power in watts. The energy density is represented by watts/cm².

LASER

Laser is an acronym for 'Light Amplification by Stimulated Emission of Radiation'. Here the *emission* of photons (radiant energy) from the excited atoms is not spontaneous but *triggered by another photon* which has a wavelength equal to the wavelength that would be emitted. Much more energy is released by the process of *amplification*.

Following are the properties of laser which make it different from other light sources.

1. Low divergence
2. Monochromatic
3. Coherent

Low Divergence

The laser rays have low divergence, i.e. the tendency of the laser rays to fall apart is much less than that of other light sources. This property increases their effectiveness and makes the application more precise and accurate.

Monochromatic

Lasers are monochromatic, i.e. they have a single colour wavelength. This makes them free from chromatic aberrations.

Coherent

Laser waves are coherent, i.e. all the waves of photons are oscillating in phase, so that some of the waves which are out of phase do not cancel each other and reduce the laser output (see Figs 2.1 and 2.2).

STIMULATED EMISSION

During stimulated emission, *release of radiant energy is triggered by another photon*. This happens when an excited atom encounters a photon of energy level equal to the difference between its excited and unexcited state. The photon triggers the release of two photons of nearly identical energy from the excited atom (Fig. 1.2).

The following steps are essential for stimulated emission to be transformed to *laser* light having sufficient energy for clinical applications.

1. Amplification
2. Population inversion

Amplification

The emitted photons can be utilized to trigger the release of four more photons from two more excited atoms and so on. This chain reaction can be amplified by surrounding the lasing medium in a cavity with mirrors so that the released photons do not escape the laser cavity immediately. They rather interact with other excited atoms within the laser cavity (Fig. 1.3).

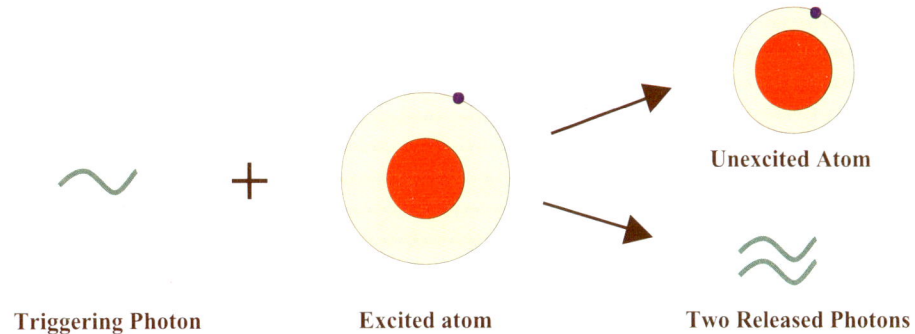

Fig. 1.2: Stimulated emission

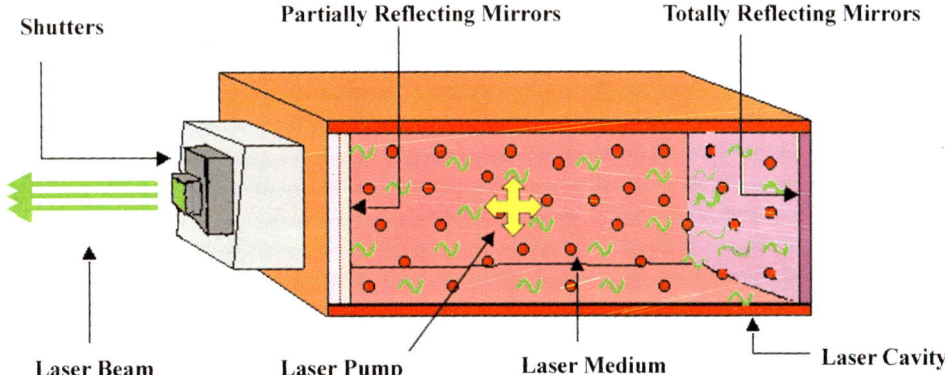

Fig. 1.3: Laser cavity

The mirrors direct the released photons backwards and forwards through the lasing media while the shutters of the lasing cavity are kept closed. The shutters are opened after sufficient laser output is build up for clinical use.

Population Inversion

At the same time the atoms are kept in an excited state by the energy delivered from a suitable laser pump. When the rate of pumping atoms to higher energy state is such that more than half of the atoms are in the excited state, it is called population inversion. This state is reverse of the one earlier described as Boltzmann's energy distribution and is maintained by the laser pump. This is a vital step for generating sufficient laser output because more atoms need to be in the excited state for stimulated emission and amplification to occur. The process continues till a balance is struck between the rate at which the laser light is allowed to leave or *coupled out* from the system and the rate which it is produced by the lasing medium.

THE LASER SYSTEM

The laser system essentially consists of the following three components:

1. Laser pump
2. Lasing medium
3. Laser cavity

LASER PUMP

The laser pump is an energy source to excite the lasing medium. It provides the required energy to raise the electrons of the atom to a higher energy level or to form the excited dimer in case of excimer lasers. Various energy sources can be used to excite the lasing medium. These are:

1. Chemical reactions
2. Electrical discharge or current
3. Electronic beams and accelerators
4. Light energy from

a. Flash lamp
b. Arc lamp
c. Another laser

Electrical discharge and flash lamps are the commonest methods used. In the excimer laser system, a very high electrical discharge with voltage around 30,000 and current 10,000 amperes is used (Table 1.1).

The Thyraton

A thyraton is a special switch which is based on the 'valve technology' to cope with the high current and fast switching. Since excimer laser pumping requires typically such high currents and rapid switching, the thyraton is a crucial device for initiating the electrical discharge during excimer laser production.

Table 1.1: Different laser pumps

Type of laser	Laser pump used
Ruby laser	Xenon flash lamp
Nd: YAG laser	Flash lamp (for pulsed delivery)
	Arc lamp (for continuous delivery)
Argon laser	High current electrical discharge
Dye laser	Flash lamp
	Argon laser (for continuous delivery)
Diode laser	Electrical discharge
Metal vapour lasers	Electrical discharge

LASING MEDIA

The lasing media are the substances which are utilized for the production of the laser. The laser wavelength produced depends on the lasing medium. Three types of lasing media can be used:

1. Gas media
2. Liquid media
3. Solid media

Gas Media

These are the most common media used for generating the lasers. The ionized gas is pulsed with electrical discharge. Example are:

1. Carbon Dioxide Laser It was the first laser to be used for corneal applications. It comprises carbon dioxide gas with some helium (10 μ or 10,000 nm).

1967: Fine et al[10] experimentally used continuous wave CO_2 laser.

1971: Beckman[11] et al used micro-second pulsed CO_2 laser.
1980: Used for thermokeratoplasty by Peyman[12].
1981: Keates et al[12] developed Q-switched nano second CO_2 laser.

2. Argon Laser (argon blue 488 nm, green 514 nm)

3. Krypton Laser (647 nm)

4. Hydrogen Fluoride Laser (2700-3000 nm)

5. Excimer Lasers

a. Argon fluoride (ArF 193 nm)
b. Krypton chloride (KrCl 222 nm)
c. Krypton fluoride (KrF 248 nm)
d. Xenon chloride (XeCl 308 nm)
e. Xenon fluoride (XeF 351 nm)

Liquid Media

The liquid media used for lasing action consist of fluorescent organic dyes dissolved in a solvent. Examples are dye lasers.

1. Dye yellow (577 nm)
2. Dye red (630 nm)

Solid Media

The solid media are advantageous for making portable laser systems. The lasers using these media are called *solid state lasers.*

Following are examples of such lasers.

1. Nd: YAG Laser Triply ionized neodymium atoms are held in place by the yttrium aluminum garnet crystals. Different available Nd: YAG lasers are:

a. Conventional Nd: YAG laser (1064 nm)
b. Frequency doubled Nd: YAG (532 nm)
c. Raman shifted Nd:YAG (2800 nm)

Solid state excimer lasers
a. Nd: YAG fifth harmonic (213 nm)
b. Nd: YLF fifth harmonic (211 nm)

2. Er: YAG/Erbium Laser (2940 nm)

3. HO: YAG/Holmium laser (2000 nm)

4. Nd: YLF Laser

5. *Ruby Laser* (694 nm)
   It was the first ophthalmic laser that was introduced by *Maiman* in 1960.

6. *Metal vapor lasers*

Two types of metal vapor lasers have been developed.

1. Gold vapor laser (628 nm)
2. Copper vapor laser (510–578 nm)

Only the copper laser has been tried in ophthalmology.

MODES OF LASER DELIVERY

Laser delivery is to be considered in relation to the following aspect.

1. With respect to time sequence
   a. Continuous wave mode
   b. Pulsed mode
      i. Conventional long (millisecond) pulse.
      ii. Ultrashort (nano and picosecond) pulse.
2. With respect to spot size and energy density
   a. Fundamental mode/monomode
   b. Multimode delivery

CONTINUOUS MODE DELIVERY

Here the photons are allowed to exit the system continuously while the laser system is operational. A study 'pumping' is required for this mode. The following lasers are operated in continuous mode:

Argon laser and Krypton laser

There are some lasers which were earlier used in continuous mode. The pulsed mode of these lasers has been developed for their newer applications, e.g.

Nd:YAG laser, dye lasers and CO_2 laser

The continuous wave lasers are suitable for photocoagulation effect but have *low peak powers* which *cannot produce* tissue effects like *photodisruption* or *photovaporization* required for their newer applications. The *collateral tissue damage* is also much more.

PULSE MODE

In this mode of delivery the photons are allowed to leave the laser system as a train of very shortpulses, grouped together, when the laser is being used. The pumping of the system is by a very short lasting energy source such a flash lamp or electrical discharge.

YAG lasers, dye lasers, metal vapor lasers, hydrogen fluoride laser, CO_2 laser and excimer lasers are used in pulsed mode.

Conventional or Long Pulse Delivery

In the conventional or long pulsed operation, the duration of the individual pulse is of the order of milliseconds. This is achieved by use of shutters which are capable of opening and closing at a very fast speed. These shutters are mechanical devices.

Ultrashort Pulse Delivery

For further shortening of pulse duration to nano- or picoseconds, special procedures are used in which devices other than the mechanical shutters are essential. This is because the mechanical shutters do not prove to be so fast responding. The two methods of producing ultrashort laser pulse are:

1. Q-switching
2. Mode locking

Q-SWITCHING

In this procedure, two special types of shutters are used to achieve shortening of the pulse duration.

Pockels Cell Polarizer Assembly This is an electrically switchable assembly. It is transparent to laser in one state but opaque in other state.

Bleachable Dye This is interposed at the shutter, either in a liquid form or as a plastic film. It becomes transmissive to the laser light only when the latter is of sufficiently high energy. With weak light the dye mold becomes opaque.

The Pockels cell polarizer is more efficient for Q-switching but is more complex and prone to malfunction. A Q-switched laser pulse is of 20–30 nanoseconds duration (billionth of a second).

MODE LOCKING

Further reduction in pulse duration to picoseconds is obtained by a method called mode locking. For this purpose two types of devices can be used.

1. Electronically controlled devices
2. Bleachable dye

Electronically Controlled Devices These devices consist of very fast opening shutters that are controlled electronically.

Bleachable Dye The dye is capable of returning to its natural state within picoseconds after being bleached and is placed very close to the partially reflective mirror as compared to the dye used in Q-switching.

The pulse duration with mode-locking is 20 to 60 picoseconds (500 times shorter than the one obtained with Q-switching).

FUNDAMENTAL MODE/MONOMODE

The 'fundamental mode' of laser delivery produces a laser spot of smallest size and highest power density. In this mode of delivery the laser cavity is so well aligned that there is a unique central path for the laser light. When the laser light traverses through this central axis, the 'electric field' distribution created is everywhere *in phase*. This results in a smallest and highly focussed laser spot with very high energy density.

MULTIMODE

Laser rays not following the above path result in an electric field distribution where the rays are not in phase everywhere. This causes cancellation of waves at some places and addition at others (Figs 2.1 and 2.2). This is called multimode delivery in which the laser spot size is large. Through the total power of this spot is higher but the power density is much lower than in case of monomode delivery.

Advantages of Making Pulse Duration very Short

1. High peak powers are achieved.
2. The high peak power is capabe of producing *optical breakdown*.
3. Shorter the pulse, lower is the energy required to achieve optical breakdown.
4. Use of lower energy causes *less collateral thermal and acoustic damage*.
5. The *picosecond photodisrupter* can therefore be used for *intrastromal photorefractive keratectomy* (ISPRK), i.e. for removing the corneal stroma without raising a corneal flap.

Suggested readings

1. Meyer Schwickrath G: Initial experiments with sunlight to produce retinal burns. Light coagulation, St. Louis: C. V. Mosby, 1960.
2. Maiman TH: Stimulated optical radiations in ruby. Nature 1960; 187: 493-494.
3. L'Esprance FA, Jr: An argon laser photocoagulation system. Trans Am Ophthal Soc 1968; 66: 827-904.
4. L'Esprance FA, Jr: Clinical photocoagulation with frequency-double Nd:YAG laser. Am J Ophthal 1971: 71: 633-638.
5. Yannuzzi LA: krypton red laser photocoagulation of ocular fundus. Retina 1982; 2: 1-14.
6. Peyman GA, Raichand M, Zeimer RC: Ocular effects of various wavelengths. Surv Ophthalmol 1984 ; 28: 391-404.
7. Marshal J: Lasers in Ophthalmology: the basic principles. Eye 1988; 2: S 98-S 112.
8. Balles MW, Puliafito CA: Semiconductor diode laser: a new laser light source in ophthalmology. Int Ophthalmol Cli 1990; 30: 452- 457.
9. Gabsay S, Kremer I, Weinberger D et al: The retinal effects of copper vapor laser exposure. Invest Ophthalmol Vis Sci 1988 Apr; 29(4):528-33.
10. Fine BS, Fine S, Peacock GR et al: Preliminary observations on ocular effects of high-power, continuous CO_2 laser irradiation. Am J Ophthalmol 1967; 64 (2): 209-222.
11. Beckman H, Rota A, Barraco R et al: Limbectomies, keratectomies and keratostomies performed with a rapid-pulsed CO_2 laser. Am J Ophthalmol 1971; 71 (6): 1277-1283.
12. Peyman GA, Larson Raichand M et al: Modification of rabbit corneal curvature with use of CO_2 laser burns. Ophthalmic surgery 1980; 11: 325-329.
13. Keates RH, Pedrotti LS, Weichel H et al: CO_2 laser beam control for corneal surgery. Ophthalmic Surgery 1981; 12 (2): 117-122.

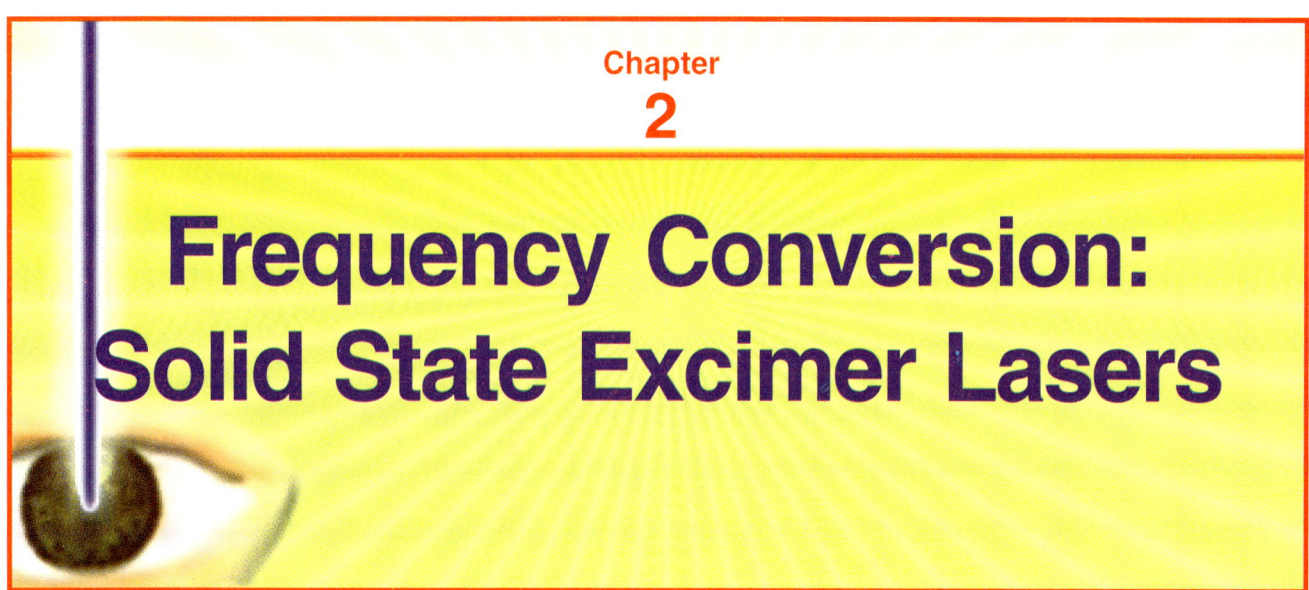

Chapter 2
Frequency Conversion: Solid State Excimer Lasers

WHAT IS FREQUENCY CONVERSION?

Frequency conversion is a technique by which higher wavelength laser is converted to a laser of lower wavelength (higher frequency). In this technique the laser output is passed through one or more **non-linear crystals** which convert it into laser light of a shorter wavelength.

HOW IT WORKS?

Normally the electrons within a transparent crystal move in phase with the electromagnetic field of the passing laser light. But the structure of the *non-linear crystal* necessitates exertion of additional forces if the movement of the electrons away from their normal position is to occur.

When the amplitude of the motion of the electrons reaches a certain level where constraints of the crystal structure do not allow it to move away any further in phase with the frequency of the passing laser, the additional forces make them oscillate at a frequency which is different from that of the original laser light, commonly at double the original frequency. The oscillating electrons emit light which is of a different wavelength.

If instead of one wavelength input, two wavelengths are passed through the non-linear crystal, this is termed **optical mixing.**

The wavelength of the emitted light (λ_3) is expressed according to the following equation:

$$\lambda_3 = \frac{\lambda_1 \lambda_2}{\lambda_1 + \lambda_2}$$

λ_1 = wavelength of first passing laser light
λ_2 = wavelength of the second passing light

Following requirements are to be fulfilled for frequency conversion to work efficiently.

1. Use of pulsed, narrow beam laser input
2. Phase matching

Use of Pulsed, Narrow Beam Laser Input

This input is intense enough to make the electrons oscillate at sufficiently high amplitude.

Phase Matching

Phase matchig is to be achieved for the following:

1. Phase matching of the emitted waves of light produced by each of the large number of different electrons.
2. Phase matching of the input and output light.

Phase matching is essential, so that the light waves do not cancel themselves out as they move through the crystal.

The light waves are said to be **in phase** if their peaks and troughs coincide with each other and thus are additive. They are out of phase if this is not the situation.

The *interference produced* due to being **out of phase** *depends on its degree*. If the phase difference is so much that the peak of one wavelength coincides with the trough of the other, complete cancellation takes place with no resultant light (Figs 2.1 and 2.2).

wavelength is half of the wavelength or double the frequency of the input.

This is called frequency doubling, for example *frequency double Nd: YAG laser* (532 nm).

Frequency Tripled Laser: Third-Harmonic Generation

Nd: YAG laser (1064 nm) is passed through one crystal to frequency-double it and then mixed with the original

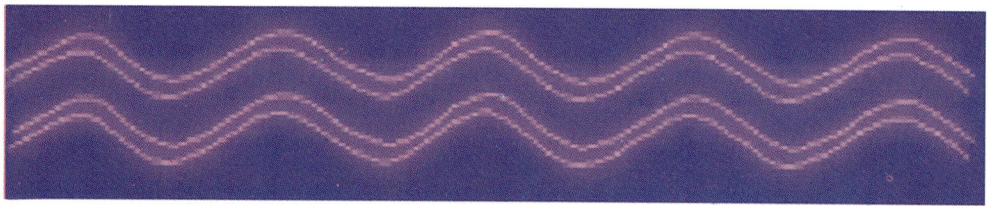

Fig. 2.1: Light waves in phase

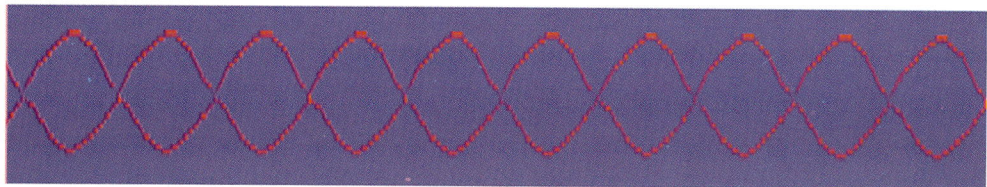

Fig. 2.2: Light waves out of phase

DISPERSION

The electrons of the crystal are forced by the incoming laser to move in phase with it, therefore the light output from them is also in phase. However, the new output falls out of phase with the input laser because *lights of different frequencies move at different speds in a medium due to dispersion and hence face attenuation or cancellation.*

This can be taken care of by a crystal having **birefringence**. Such crystals have a *non-symmetrical matrix* which allows light to move at faster speed in one plane than in the opposite plane. This crystal can be placed at such an angle, with respect to the incoming wavelength of the laser light, so that the dispersion and birefringence cancel each other.

Frequency Doubling: Second-Harmonic Generation

If only one laser wavelength is being passed through, then $\lambda_1 = \lambda_2$ and therefore $\lambda_3 = \lambda_{1/2}$, i.e. the resultant

wavelength (1064) before passing them through a second crystal. This results in production of 353 nm laser wavelength according to the above equation.

Frequency Quadrupling: Fourth-Harmonic Generation

Here a laser having wavelength in the upper visible spectrum is frequency-doubled twice to produce a frequency-quadrupled wavelength close to 193 nm.

Frequency Quintupling: Fifth-Harmonic Generation

This technique of frequency conversion is employed to produce laser output in the ultraviolet range (that of the excimer lasers). The *lasing media* used is *solid* instead of the gas medium of the conventional excimer lasers, therefore these lasers are called **solid state excimers**. Following are the examples of solid state examer lasers.

1. **Fifth harmonic Nd: YAG (213 nm)**
   This is a three-stage procedure. The Nd: YAG laser (1064 nm) is frequency-doubled twice and then mixed with the original wavelength (1064) and passed through a second crystal. This generates the fifth harmonic at 213 nm. This wavelength can be used to obtain effct similar to that of ArF laser.

2. **Fifth harmonic Nd: YLF (211 nm)**
   Using the similar technique as described above for Nd: YAG laser, the fifth harmonic from the Nd: YLF laser at 1053 nm can be generated to produce a solid state excimer wavelength at 211 nm.

These solid state excimer lasers are under extensive investigations for clinical applications in corneal surgery.

Clinical Applications of Frequency Conversion

1. Frequency conversion produces entirely different laser wavelength from the wavelength utilized.
2. The tissue effect of the laser depends on its wavelength. For example the *Nd: YAG laser at 1064 nm causes 'photodisruption' but the frequency-doubled Nd: YAG causes photo-coagulation*. This is utilized for replacing *argon laser* for retinal applications.
3. Similarily solid state *'frequency converted'* 193–213 nm wavelengths, which truly are not *excimer lasers*, have been used for corneal applications in an attempt to replace the 'gas media' excimer lasers. This is because the latter are *difficult to maintain* and are *not portable*.

Suggested readings

1. Gailitis RP, Ren QS, Thompson KP, Lin JT et al: Solid state ultraviolet laser (213 nm) ablation of the cornea and synthetic collagen lenticules. Lasers Surg Med 1991;11(6): 556-62.
2. Wu TM, Brown DW et al: Quantum theory of solid-state excimers: Eigenstates and transition rates. Physical Review. B. Condensed Matter. 1993 Apr 15;47(16): 10122-10134
3. Dair GT, Pelouch WS, van Saarloos PP et al: Investigation of corneal ablation efficiency using ultraviolet 213-nm solid state laser pulses. Invest Ophthal Vis Sci 1999 Oct;40(11): 2752-6.
4. Ren Q, Simon G, Parel JM: Ultraviolet solid-state laser (213-nm) photorefractive keratectomy; in vitro study, Ophthalmology 1993; 100: 1828–1834.

Chapter 3

Effect of Different Lasers on the Ocular Tissue

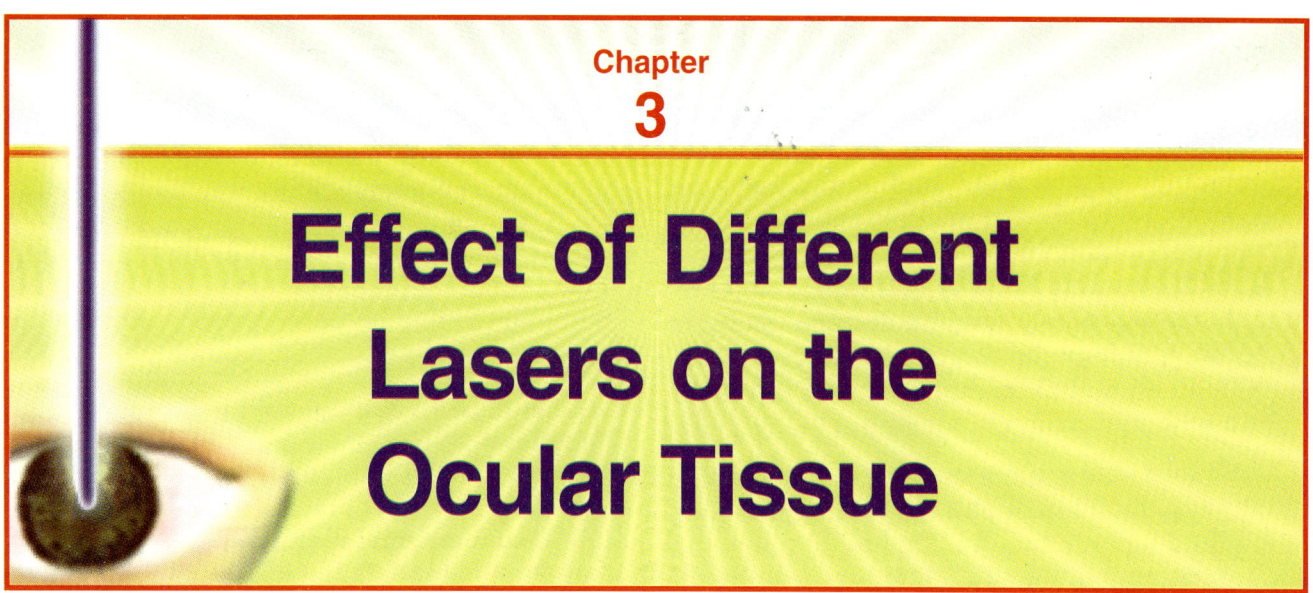

The interaction of various ophthalmic lasers on the ocular tissues can be grouped under the following headings.

1. Photothermal
   a. Photocoagulation
   b. Photothermal tissue shrinkage
2. Photodisruption (optical breakdown)
3. Photovaporization
4. Photochemical
   a. Ablative photodecomposition
   b. Photodynamic
   c. Transpupillary thermotherapy (TTT)

PHOTOTHERMAL EFFECTS

This is the most commonly used tissue interaction of ophthalmic lasers. Two types of photothermal effects are utilized in ophthalmology, the first one being the commonest.

1. Photocoagulation
2. Photothermal tissue shrinkage

Photocoagulation

This is the effect produced by coagulation of proteins of the tissue, when a rise of 10–20° C temperature occurs as the tissue absorbs the laser energy. Clinically, it is seen as tissue whitening, which is proportional to the magnitude and duration of the increase in temperature.

Chromophores

The effect of the laser is augmented by certain substances which absorb the laser energy. They are called *chromophores*. The *tissue pigments* such as melanin, xanthophylls and hemoglobin act as chromophores for photocoagulation. Melanin present in the retinal pigment epithelium, choroid and pigment epithelium of the iris absorbs most of the laser energy to produce the photocoagulation effect.

The energy absorption characteristics of these chromophores at different laser wavelengths differ and this should be suitably utilized when treating different disorders by photocoagulation (Table 3.1).

For example xanthophyll present in the macular area absorbs blue wavelength maximally. Therefore treatment in this area by the argon blue laser would result in sever macular burn. *Hence photocoagulation in the macula region by argon blue wavelength is contraindicated.*

The presence of vitreous blood does not hamper the penetration of the red wavelengths. *Hence red wavelengths are ideal for retinal photocoagulation in the presence of mild to moderate vitreous hemorrhage.*

Lasers in the visible and infrared range (488–810 nm) are utilized for treating various *retinal disorders, intraocular tumors* and *glaucoma* by photocoagulation effect.

Table 3.1: Different lasers, their absorption by chromophores and other characteristics

Laser wavelength	Absorption by		Penetration through		Other comments
	Xanthophyll	Hemoglobin	Blood	Media opacity	
Argon blue (488 nm)	++++	+++	poor	poor	- **contraindicated for macular photocoagulation** - Xanthophyll absorption leads to inner retina damage - formation of macular cyst, hole, epiretinal membrane - high scattering, less precise focusing
Argon green (514 nm)	nil	+++	poor	fair	- **most commonly used laser for photocoagulation** - absorbed by blood, treating over retinal or preretinal hemorrhage may results in inner retinal damage
Nd:YAG green (532 nm) (Frequency-doubled)	nil	++++	least	fair	- used as pulsed output, effect similar to Argon green - lasing medium hence more reliable - **safe for macular photocoagulation**
Dye yellow (577 nm)	nil	++++	least	fair	- useful in **pale fundi** as absorbed by choroidal vessels - excellent hemoglobin absorption hence most useful for treating retinal and choroidal vasculature abnormalities - but less useful in presence of vitreous, pre-retinal subretinal hemorrhage
Dye red (630 nm)	nil	+	fair	good	- uses and effects similar to those of Krypton red
Krypton red (647 nm)	nil	+	fair	good	- **painful** as other red wavelengths - **excellent** for macular lesions such as juxtafoveal choroidal neovascularization - **poor absorption by hemoglobin, less useful for treating vasculature abnormalities** - cannot penetrate through very thick hemorrhage
Semiconductor-Diode (810 nm)	nil	nil	good	good	- no sensation of light flashing being near infra-red - small, portable, cheap, air cooled system - **most useful for** studying and treating CNVM in macular region, **guided or enhanced by ICG dye** - **preferred** for ROP, **cyclodestructive** procedures, **endolaser** and transpupillary thermotherapy

Delivery System for Laser Photocoagulation

Slit-lamp Delivery

It is the commonest system for laser delivery, e.g. argon laser, Nd: YAG laser.

Contact lenses such the *Mainster standard lens* for posterior pole and *Volk quadraspheric lens* for midperiphery treatment provide globe fixation, magnified view and proper delivery at the desired site.

The *Peyman convex contact lens* is used for Nd: YAG laser surgery (*vitreolysis*).

Goldmann three mirror lens for panretinal and the *Volk super macula* for macular treatment are other lenses.

Delivery Through a Probe

The fiber-probe delivery system is used for endophotocoagulation with diode laser during retinal surgeries, for 'contact thermokeratoplasty' and for cytophotocoagulation.

Table 3.2 gives a brief summary of the protocol for photocoagulation of various retinal diseases.

Laser Indirect Ophthalmoscope (LIO)

Uses the indirect ophthalmoscope combined with diode laser for treating retinopathy of prematurity (ROP), Coats' disease, pars planitis and retinal breaks, etc.

Photothermal Tissue Shrinkage

This effect has been *utilized for treating hyperopia and astigmatism* by the procedure termed as *laser thermal keratoplasty (LTK)*. This procedure shrinks the corneal stromal collagen without causing any thermal necrosis,

Table 3.2: Protocol for photocoagulation of different retinal conditions

Condition	Spot size	No. of spots	Burn duration	Power /Burn intensity	Other considerations

Diabetic Proliferative Retinopathy (scatter/panretinal photocoagulation)	500µ	1500-2000	0.1 to 0.5 sec.	**Moderate intensity** (Opaque/dirty white)	• treatment given in three sessions spread over weeks
					• preceded by macular grid
					• placed one burn width apart
					• posterior limit-
					  - 500µ nasal to disc
					  - 3000µ above, temporal and below the macular center
					• anterior limit-
					  just anterior to the equator
					• retinal hemorrhage, major vessels, papillomacular bundle, previous scars avoided
					  - treating these results in damage

Indications: 1. Proliferative diabetic retinopathy with 'high-risk characteristics' (PDR with HRC) 2. PDR without HRC 'Severe NPDR' if follow up not sure					
Dia. Macular Edema 1. Macular grid	100-200µ		0.1 sec.	**Light burns** (*barely visible*)	• three rows of laser burns 500µ to 3000µ from macular center • one burn width apart • papillomacular bundle treated
2. Focal Treatment	50-100 µ	to cover the focal lesion	0.05–0.1 sec.	**Moderate to heavy** (dark white)	
BRVO (branch retinal vein obstruction) Grid for macular edema	100 µ		0.1 sec.	**Mild** (faint white)	
Neovascularization	200-500µ	sector scatter	0.1 sec.	**Moderate burns**	• treats the sector involved
CRVO (central retinal vein obstruction) Iris neovascularization Posterior segment neovascularisation	500-1000µ	panretinal	0.1-0.5 sec.	**Moderate intensity**	
Idiopathic CSR (Central serous retinopathy)	100-200µ	focal	0.1-0.2 sec.	**Light burns**	
Choroidal Neovascular Membranes	200-500µ	covers the entire lesion	0.2-0.5 sec.	**Mild reaction**	
Intraocular Tumors	200-500µ	confluent burns	0.5-1.0 sec.	**Heavy burns**	
Retinal Breaks	200-500µ	2-3 confluent rows	0.1-0.2 sec.	**Moderate**	

unlike the previously used **'radial TKP'** developed by Fyodorov in which he used nichrome wire probes heated at 600° C to purpose.

This topic is covered in detail in Chapter 10 on refractive procedures.

The following lasers have been utilized for thermal keratoplasty.

1. The CO_2 laser (continuous mode)
2. Cobalt-magnesium fluoride laser
3. Holmium: YAG laser
4. Diode laser at 1870 nm (continuous wave)

PHOTODISRUPTION/OPTICAL BREAKDOWN (IONIZING EFFECT)

Sufficiently high peak powers are required for producing this tissue effect. There are three major events during optical breakdown:
1. Plasma formation
2. Shock wave generation
3. Gas bubble cavitation

Plasma Formation

Laser pulse causes localized formation of high-temperature ionized gas in the tissue called the plasma.

Plasma Shielding Effect The plasma formed by the laser action on the tissue leads to more absorption of the incident energy. This absorption of energy leads to further expansion of the plasma.

Shock Wave Generation

Plasma formation is associated with high temperature and localized heating. This generates a shock wave which propagates in the tissue.

Cavitation or Gas Bubble Formation

Creation of plasma produces a gas-liquid phase leading to cavitation or gas bubble formation, which rapidly expands within microseconds and then collapses, causing secondary shockwaves. The gas bubbles are a mixture of CO_2, water vapor and carbon monoxide. These are clinically noticed during the procedure. Later they diffuse out of the tissue.

Lasers Causing Photodisruption

1. **Nd: YAG laser (Q-switched, mode locked)** This laser is used for YAG iridotomy, capsulotomy and intrastromal PRK.

    Intrastromal photorefractive keratectomy is removal of the corneal stroma without making a corneal flap. For this application, *picosecond and femtosecond* pulsed YAG lasers are used. It avoids violation of the corneal surface and the Bowman's layer and is *being investigated as an alternative to excimer laser refractive surgery.*

2. **Nd: YLF (Yttrium lithium fluoride 1053 nm)** This picosecond and femtosecond photodisrupter is also being extensively investigated for its application to perform intrastromal PRK.

PHOTOVAPORIZATION/PHOTOTHERMAL ABLATION

This effect needs *water* acting as the *chromophore*, which absorbs the laser energy and results in heating greater than 100° C. Consequently boiling and volatilization occurs at the site, bordered by an area of thermal damage measuring 10 µ to 120 µ, depending on the laser used. This effect can be produced by lasers in the *longer infrared* spectrum. The *absorption peak for water is around 2900 nm*, therefore only laser wavelengths near this and having sufficient energy are best utilized for photovaporization.

The following lasers can produce photovaporization:

1. **CO_2 Laser (10,600 nm)**
    a. **Continuous wave** laser produces gross area of charring around the vaporized zone (thermal charring).
    b. **Microsecond pulsed delivery** also result in a collateral thermal damage of few hundred microns.
    c. **Q-Switched nanosecond** (500 ns) pulsed laser further reduces the collateral damage zone. But the penetration depth is 20 µ.

2. **Er:YAG Laser (2940 nm)**
    This produces precise and reproducible excision with 10–50 µ zone of collateral thermal damage and only 1.3 µ of penetration depth. It is currently most extensively studied laser for newer applications like *laser vitreoretinal surgery* and laser cataract surgery *(laser phaco)*. Penetration is minimum (1.3 µ), even less than that for excimer laser (3–4 µ). It is best suited for very fine *cutting of epiretinal membranes,* etc.

3. **Hydrogen Fluoride Laser**
    This laser (2900 nm) causes 10 to 50 µ of collateral damage with 1–2 µ deep incision.

4. **Raman shifted Nd: YAG (2800 nm)**
    The collateral damage is about 1.5–10 µ with this laser.

PHOTOCHEMICAL EFFECT

This effect is produced by ultraviolet and visible wavelengths through *breaking* or *formation* of chemical bonds. Three types of photochemical effects are as follows:

1. Naturally occurring photochemical reactions
2. Ablative photodecomposition
3. Photodynamic effect

Naturally Occuring Photochemical Reactions

Naturally occurring photochemical reactions are *photosynthesis, bleaching of rhodopsin* and *free radical* formation.

Ablative Photodecomposition

Ablative Photodecomposition is a laser-tissue interaction in which the *excimer laser* photons break the co-valent bonds between the molecules. The remaining energy of the photons causes ejection of the products, thus producing precise, repeatable and smooth incisions or tissue removal.

The collateral damage zone is narrow and less with shorter wavelengths in comparison to the more damaging effects of longer wavelengths. Table 3.3 shows the zone of collateral damage (thermal in case of longer wavelengths) produced by different lasers.

Table 3.3: Zone of collateral thermal damage by excimer lasers

Excimer laser		Zone of collateral thermal damage
Argon Fluoride	(193 nm)	0.070 µ to 0.100 µ
Krypton Fluoride	(248 nm)	10 µ
Xenon Chloride	(308 nm)	10-20 µ
Xenon Fluoride	(351 nm)	large zone

Photodynamic Effect

This effect is produced when a photosensitizing agent transfers the energy from the incident laser of a specific wavelength, to tissue oxygen that liberates highly reactive singlet oxygen species. These reactive species destroy the membranes of cells that contain the photosensitive dye. In addition platelet activation and subsequent thrombosis and occlusion of the new vessels and blood supply to the neoplasm leads to destruction of the lesion.

The dye has affinity for the lipoproteins, which are taken up by the dividing cells in high concentrations in comparison to the normal surrounding tissue. Laser energy is delivered directly to the abnormal area which selectively destroys the lesion where the dye is present in more concentration.

The energy required to produce this effect is low, which again avoids unnecessary collateral damage. Photodynamic therapy has been used for treatment of the following conditions.
1. Retinoblastoma
2. Malignant melanoma
3. Subfoveal neovascular membranes

Two types of photosensitizing agents can be utilized for this effect. These are:
1. Protoporphyrin derivatives
2. Benzoporphyrin derivatives

Protoporphyrin Derivatives

Hematoporphyrin derivatives (e.g. HPD 2.5 to 5.0 mg per kg) are slowly excreted They remain in the body and skin for about one month. Their use require indoors confinement for the same period to avoid sunburns.

Benzoporphyrin Derivatives

Verteprofin (Visudyne) is rapidly excreted from the body. Clinical trials of photodynamic therapy for treating '*subfoveal choroidal neovascular membranes*' have shown its utility because it causes less vision loss in comparison to placebo, when photocoagulating the lesions in the subfoveal location. The dose is 6 mg /m^2 at the rate of 3 ml/minute. The diode laser at wavelength of 689 nm, energy 50 J/m^2 and intensity of 600 m W/cm^2 is used. It is delivered for 83 seconds after 15 minutes of infusion of Verteprofin.

Transpupillary Thermotherapy (TTT)

Transpupillary thermotherapy is a newer modality of treatment of age related macular degeneration specially aimed for **subfoveal, occult** and **large neovascular membranes.** In these situations the photocoagulation with the conventional argon laser therapy results in precipitous fall in visual acuity due to damage to the neuroretina when closure of the neovascular membrane is attempted.

Moreover, the closure rate of the occult and large membranes is low and recurrence rate frequent with the argon laser.

Transpupillary thermotherapy acts by closing the neovascular membranes through vascular occlusion due to *thrombosis* of the vessels. The action is thought to be mediated by the release of cytotoxic *free radicals* from the irradiated tissue *rather than by the photocoagulation effect* of the laser. This is substantiated by the fact that no visible reaction is seen on the retina that occurs during photocoagulation as whitening of the retina.

The maximum chorioretinal temperature rise during this therapy is about 10°C (range 4–10°C) as compared to 20°C measured during the conventional photocoagulation. This is achieved due to the **low irradiance, large spot size and prolonged exposure time** protocol of the this therapy using the infrared laser.

A typical protocol for *lightly-pigmented fundi* is 800 mW, 3 mm retinal diameter, 60 seconds exposure with 810 nm diode laser (c.f. 200–500 micron spot size,

0.2–0.5 seconds exposure burns of argon or Krypton laser). For Indian eyes with pigmented fundi the power used is less in the range of 300–500 mW. The spot should encompass the whole lesion to be treated. Multiple laser deliveries are made centered on the first application site. Table 3.4 lists different laser used in ophthalmology.

Table 3.4: Different lasers and their use in Ophthalmology

Laser	Wavelength	Ophthalmic tissue-interaction	Clinical use
Fifth harmonic			
Nd: YLF	211 nm	Photoablation	Solid state excimer lasers
Nd: YAG	213 nm	Photoablation	
ArF Excimer laser	193 nm	Photoablation	Phototherapeutic keratectomy (PTK)
			Photorefractive surgeries
			—PRK, LASIK, LASEK, C-LASIK
			Sclerostomy
			Partial external laser trabeculoplasty
Argon laser (blue)	488 nm	Photocoagulation	not in common use
Argon laser (green)	514 nm	Photocoagulation	Retinal photocoagulation
			Iridectomy
			Trabeculoplasty
			VR surgery
			Retinal/choroidal tumors
			Treating corneal vascularization
Nd: YAG (Frequency-doubled)	532 nm	Photocoagulation	Similar to argon green
Dye yellow	577 nm	Photocoagulation	Retinal photocoagulation
Dye red	630 nm	Photodynamic	Destruction of melanoma, retinoblastoma
Krypton red	647 nm	Photocoagulation	Foveolar photocoagulation
Semiconductor-Diode	810 nm	Photocoagulation	Retinal photocoagulation
			Foveolar photocoagulation: TTT
			Endolaser in VR surgery
			ICG angiography
			Treatment of CSR
			Diode laser cytophotocoagulation: DLCP
Nd: YAG (picosecond)	1,064 nm	Photodisruption	Capsulotomy
			Iridectomy
			Cytophotocoagulation
Titanium: sapphire (femtosecond)	785 nm	Photodisruption	**Intrastromal PRK**
Nd: YAG (nanosecond)	1,064 nm	Photodisruption	**Intrastromal PRK**
Nd: YLF (picosecond)	1,053 nm	Photodisruption	**Intrastromal PRK**
Holmium: YAG	2,000 nm	Photothermal	**Laser thermokeratoplasty**
			Laser sclerostomy
Er: YAG	2,940 nm	Photovaporization	**Laser cataract surgery**
			Laser vitreoretinal surgery
Hydrogen fluoride	2,900 nm	Photovaporization	
Raman shifted			
Nd: YAG	2,800 nm	Photovaporization	
CO2 (Continuous wave)	10,060 nm	Photothermal	
CO2 (Pulsed nanosecond)	- do -	Photoevaporization	Blephroplasty
			Intraocular tumors
			Filtering surgeries
			Capillary hemangiomas

Suggested readings

1. Aron Rosa D, Aron JJ et al: Use of the Nd: YAG laser to open the posterior capsule after lens implant surgery: a preliminary report. J Am Intraocl Implant Soc 1980; 6: 352-354.
2. Peyman GA, Raichand M, Zeimer RC: Ocular effects of various wavelengths. Surv Ophthalmol 1984; 28: 391-404.
3. Lin CP: Laser tissue interaction: Basic principles. Ophthalmol Cli North Am 1993; 6: 381-391.
4. Mainster MA: Wavelength selection in macular photocoagulation. Ophthalmology 1986; 93: 952-58.
5. Johnson MW, Hasan TS, Elner VM: Laser photocoagulation of the choroid. Arch Ophthalmol 1995; 113: 516-527.
6. Geerling G, Koop N et al: Diode laser thermokeratoplasty. Initial clinical experiences. Ophthalmologe 1999 May; 96(5):306-11
7. Mechini U, Trabuchi G et al: Can diode laser (810 nm) effectively produce chorioretinal adhesions?, Retina 1992; 12: S 80-S 86.
8. Luke K, Steinmaatz M et al: Diode laser retinal photocoagulation. Laser Light Ophthalmol 1990; 3:167- 172.
9. Bandello F, Brancato R et al: Diode versus argon laser panretinal photocoagulation in proliferative diabetic retinopathy, A randomized study in 44 eyes with a long follow up. Graefe's Arch Cli Exp Ophthalmol 1993; 231:491-494.
10. Ulbig MW, McHugh DA, Hamilton AMP: Diode laser photocoagulation for diabetic macular edema. Br J Ophthalmol 1995; 79: 318-321.
11. Reichel E, Puliafito CA et al: Indocyanine green dye-enhanced diode laser photocoagulation of poorly defined subfoveal neovascular membranes. Ophthalmic Surgery 1994; 25: 195-201.
12. McHugh DA, Schwartz S et al: Diode laser contact transscleral retinal photocoagulation. Br J Ophthalmol 1995; 79: 1083-1087.
13. Macular Photocoagulation Study (MPS) Group: Evaluation of argon green versus krypton red laser for photocoagulation of subfoveal choroidal neovascularization in the macular photocoagulation study, Arch Ophthalmol 1994; 112:1176-1184.
14. Shields CL, Shields JA et al: Treatment of Retinoblastoma with indirect ophthalmoscope laser photocoagulation. Pediatr Ophthalmol Strabismus 1995; 32: 317-322.
15. Augusberger JJ, Faulkner CB et al: Combined iodine-125 plaque irradiation and indirect ophthalmoscope laser therapy of choroidal malignant melanomas. Graefe's Arch Cli Exp Ophthal 1993; 231:500-507.
16. Bressler NM: Photodynamic therapy of subfoveal choroidal neovascularization in age related macular degeneration with Verteprofin:2 year randomized clinical trials-tap report 2. Arch Ophthalmol 2001; 119(2): 198-207.
17. Schmidt-Eefurth U, Hasan T: Mechanism of action of photodynamic therapy with vertiprofin for the treatment of age related macular degeneration. Surv Ophthalmol 200; 45(3): 195-214.
18. Atul Kumar, Nainiwal S: Age related macular degeneration: Fluorescein and Indocyanin-green angiography. DOS Times 2002; 7 (4): 3-12.
19. Azad R, Chandra P: Photodynamic therapy. DOS Times 2002; 7 (4): 16-18.
20. Obana A, Gohoto Y et al: A retrospective study of ICG enhanced diode laser photocoagulation for subfoveal choroidal neovascularization associated with age related macular degeneration. Jpn J Ophthalmol 2002; 44(6): 668-676.
21. Newsom RS, McAlister JC et al: Transpupillary Thermotherapy for choroidal neovascularization. Ophthalmol 200; 85(2): 173-178.
22. Verma Lalit, Tewari K et al: TTT in CNVM: Initial experience, DOS Times 2002; 7 (4): 19-22.
23. Diabetic Retinopathy Study Research Group. Indications for treatment of diabetic retinopathy: Report no. 14. Int Ophthal Clin 1987; 27: 239-253.
24. Early Treatment Diabetic Retinopathy Study Research Group. Techniques for local and scatter photocoagulation. Report no. 3. Int Ophthal Clin 1987; 27: 254-264.
25. Early Treatment Diabetic Retinopathy Study Research Group. Early photocoagulation for diabetic retinopathy. Report no. 9. Ophthalmology 1991; 98: 766-785.
26. Early Treatment Diabetic Retinopathy Study Research Group. Photocoagulation for diabetic macular edema Report no. 4. Int Ophthal Clin 1987; 27: 265-272.
27. Branch Vein Study Group. Argon laser photocoagulation for macular edema in branch vein occlusion. Am J Ophthalmol 1984; 98: 271-282.
28. Branch Vein Study Group. Argon laser photocoagulation for macular edema in branch vein occlusion. Am J Ophthalmol 1985; 99: 218-219.
29. Branch Vein Study Group. Argon laser photocoagulation for prevention of neovascularization and vitreous hemorrhage in branch vein occlusion: A randomized clinical trial. Arch Ophthalmol 1986; 104: 34-41.
30. Hayreh SS, Klugman MR et al: Argon laser photocoagulation in ischemic CRVO. Graefe's Arch Cli Exp Ophthalmol 1990; 228: 281-296.
31. Central Vein Study Group. Evaluation of grid pattern photocoagulation for macular edema in central retinal vein occlusion: the Central Vein Study Group M report. Ophthalmology 1995; 102: 1425-1433.
32. Central Vein Study Group: A randomized clinical trial of early panretinal photocoagulation for ischemic central retinal vein occlusion. Ophthalmology 1995; 102: 1434-1444.
33. Robertson DM, Ilstrup D: Direct, indirect and sham laser photocoagulation in the management of central serous chorioretinopathy. Am J Ophthalmol 1983; 95 457- 491.

34. Slusher MM: Krypton red laser photocoagulation in selected cases of central serous chorioretinopathy. Retina 1986; 6: 81-84.
35. Yannuzzi LA, Slakter JS, Gupta K et al: Laser treatment of diffuse retinal pigment epitheliopathy. Europ J Ophthalmol 1992; 2: 103-114.
36. Annesley QH, Augusberger JJ: Ten year follow up of photocoagulated central serous chorioretinopathy. Trans Am Ophthalmol Soc 1981; 79: 335-346.
37. Brancato R, Scialdone A et al: Eight year follow up of photocoagulated central serous chorioretinopathy. Graefe's Arch Cli Exp Ophthalmol 1990; 228: 305-309.
38. Weinberger D, Kremer I et al: The treatment of foveal central serous chorioretinopathy by krypton red laser. Ann Ophthalmol 1990; 22: 35-38.
39. Piccolino FC: Laser treatment of eccentric leaks in central serous chorioretinopathy resulting in disappearance of untreated juxtafoveal leaks. Retina 1992; 12: 96-102.
40. Peyman GA, Koch N: Effects of Erbium : YAG laser on ocular tissues. Int Ophthalmol 1987; 10: 245-53.
41. Peyman GA, Bayer C et al: Long term effects of Erbium: YAG (2.9.4 μm) laser ablation on primate cornea. . Int Ophthalmol 1991; 15: 249-258.
42. Wolbrast MK, Foulks GN et al: Corneal surgery with an Erbium: YAG laser at 2.9.4 μm. Ophthal Vis Sci 1991; 27 (Suppl): 93.
43. Ross BS, Puliafito CA: Erbium: YAG laser photoablation of normal and cataractous lens in rabbits: preliminary report. J Cataract Ref Surg 1995; 21: 282- 286.
44. Berger JW, Kim SH et al: Er :YAG laser drilling of the lens tissue: Predicting the ablation rate with a simple model. Proc Society of Photo-Optical Instrumentation Engineering 1995; 148: 2393.
45. Stevens G Jr, Long B et al: Erbium: YAG laser assisted cataract surgery. Ophthalmic Surg and Lasers 1998; 29: 185-189.
46. D'Amino DJ, Blumenkranz MS et al: Multicenter clinical experience using an Er: YAG laser for vitreoretinal surgery. Ophthalmology 1996; 103: 1575.
47. Schmidt Petersen H, Mrochen M et al: Er: YAG laser vitrectomy. ARVO Abstracts. Invest Ophthalmol Vis Sci 1997; 38 (suppl): S 86.
48. Planker D, Hemo I et al: Vitreoretinal ablation with the 193 nm excimer laser in fluid medium. Invest Ophthalmol Vis Sci 1994; 35: 3835.
49. Stern D, Shoenlein R wet al: Corneal ablation with nanosecond, picosecond and femotosecond laser at 532 and 625 nm. Arch Ophthalmol 1989; 107: 587-92.
50. Zyset B, Puliafito CA et al: Picosecond optical breakdown: tissue effects and reduction of collateral damage. Laser Surg Med 1989; 9: 193.
51. Niemz MH, Kancnik EG et al: Plasma mediated ablation of the corneal tissue at 1053 nm using a Nd: YAG oscillator/ regenerative amplifier laser. Laser Surg Med 1991; 11:426- 431.
52. Freuh BE, Bille JF et al: Intrastromal relaxing incisions in rabbits with a picosecond infrared laser. Laser Light Ophthalmol 1992; 4:165-168.
53. Remmel RM, Dardenne CM et al: Intrastromal tissue removal using an infrared picosecond Nd: YLF ophthalmic laser operating at 1053 nm. Laser Light Ophthalmol 1992; 4:169-173.
54. Niemz MH, Hopler TP et al: Intrastromal ablation for refractive corneal surgery using picosecond infrared laser pulse. Laser Light Ophthalmol 1993; 5:149-155.
55. Juhasz T, Speaker MG et al: Refractive effects of myopic ablation of cat cornea the Nd: YLF ophthalmic picosecond laser. Invest Ophthalmol Vis Sci 1994; 35 (suppl): 2026.
56. Juhasz T, Hu XH et al: Dynamics of shock wave cavitation generated by picosecond laser pulses in corneal tissue and water. Laser Light Ophthalmol 1996.
57. Srinivasan R, Sutcliffe E: Dynamics of ultraviolet ablation of the corneal tissue. Am J Ophthalmol 1987; 103: 470-471.
58. Ren Q, Simon G et al: Ultraviolet solid state laser (213nm) photorefractive keratectomy: in vitro study. Ophthalmology 1993; 100: 1828-1834.
59. Hu XH, Juhasz T: Experimental study of picosecond laser ablation at 211nm and 263 nm. Ophthalmologic technologies, editorial Parel JM 1994.
60. Krueger RR, Quantock AJ, Juhasz T et al: Ultrastructure of picosecond laser intrastromal photodisruption. J Refract Surg 1996 Jul-Aug;12(5): 607-12.
61. Condon PI, Mulhern M, Fulcher T et al: Laser intrastromal keratomileusis for high myopia and myopic astigmatism. Br J Ophthalmol 1997 Mar;81(3): 199-206.
62. Lubatschowski H, Maatz G, Heisterkamp A, et al: Application of ultrashort laser pulses for intrastromal refractive surgery. Graefes Arch Clin Exp Ophthalmol 2000 Jan; 238(1): 33-9.
63. Kurtz RM, Horvath C, Liu HH, Krueger RR et al: Lamellar refractive surgery with scanned intrastromal picosecond and femtosecond laser pulses in animal eyes. J Refract Surg 1998 Sep-Oct; 14(5): 541-8

Section II
Excimer Lasers

Chapter 4

Excimer Lasers: History

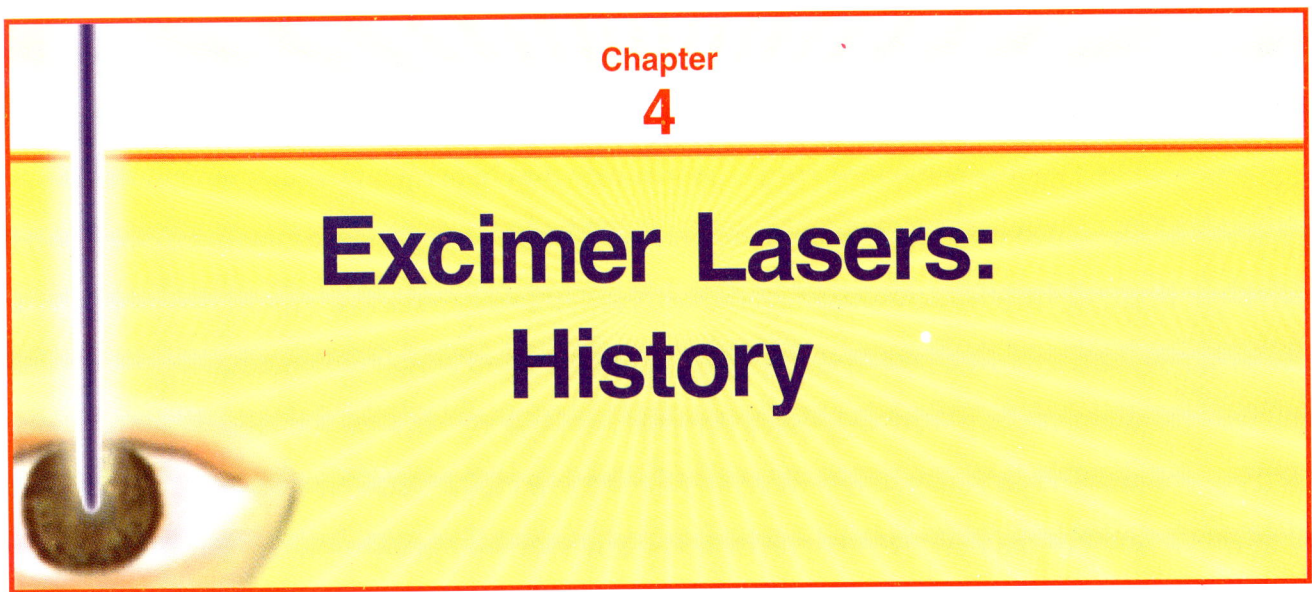

Velazco et al discovered excimer lasers using xenon (Xn), a noble gas and halogen gases in 1975.

Searles et al discovered laser action with xenon and krypton chloride and fluorides in 1975. Only XeCl with sufficient energy output has found its use in angioplasty, excimer laser trabeculectomy and endarterectomy.

Hoffman et al reported laser action at 193 nm wavelength from argon fluoride molecule in 1976. It had photons of 6.4 eV of energy and a pulse duration of 10–15 ns.

Taboada et al studied the effect of these laser on rabbit cornea in 1981.

Stephens Trokel, John Marshall and Srinivasan studied the histopathology and ultrastructural changes in ablated cornea during 1984-1985.

Munnerlyn et al were the first to use the term photorefractive keratectomy in 1984. They showed quantitative relationship between the amount of corneal tissue removed and the change in refraction. They also showed that removal of 5 μ of tissue from the central 6 mm zone of corneal surface would flatten the cornea by one diopter.

Kruger et al determined the thresholds, ablation rates, healing patterns, ablation parameters and ultrastructural changes in the ablated corneal tissue during 1984-1985.

Serdarevic et al performed first experimental PTK to treat candidial keratitis in rabbit cornea in 1984.

Berlin, Bende and Seiler were the first to use PTK clinically in 1988. They excised superficial diseased corneal tissue with excimer laser.

Seiler and Bende performed first photoastigmatic keratotomy (PARK) in 1988. They treated astigmatism by giving relaxing keratotomy incisions using excimer laser in human eyes.

McDonnell and Kaufman first described PRK on blind human eyes in 1987. In 1988 they reported the first series of PRK on sighted human eyes.

Gartry et al reported the first series of PTK in 25 sighted human eyes in 1990.

Pallikaris et al introduced Laser in-situ keratomileusis (LASIK) in 1990.

Seiler et al introduced wavefront-guided LASIK in 1999.

Velazco and his colleagues discovered the excimer lasers in 1975. They suggested that if xenon (Xn), a noble gas is made to react with halogen gases, an unstable compound would be formed. This compound, called noble gas halide compound would rapidly dissociate to ground state with the release of energetic photons in the range of ultraviolet (UV) wavelength. These emissions were termed excimer laser (Fig. 4.1).

The term excimer laser is a misnomer because it stands for *excited dimer*, i.e. an energized molecule with two identical components, whereas the rare gas-halide compound consists of two different components.

Searles and other researchers, in 1975, demonstrated laser action with xenon and krypton chloride and fluorides. Only XeCl with sufficient energy output has found use in angioplasty and endarterectomy.

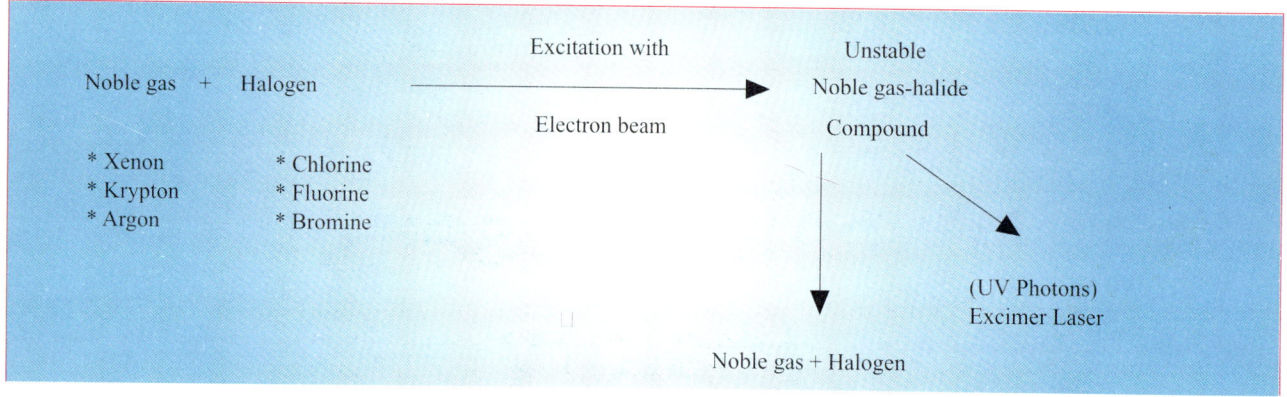

Fig. 4.1: Genesis of excimer laser

Hoffman and co-workers, in 1976, reported laser action at 193 nm wavelength from argon fluoride molecule having photons of 6.4eV of energy and a pulse duration of 10–15 ns. Table 4.1 shows the various 'excimer lasers', their wavelengths and the photon energy.

Table 4.1: Excimer lasers, their wavelengths and energy of photons

Excimer laser	Wavelength	Photon energy
Argon fluoride (ArF)	193 nm	6.4 eV
Krypton chloride (KrCl)	222 nm	5.59 eV
Krypton fluoride (KrF)	248 nm	4.99 eV
Xenon chloride (XeCl)	308 nm	4.03 eV
Xenon fluoride (XeF)	351 nm	3.53 eV

Srinivasan, in 1983, at Watson Laboratory studied the mechanism of action of 193 nm ArF excimer laser on organic materials such as plastics and human hair. He proposed the **photochemical** nature of interaction of 193 nm. ArF laser with organic molecules, different from photothermal damage produced by other conventional surgical lasers.

He proposed that the high energy (6.4 eV) photons of ArF laser broke the covalent bonds of organic molecules in a short time. He used the term **ablative photodecomposition** for this process (Fig. 4.2).

The broken fragments occupy a larger volume, rapidly expand and are ejected from the ablated surface at a supersonic speed in the form of a plume.

The kinetic energy for ejection of the fragments is provided by the unused energy of ArF laser photons and

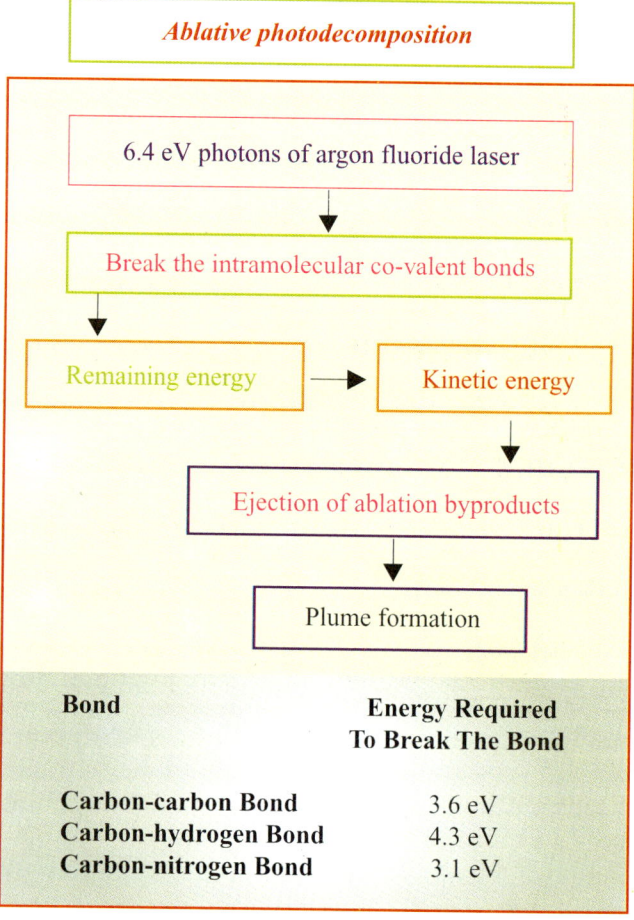

Fig. 4.2: Ablative photodecomposition

the latent energy of the covalent bonds of organic molecules (Fig. 4.3). He also reported that there was a threshold for this ablative photodecomposition which was independent of the laser firing rate.

Stephens Trokel with *Srinivasan* and coworkers studied the ablation interaction of ArF excimer laser on

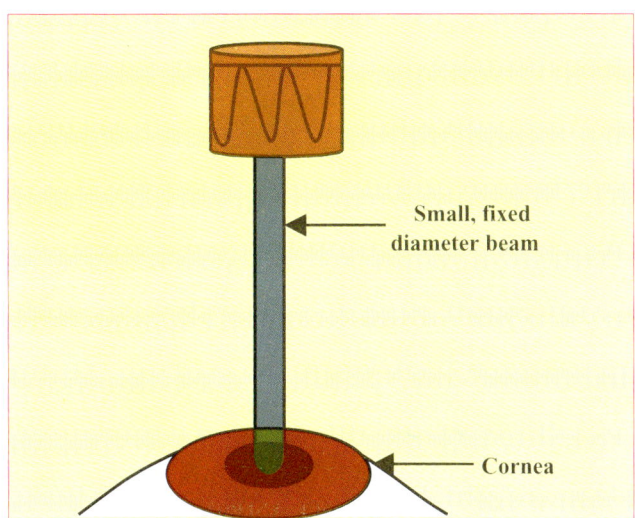 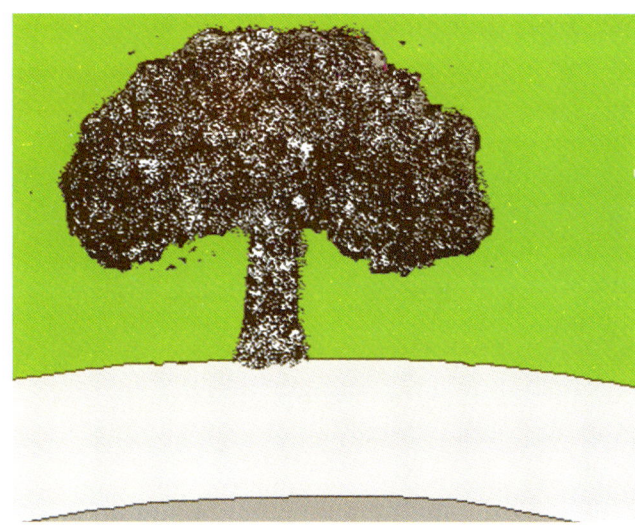

Fig. 4.3: Excimer laser ablation of cornea and ejection of ablation by-products (plume formation)

bovine eyes. The ablation produced trench on corneal surface with crispy edges, with no deformation of adjacent corneal tissue. Histopathology showed no significant collateral damage. Each pulse removed fraction of a micron of corneal tissue. The resulting surface was extremely smooth and uniform.

They demonstrated that the **long held axiom** and clinical observation **that the presence of Bowman's layer was essential for uniform corneal topography and transparency, was not true**. The conventional corneal surgeries such as lamellar keratectomy and keratomileusis failed in producing clear corneas because these produced an uneven and rough surface at the site of incision in terms of optical standards, even if incisions were made with diamond blades.

On the contrary, when they used 193 nm ArF excimer laser, the tissue removal was with submicron precision with a smoothness of better than one third to half the wavelength of visible light (0.4–0.8 μm) The healed cornea was clear and smooth. They suggested a surgical application of the 193 nm ArF excimer laser, either to give an incision or to remove large areas of corneal tissue as *controlled lamellar keratectomy* or to reshape the corneal curvature.

They studied the ultrastructural changes in ablated cornea of animals, using scanning electron microscope (SEM) and transmission electron microscope (TEM). The ablated stromal surface showed extreme smoothness. The healed reepithelised surface appeared similar to the adjacent unablated surface. The *damage zone* was limited to less than 100 nm (0.1 μm), forming a uniform electrondense condensation. They called it *pseudomembrane*, which seemed to maintain the integrity of the severed cells and stromal surface. There was no conductive damage to stromal lamellae adjacent to the pseudomembrane.

EXCIMER LASER PARAMETERS AND DEFINITIONS

Irradiance

Irradiance is the laser energy *per unit area*. It is the density of photons striking the cornea per pulse per unit area and is the function of energy output and the beam diameter.

Fluence

It is the laser energy used *per unit volume* of the ablated tissue.

Repetition Rate

It is the number of laser pulses delivered per second and is usually about 10 Hz.

Higher irradiance and repetition rate could generate more acoustic shock waves and might be associated with increased thermal hazards. The repetition rate higher than 40 Hz may cause irreversible damage to the cornea, endothelium and the Descemet's membrane.

Ablation Threshold

Ablation threshold is the minimum laser energy (irradiance) required to produce photoablation. *It varies depending on the following variables.*

1. Excimer laser wavelength
2. Different ocular tissue and the species
3. Laser firing rate

Excimer Laser Wavelength

Ablation threshold is lowest for 193 nm ArF excimer laser and increases logarithmically with increasing wavelengths.

Different Ocular Tissue and the Species

Ablation threshold for *human cornea* it is *about* 50 mJ/cm^2 and for *bovine cornea* 20 mJ/cm^2 in case of 193 nm ArF excimer laser. It is different for epithelium, stroma and scarred corneal tissue of the same species.

Laser Firing Rate

The ablation threshold is independent of laser firing rate only at 193 nm and 351 nm. Other wavelengths show a *decrease in the threshold with increasing pulse frequency* (firing rate). This decrease in ablation threshold is maximum with 248 nm wavelength. The cause of decrease in the threshold is associated thermal damage with other excimer lasers.

Ablation Rate (Ablation Depth)

The ablation depth per pulse is *dependant on the irradiance.* For 193 nm ArF excimer laser it is predictable and increases smoothly on increasing the energy (Table 4.2).

In contrast, the ablation depth with other excimer laser wavelengths show greater variation with smaller changes in irradiance energy and had poor predictability of ablation (Fig. 4.4).

Table 4.2: Laser irradiance and ablation depth

Irradiance	Ablation depth*
100 mJ/cm^2	0.10 µ
150 mJ/cm^2	0.20 µ
180 mJ/cm^2	0.26 µ
200 mJ/cm^2	0.45 µ

*The above figures may vary slightly depending on the laser system used due to variation in the energy profile of the laser beam

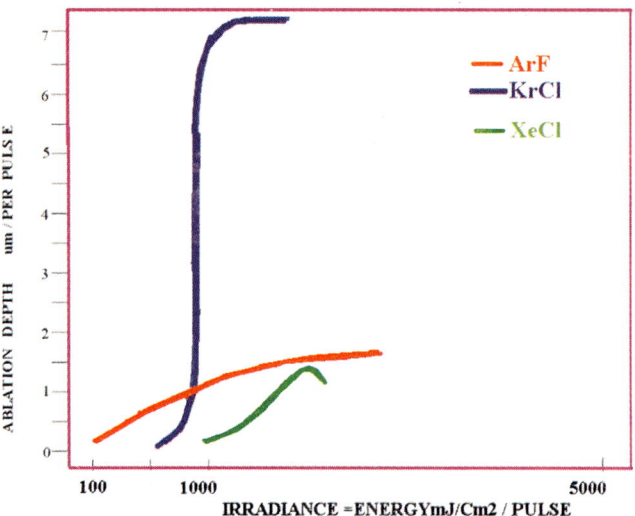

Fig. 4.4: Ablation rate of three different excimer lasers at different energy levels

Following are the known factors associated with change in the ablation rate.

Tissue Hydration

Ablation rate depends on tissue hydration. Dehydration of the tissue such as by dry gas blowing, leads to deeper (increased) ablation of the tissue.

State of the Cornea

Abnormal cornea has different ablation rate than a normal cornea. Corneal scars and calcified areas have much lower ablation rate and could be even resistant to ablation.

Different Layers of Cornea

The ablation rate is more for epithelium than for stroma and is least for the Bowman's layer, at a given irradiance.

Suggested readings

1. Velazco JR, Setser DW et al: Bound-free emission spectra of diatomic xenon halides, J Chem. Phys 1975; 62: 1990-1991.
2. Taboada J, Mikesell GW, Reed RD: Response of the corneal epithelium to KrF excimer laser pulses, Health Phys 1981.
3. Taboada J, Archibal CJ et al: An extreme sensitivity in corneal epithelium to far UV ArF excimer laser pulses,

proceedings of the Scientific Program of the. Aerospace Medical Association, San Antonio, Texas, 1981.
4. Trokel SL, Srinivasan R, Braren B: Excimer Laser Surgery of the Cornea. Am J Ophthalmol 1983; 96: 749-58.
5. Trokel S: Evolution of excimer laser corneal surgery. J Cataract Refract Surg 1989; 15: 373-83.
6. Srinivasan R: Kinetics of the ablative photodecomposition of organic polymers in the far-ultraviolet. J Vac Sci Techno B1 1983; 4: 923-926.
7. Searles SK, Hart GA: Bound free emission spectra of xenon halides. Appl. Phys Lett 1975; 27: 243.
8. Seiler T, Bende T, Trokel S, Wollensak J: Excimer laser keratectomy for correction of astigmatism. Am J Ophthalmol 1988; 105:117-24.
9. Srinivasan R. Sutcliffe E: Dynamics of the ultraviolet laser ablation of corneal tissue. Am J Ophthalmol 1987; 103: 470-471.
10. Puliafito CA, Steiner RF, Oeutsch TF, Adler CM: Excimer laser ablation of the cornea and lens. Ophthalmology 1985; 92: 741-8.
11. Marshall, J Trokel SI, Rothery S, Krueger R: A comparative study of comea incisions induced by diamond and steel knives and two ultraviolet radiations from excimer laser. Br J Ophthalmol 1986; 70: 482-501.
12. Munnerlyn CR, Koons SJ, Marshall J: Photorefractive keratectomy: a technique for laser refractive surgery. J Cataract Refractive Surg 1988; 14: 46-52.
13. Marshall J, Trokel S, Rothery S et al: Photoablative reprofilling of the cornea using an excimer laser: photorefractive keratectomy. Lasers in Ophthalmol 1986; 1: 21-48.
14. Munnerlyn CR, Koons SJ, Marshall J: Photorefractive keratectomy: a technique for laser refractive surgery. J cat Refract Surg 1988; 14: 46-52.
15. Marshall J, Trokel SL, Rothery S et al: Long term healing of the centra cornea after photorefractive keratectomy using an excimer laser. Ohthalology 1988; 95: 1411-1421.
16. McDonald MB, Beureman R, Falzoni W et al: Refractive surgery with the excimer laser. Am J Ophthalmol 1987; 103: 469.
17. McDonald MB, Kaufman HE et al: Excimer laser ablation in a human eye. Arch Ophthalmol 1989; 107: 641-642.
18. McDonald MB, Liu JC, Byrd TJ et al: Central photorefractive keratectomy for myopia. Partially sighted and normally sighted eyes. Ophthalmology 1991; 98: 1327-1337.
19. Krueger RR, Trokel SL, Schubert HD: Interaction of Ultraviolet Laser Light with the cornea. Invest Ophthal Vis Sci 1985; 26: 1455-64.
20. Krueger RR, Trokel SL: Quantification of Corneal Ablation by Ultraviolet Laser. Arch Ophthalmol 1985; 103: 1741-1742.
21. Berlin T, Bende T, Seiler T: Corneal resurfacing by excimer laser ablation. ARVO Abstracts. Invest Ophthalmol Vis Sci 1988; 29 (suppl) : 310.
22. Pallikaris IG, Papatazanaki ME et al: Laser in situ keratomileusis. Laser Surg Med 1990; 10: 463-8.
23. Mrochen M, Kaemmerer M, Seiler T: Wavefront-guided laser in situ keratomileusis: early results in three eyes. J Refract Surg 2000 Mar-Apr;16(2):116-121.
24. Seiler T, Mrochen M, Kaemmerer M: Operative correction of ocular aberrations to improve visual acuity J Refract Surg 2000 Sep-Oct;16(5): S619-622.
25. Van Saarloos PP, Constable IJ: Bovine corneal stroma ablation rate with 193-mm excimer laser radiation: Quantitative measurement. Refract Corneal Surg 1990; 6: 424-429.
26. Serdarevic O, Darrell RW, Krueger RR, Trokel SL: Excimer Laser Therapy for Experimental Candida Keratitis. Am J Ophthalmol 1985; 99:534-8.
27. Seiler T, Kriegerowski M, Schnoy N, et at: Ablation rate of human corneal epithelium and Bowman's layer with the excimer laser (193 nm), Refract Corneal Surg 1990; 6: 99-102.
28. Krueger RR, Campos M, Wang X, et at: Corneal surface morphology following excimer laser ablation with humidified gases. Arch Ophthalmol 1993; 111: 1131-1137.
29. Campos M, Cuevas K, Garbus J, et 31: Corneal wound healing after excimer laser ablation: effects of nitrogen gas blower. Ophthalmology 1992; 99: 893-897.

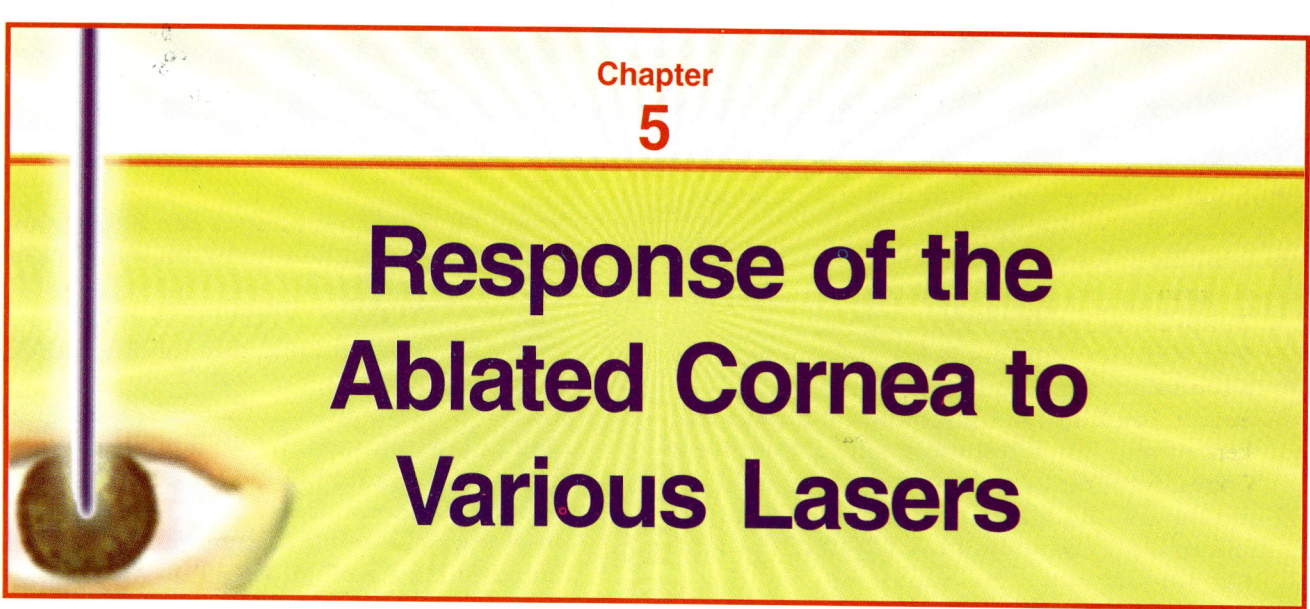

Chapter 5

Response of the Ablated Cornea to Various Lasers

Various corneal tissues show the following changes after excimer laser photoablation:

COLLATERAL DAMAGE AND THERMAL EFFECT

Only 193 nm ArF laser shows sharp, crisp and smooth edges of the ablated tissue without any significant collateral tissue damage. *Other wavelengths show increasing thermal damage,* charring, vacuolation and shrinkage of stromal lamellae, as the wavelength increases. The excised edges/surface has irregular and jagged margins.

Moreover, progressive increase in the irradiance of laser causes more coagulative changes in corneal tissue and stromal clouding of the exposed cornea. This is seen with all other excimer wavelengths except 193 nm and is because of increase in the thermal component with increase in the energy (Table 5.1).

Table 5.1: Zone of collateral damage with different lasers

Laser	Wavelength	Zone of collateral damage
Argon Fluoride	(193 nm)	0.070 µ to 0.100 µ
Frequency Quintupled		
Nd: YLF	(211 nm)	< 0.100 µ to 0.600 µ
Nd: YAG	(213 nm)	< 0.600 µ
Krypton Fluoride	(248 nm)	10 µ
Xenon Chloride	(308 nm)	10-20 µ
Xenon Fluoride	(351 nm)	large zone

1. No thermal component occurs with 193 nm ArF laser, which has purely photochemical interaction with the tissue.
2. The frequency quintupled 'solid state excimer lasers' show very similar excision profile to that of 193 nm ArF laser.
3. Only 193 nm ArF laser removes tissue with great smoothness of the ablated surface/edges, precision and predictability over increasing energies for ablation and causes least collateral thermal damage. *Therefore, presently it is the only excimer laser in clinical use for corneal surgeries.*

FORMATION OF PSEUDOMEMBRANE

After excimer laser photoablation of cornea, an electrondense, ultrathin zone called *pseudomembrane* is formed, which covers the unablated corneal tissue. It serves the following functions:

1. Membrane like function in maintaining the integrity of the ablated corneal surface.
2. It acts as a protective barrier to water transportation into the lamellae and prevents corneal swelling and haze.
3. It directs the new migrating hyperplastic epithelial cells to fill in the wound, *serving as a template* for re-epithelization and helps in creating a smooth epithelial surface.

Dehydration (as occurred due to dry gas blowing for removing ablation by-products previously) during ablation has detrimental effect, resulting in thicker, less dense, discontinuous pseudomembrane formation with detached fragments on its surface. *This is responsible for increased incidence of corneal haze.*

Optimal hydration (at physiological level) of the cornea results in formation of a uniform and thin pseudomembrane.

A thicker pseudomembrane (up to 250 nm) is formed as the irradiance increases. The thickness increases almost in a linear manner with increasing energy used for ablation. This suggest that it might be a thermal effect.

EPITHELIAL RESPONSE

Large number of clinical studies on human corneal ablation with 193 nm excimer laser have shown re-epithelization of the ablated surface within 3–5 days. Epithelial healing begins after 4–6 hours of the surface ablation of the cornea and the corneal surface is fully covered by new epithelium within 3–5 days. Rarely an epithelial deffect my be seen beyond the 7th day.

Initially, the epithelium consists of three to five layers. *It continues to thicken* over the next 6–18 months *so that the epithelium is thicker over the central ablated zone* after PRK than over the untreated area. It is thickest at the site which is ablated most deeply. This difference in the epithelial thickness can be documented by the modified optical pachymeter and more recently by the technique of '*Confocal microscopy through-focussing* (CMTF)'. The epithelial hyperplasia takes place in an attempt to restore the original corneal surface contour.

During the early period, the epithelial thickening is non-uniform. This is the reason why a good quality map of corneal topography is difficult to obtain after PRK during this period.

Factor Governing the Epithelial Healing Response

1. The removal of epithelium results in release of *growth factors* from the limbal area near the epithelial defect. These growth factors, mainly epidermal growth factor and fibroblastic growth factor, are responsible for stimulation of proliferation of epithelial cells and fibriblasts even if present in microquantities.
2. The degree of epithelial hyperplasia is dependent on the shape of the excised tissue or the excision profile. After PTK, it is thickest at the junction of the ablated and non-ablated zones *if tapering of the ablation is not done*. This results in greater hyperopic shift.
3. In PRK, the single profile (transitionzone ablation) and smaller diameter (< 5 mm) ablations lead to greater hyperplasia compared to larger area and multi-profile ablations (multizone ablation using 4 mm, 5 mm and 6 mm diameters in succession). *Early regression of refractive effect after PRK is due to this epithelial hyperplasia.*

ADHERENCE OF NEWLY FORMED EPITHELIUM TO THE STROMA

Anchorage of the new epithelium to the underlying stroma through reformation of normal type III collagen (anchoring fibrils), epithelial hemidesmosomes ($beta_4$-integrin) and basement membrane (type IV collagen) occurs during the first week. Rarity of recurrent epithelial erosions following 193 nm excimer laser ablation indicates normal adherence of the epithelium to the ablated stroma.

BOWMAN'S LAYER RESPONSE

Many studies, comparing corneal ultrastructural changes after conventional surgery and 193 nm excimer laser photoablation, have shown that **Bowman's layer is not necessary for corneal clarity** and for the formation of normal epithelial attachment complexes.

STROMAL RESPONSE AND CORNEAL HAZE

After ablation the collagen fibers under the pseudomembrane are normal. Stromal wound healing begins within 24 hours after the pseudomembrane disappears.

After initial disappearance during first 3 days, keratocytes repopulate and increase in number over next two weeks and a healing response is mounted. Keratocytes are activated by various growth factors that are released due to a break in the epithelium (see above). They form *new collagen, proteoglycan matrix* and vacuoles filled with proteoglycan debris. These are responsible for corneal haze, which appears as early as 1 week after photoablation, becomes maximum after 1–3 months and decreases thereafter as the stromal remodeling ensues.

These healing changes in the form of estracellular matrix, laying down of disorganized as well as type III new collagen and the ensuing stromal remodelling *collectively contribute to the myopic regression* after PRK, in addition to *corneal haze*. These two finding are commonly seen to occur together.

The activity of keratocytes may sometimes persist for up to 1½ year, necessitating use of low potency steroids and NSAIDs for long period to improve corneal clarity as well as minimize the regression of effect after PRK. Use of these agents during the postoperative period has been advocated by many clinical studies due to their effect on stromal remodeling. Many other agents like mitomycin-C and plasminogen-inhibitors, etc. also have been tried for modulation of stromal healing in an attempt to reduce corneal haze as well as the refractive changes after PTK and PRK.

LASIK surgery does not breach the epithelium. Therefore the activation of the stromal keratocytes by the growth factors and significant healing response does not occur after LASIK.

Visually significant corneal haze is found in 3–11% of the patients undergoing moderate photoablation. The incidence is 10–40% in patients with higher depth of ablation. Other factors contributing to greater level of corneal haze are male subjects, non compliance with postoperative steroid medication and intraoperative dehydration (see under complications).

Slit-lamp examination to evaluate haze is the most practical way of grading the level of haze. Corneal haze is graded according to Gartry et al as shown in Table 5.2.

Table 5.2: Grading the level of corneal haze

Grade	Description
Grade 0	Totally clear cornea
Grade 0.5	Barely perceptible, seen only with indirect broad tangential, illumination.
Grade 1	Trace haze of minimal density seen with direct and diffuse illumination.
Grade 2	Mild haze, easily visible with direct focal slit illumination.
Grade 3	Moderate haze that partially obscures iris details
Grade 4	Server haze that completely obscures iris details

Based on the postoperative refraction and the slit-lamp finding of corneal haze during 6 month after PRK, the healing response of stroma has been claffified into three subgroups by Durrie et al.

Normal Healers (Type I Healing, 85%)

In normal healers refraction is slightly hyperopic. It reverts to emmetropia as the subepithelial faint and reticular haze appears causing corneal steepening.

Inadequate Responders (Type II Healers)

Corneal haze is absent and refraction remains hyperopic indefinitely. The topical steroid drops are discontinued in these patients.

Aggressive Responders (Type III Healers)

They demonstrate dense subepithelial haze which produces myopic regression and also compromises the vision. Haze respond quickly to topical steroids with-reversal of the regression within 1 week to 1 month.

DESCEMET'S MEMBRANE RESPONSE

An unusual fibrillar response has been seen in the mid to anterior one third of Descemet's membrane in rabbit cornea following PRK mode of photoablation similar to that seen after manual lamellar keratectomy in animal studies[19,38]. One study has found similar fibrillar change in single human eye specimen[39]. No clinical significance has been found associated with this response.

ENDOTHELIAL RESPONSE

Zero to 13% endothelial loss has been found by different PRK studies where wide area ablation is used. The loss is limited to corneal periphery. These changes, however, are short-lived and of doubtful clinical significance.

Loss of endothelium *increases proportionately to attempted depth of ablation* and is *significant only with deeper ablation*. Unless the excimer beam approaches up to 40 μm of endothelium (>90% of corneal depth), there is *no direct risk* to corneal endothelium. It is theoretically possible to reach this level in case of extreme myopic LASIK; because the ablation is under a 160 μ corneal flap.

Wide area ablation, though only removing 10% of corneal thickness, may be followed by changes in endothelium such as vacuolation. This effect on endothelial cells could be possibly due to acoustic waves associated with wide area ablation such as during PTK and PRK. No significant endothelial loss has been reported after any LASIK surgery till date.

CORNEAL SENSITIVITY

After excimer laser photoablation of cornea, there is an immediate heightened pain response and increase in PGE_2 levels. This is followed by decrease in corneal sensitivity to about 50% during first month. Corneal sensitivity returns to normal by 3 months in almost all cases.

The loss of corneal sensitivity is related to removal of subepithelial nerve plexus after ArF excimer laser photoablation. Reappearance of the nerve plexus takes place at 1 month, which is initially disorganized morphologically. Regeneration of the nerve plexus continues up to 4 months.

Suggested readings

1. Marshall, J Trokel SI, Rothery S, Krueger R: A comparaive study of Comeal. incisions induced by Diamond and Steel Knives and two ultraviolet radiations from and Excimer Laser. Br J ophthalmol 1986; 70: 482-501.
2. Campos M, Wang X et al: Ablation rate and surface Ultrastructure of 193nm excimer laser keratectomies. Invest Ophthalmol Vis Sci 1983; 34: 2493-2500.
3. Krueger RR, Campos M, Wang X, et at: Corneal surface morphology following excimer laser ablation with humidified gases. Arch Ophthalmol 1993; 111: 1131-1137.
4. Trokel S: Evolution of excimer laser corneal surgery. J Cataract Refract Surg 1989; 15: 373-83.
5. Tuft SJ, Zabel RW et al: Corneal repair following keratectomy. A comparison between conventional surgery and laser photoablation. Invest Ophthal Vis Sci 1989; 30: 1769-77.
6. Seiler T, Wollensak J: Myopic PRK with the excimer laser. One year follow-up. Ophthalmology 1991; 98:1156-1163.
7. Sher NA, Chen V, Bowers RA, et al: The use of the 193-nm excimer laser for myopic photorefractive keratectomy in sighted eyes. A multicenter study. Arch Ophthalmol 1991; 109: 1525-1530.
8. Campos M, Cuevas K, Shieh E et al: Corneal wound healing after excimer laser ablation in rabbits. Refract Corneal Surg 1992; 8: 378-381.
9. Fantes F, Hanna D, Waring CO III, et al: Wound healing after excimer laser keratomileusis (photorefractive keratectomy) in monkeys. Arch Ophthalmol 1990; 108: 665-675
10. Fantes F, Manna K, Waring GO III: Myopic laser keratomileusis on monkeys. Clinical microscopic and ultrastructural observations, Invest Ophthalmol Vis sci 1989; 30 (8uppl): 217.
11. Renard G, Hanna K, Saragoussi JJ, et al: Excimer laser experimental keratectomy: ultrastructural study. Cornea 1987; 6: 269-272.
12. Rawe I, Zabel R, Tuft S: A morphological study of rabbit corneas after laser keratectomy. Eye 1992; 6: 637-642.
13. Ahmad O, Green R, Stark W, et al: Excimer laser keratectomy: morphometric analysis of epithelial basement membrane and hemidesmosome reformation, Invest Ophthal- mol Vis Sci 34 (Suppl): 703, 1993.
14. Paallysaho T, Twrvo K, Van Setten G et al: Distribution of integrins alpha-6 and beta-4 in the rabbit corneal epithelium after anterior keratectomy. Cornea 1992; 11: 523-58.
15. Binder PS, Anderson J et al: The morphological features of human excimer laser corneal ablation. Ophthalmology 1994; 101 (6): 979-989.
16. Seiler T, Kriegerowski M, Schnoy N, et at: Ablation rate of human corneal epithelium and Bowman's layer with the excimer laser (193 nm). Refract Corneal Surg 1990; 6: 99-102.
17. Kerr-Muir M, Trokel S, Marshal J: Ultrastructural comparison of conventional surgical and ArF excimer laser keratectomy. Am J Ophthal 1987; 103: 448-453.
18. Marshall, J Trokel SI, Rothery S, Krueger: A comparative study of comeal incisions induced by Diamond and Steel Knives and two ultraviolet radiations from excimer laser, Br J ophthalmol 1986; 70: 482-501.
19. Hanna KD, Pouliquen Y, Waring GO et al: Corneal stromal. wound healing in rabbits after 193-nm excimer laser surface ablation. Arch Ophthalmol 1989; 107: 895-901.
20. Caubert E: Cause of sub-epithelial comeal haze over 18 months after photorefractive keratectomy for myopia. Refract Corneal Surg 1993; 9 (Suppl): S65-S70.
21. Tuft S, Marshal J et al: Stromal remodeling after PRK. Laser Ophthalmol 1987; 1: 177-183.
22. Lobmann C, Gartry D, Kerr-Muir M et al: Haze in photorefractive keratectomy: its origins and consequences. Lasers Light Ophthalmol 1991; 4:15-34.
23. Hanna KD, Pouliquen YM, et al: Corneal wound healing in monkeys after repeated excimer laser photorefractive keratectomy, Arch Ophthalmol 1992; 110: 1286-1291.
24. Aquavella J, Gasset .A, Dohlmann C: Corticosteroids in corneal wound healing. Am J Ophthalmol 1964; 58: 621-626.
25. Gartry Ds, Kerr Muir MG, Marshall J: The effect of topical corticosteroids on refraction and corneal haze following excimer laser treatment of myopia: an update. A prospective, randomized, double masked study. Eye 1993; 7: 584-90.
26. Sher NA, Frantz JM, Talley A, et al: Topical diclofenac in the treatment of ocular pain after excimer photorefractive keratectomy. Refract Corneal Surg 1993; 9: 425-436.

27. Nassaralla SA, Szerrenyi K, Wang XW et al: Effect of diclofenac or corneal haze after PRK in rabbits, Ophthalmology (1995) 102: 469-74.
28. Morlet N, Gillies MC, Crouch R, et al: Effect of topical interferon-alpha 2b on corneal haze after excimer laser photorefractive keratectomy in rabbits. Refract Corneal Surg 1993; 9: 443-451.
29. Talamo J, Collamudi S, Green W, et al: Modulation of corneal wound healing after excimer laser keratomileusis using topical mitomycin C and steroids. Arch Ophthalmol 1991; 109: 1141-1146.
30. Lohmann CP, Marshall J: Plasmin and plasminogen-activator inhibitors after excimer laser photorefractive keratectomy: new concept in prevention of postoperative myopic regression and haze, Refract Corneal Surg 9:300-302, 1993.
31. Lohmann CP, Obart D, Patmore A et al: Plasmin-inhibitors and plasminogen-activator inhibitors after excimer laser PRK: new concept in prevention of myopic regression and haze. Invest Ophthalmol Vis Sci 1993; 34 (suppl): 705.
32. Phillips AF, Szerrenyi K, Campos M et al: Arachidonic acid metabolites after excimer laser corneal surgery. Arch Ophthalmol 1993; 1: 1273-1278.
33. Fitzsimmons T, Fagerholm P, Harfstrand A et al: Steroids after excimer surgery decrease corneal hydraulic acid conten. Invest Ophthalmol Vis Sci 1992; 33 (Suppl): 766.
34. Amano S, Shimizu K: Corneal endothelial changes after excimer laser photorefractive keratectom. Am J Ophthalmol 1993; 11: 692-694.
35. Carones F, Brancato R, Venturi E et al: The corneal endothelium after myopic excimer laser photorefractive keratectomy. Invest Ophthalmol Vis Sci 1993; 34 (suppl): 804.
36. Beldavs R, Thompson K, Waring GO III et al: Quantitative microscopy after PRK (abst). Ophthalmology 1992; 99: 125.
37. Binder P, Anderson J, Lambert R et al: Endothelial cell loss associated with excimer laser. Ophthalmology 1993; 97: 107.
38. Gaster RN, Binder PS, Goalwell K et al: Corneal surface ablation by 193 nm excimer laser and wound healing in rabbits. Invest Ophthalmol Vis Sci 1989; 30: 90-97.
39. Wu WCS, Stark WJ: Corneal wound healing after 193-nm excimer laser keratectomy. Arch Ophthal 1991; 109: 1426-32.
40. Campos M, Hertzog L, Grabus JJ, et al: Corneal sensitivity after PRK. Am J Ophthalmol 1992; 14: 51-54.
41. Trabuchi G, Brancato R, Verdi M et at: Corneal nerve damage and regeneration after excimer laser photorefractive keratectomy in rabbit eyes. Invest Ophthalmol Vis Sci 1994; 35: 229-235.
42. Edelhauser HF: The resiliency of the corneal endothelium to refractive and intraocular surgery. Cornea 2000 May; 19(3): 263-73.
43. Durrie DS, Lesher MP et al: Classification of variable clinical response after PRK for myopia. J Ref Surg 1995; 1: 341-7.

Chapter 6
Hazards of Excimer Laser Radiations

Though concern has been raised regarding possibility of compromization of structural integrity of cornea and risk of mutagenesis, photokeratitis and cataractogenesis, etc. that might be caused by primary or secondary phenomenon associated with the excimer laser ablation of cornea; extensive studies have reported that no such risk exists clinically.

RISK TO THE LENS AND PHOTOTOXICITY

Absorption vs. Transmission of Laser

When considering whether a laser light used for corneal surgery could pose any danger to the deeper ocular structures, the following factors are to be considered.

1. Absorption coefficient of the laser/penetration depth
2. Associated secondary phenomenon.

Wavelengths of lasers between 400-1400 nm are generally transmitted through the cornea. Wavelengths in the far-ultraviolet (<300 nm), e.g. ArF excimer laser, mid-infrared (3000–6000 nm), e.g. Erbium YAG laser and far-infrared regions (> 10,000 nm), e.g. CO_2 laser have a *high absorption coefficient and low penetration depths*. Therefore *direct damage to the deeper ocular structures is not possible*. Such characteristics of these lasers make them suitable for corneal surgical applications[1].

The high *absorption* of these lasers by cornea is *through the macromolecules* in case of the UV wavelengths *and by water* in case of the infrared wavelengths. It can be seen from Table 6.1 that Er: YAG laser has the least penetration depth into the cornea, even less than that of the ArF excimer laser[1].

Table 6.1: Penetration depths of different lasers

Lasers		Penetration Depth
1. Excimer Lasers		
• Argon Fluoride	(193 nm)	3-4 µ
• Krypton Fluoride	(248 nm)	10 µ
• Xenon Chloride	(308 nm)	300 µ
2. Nd: YAG Laser (Frequency Quintupled)	(213 nm)	2 µ
3. Holmium YAG	(2060 nm)	330 µ
4. Hydrogen Fluoride	(2910 nm)	1.5 µ
5. Erbium YAG	(2940 nm)	0.75 µ
6. Raman Shifted YAG	(2800 nm)	1.5 µ

Scattering of the Laser into the Tissue

The laser may have a low penetration but may show scattering at the site of application. This causes local heat production and decrease in the desired effect of the laser on the tissue.

Excimer Lasers

The peak absorption for the UV wavelength by cornea is around 190 nm, making ArF laser most suitable for corneal surgery. ArF excimer laser has high absorption and low penetration (less than 4 µm) into the corneal tissue.

Moreover, *scattering* of this wavelength and hence the conversion of the laser energy into heat is insignificant, unlike the CO_2 laser. The krypton fluoride excimer laser also has some heat element associated with it, which causes more collateral damage.

Secondary Fluorescence

Secondary fluorescence is a phenomenon in which light of longer wavelengths (in the range of 260-500 nm, mainly the UVB range) is produced by the excimer laser as it strikes the corneal tissue.

These longer wavelengths are partially transmitted by cornea. They can reach the deeper intraocular tissue and could be absorbed by the lens (peak absorption 320 nm). But these **are clinically insignificant** because it has been worked out that energy converted into this fluorescent light of longer wavelength is **as low as 0.001% of the incident energy**.

Even if 400 pulses of 160 mJ/cm^2 are given to cornea, the UVB produced and reaching the lens would be 10–80 µJ/cm^2, which would be 250-2000 times less than that required to produce cataract experimentally in rabbit and 1250–10000 times less than the annual average solar UVB exposure of a human eye[2-6].

For this reason and due to the hindrance to these wavelengths for further penetration by the lens, the risk of *phototoxicity* is also non existent.

The peak fluorescence produced at the corneal epithelium is about 460 nm and at the stroma is about 320 nm. The former comes into the visible spectrum and can be clinically seen as bluish glow while ablating the epithelium. No such fluorescence is seen when the excimer laser is working on the stroma. This is used as an indicator to decide the end point of laser removal of epithelium during PRK and PTK.

INTEGRITY OF THE CORNEA

The possibility of compromising the ocular integrity after excimer laser corneal surgeries (keratorefractive or phototherapeutic) has been a crucial area of concern for the ophthalmologist as well for the patient undergoing such a procedure. This risk to the otherwise *apparently normal eye* may occur in the following three ways.

1. Increased susceptibility to traumatic rupture of the globe
2. Corneal ectasia
3. Forward shift of both corneal surfaces

Susceptibility to Traumatic Rupture

Till date there has been no report of an eye developing corneal rupture after an uneventful excimer laser procedure. This has occurred after manual corneal incisional and lamellar surgeries[7, 8].

The possibility of such a hypothetical eventuality occurring after excimer laser surgery was examined under laboratory conditions[9].

Porcine eyes, on which RK, PRK or PTK had been performed using different ablation depths and normal eyes without any such procedures were subjected to globe compression of similar magnitudes. The following results emerged after these experiments.

1. Rupture occured at the site of incision in all RK eyes.
2. Eyes undergoing -12 D of PRK correction ruptured along the sclera, similar to the normal eyes.
3. Only the eyes that underwent PTK involving more than 40% of the corneal thickness showed corneal rupture.

In another experimental study[10] on human eyes from eye bank, ablated with ArF laser, central steepening of corneas was noticed only if ablated to more than 150 µ. Normally a flattening of cornea has been reported after corneal surface ablation. This steepening and increase in curvature of cornea represents a structural weakening of the corneal lamellae after deeper ablation that might lead to ectasia or corneal rupture on pressure of the globe.

An experimental model by Bryant et al also has found more than 40% ablation depth to be associated with increasing corneal ectasia in proportion to further ablation using 6 mm ablation zone[11].

Corneal Ectasia

PRK and Corneal Ectasia/Forward Shift

No case of corneal ectasia has been reported till date following PRK. However cases of forward shifting of corneal curvature are common. This change is not progressive and does not lead to corneal ectasia, which is a progressive protrusion of the cornea requiring keratoplasty. However this forward shift is responsible for the *regression* of refractive effect.

Miyata et al studied 65 eyes with PRK and found significant forward corneal shift (36.6 ± 23.3 µ at 1 week and 55.1±46.1 µ at 1year). The change was maximum between 1 week and 6 month and stabilized thereafter. No progression occurred to suggest true ectasia[12]. A positive relation was noticed with myopic regression. This change in corneal curvature was more in case of:

1. Thinner corneas
2. Higher myopia/greater ablation depth.

LASIK and Corneal Ectasia

As for LASIK is concerned, ectasia has been reported following this procedure. Two factors are of prime importance in deciding the maximum limit of safe ablation to avoid corneal ectasia. These are:

1. Corneal flap thickness
2. The residual stromal bed thickness (RBT)

Corneal Flap Thickness

Corneal flap thickness is an important consideration in calculating the safe margin for stromal ablation. The *flap thickness varies depending on the microkeratome* used because of the following three reasons.

1. Different Depth plate setting (the intended flap thickness), for example:

The Automated Corneal Shaper (ACS) 160 μ depth plate setting

The Nidek MK 2000 microkeratome 130 μ depth plate setting

The Hansatome 160 μ depth plate setting
180 μ depth plate setting

2. The difference between the intended flap thickness (as expected from the depth setting) and the actual flap thickness cut by the microkeratome.
3. Variability in the flap thickness, cut by the same microkeratome, in two eyes of the same patient as well as the interpatient variability.

The last two factors may lead to fatal errors of calculations to jeopardize the planned ablation depth and residual bed thickness thereby resulting in postoperative surprises. Therefore measurements of the flap and the stromal bed thickness by intraoperative pachymetry is of paramount importance for desirable results.

Some recent studies in 2002 have highlighted these facts. Shemesh G et al have found that the ACS and the Hansatome both made flaps much thinner than the expected thickness as well as showed statistically significant variation in the flaps of the two eyes of the same patient. The Nidek MK 2000 microkeratome showed no statistically significant flap thickness variation in same patient's eyes. It also made flaps that were close to the expected thickness[13].

Gokmen et al found that the Hansatome made flaps varying in thicknesses from 141-209 μ and the ACS made 120-150 μ flaps, the intended thickness being 160 μ in both the cases[14].

Spadea et al reported one case developing corneal ectasia in both eyes after LASIK. Corneal specimen taken after keratoplasty revealed the flap to be 260 μ instead of the intended 120 μ, using the Moria-manually guided MDCS[15].

Residual Stromal Bed Thickness (RBT)

Although the thickness of corneal flap is an inseparable constituent in the mathematics of LASIK ablation, *it is the thickness of remaining unablated corneal stromal bed which is crucial in maintaining the integrity of the cornea.* This is due to the fact that after LASIK the corneal flap does not act in an integrated manner with the residual stroma to contribute to the corneal strength since bridging between the two is not strong enough for many months[16].

Based on their experience with corneal lamellar surgeries, Probst et al opined that 250 μ of the residual stromal thickness is mandatory to preserve corneal integrity. Because an average corneal flap is about 160 μ thick, an ablation of >140 μ of issue should not be attempted to preserve 250 μ RBT as the average corneal thickness is about 550 μ[17].

Many other clinical studies on LASIK have concurred with the above concept of residual bed thickness of 250 μ, above which no cases of 'kreactesia' were reported during the follow up of these studies[18-20].

Question about this **apparently safe figure of 250 μ RBT** was raised by Seitz et al[21]. Rao et al noticed severe ectasia on first postoperative day after LASIK in one eye of a patient who had preoperative mild inferior steepening in both eyes without any evidence of keratoconus, although the RBT was 314 μ[22].

Pallikaris et al, in a recent review of 2873 eyes that underwent LASIK for different degree of myopic correction, reported 19 cases of corneal ectasia after a mean follow up period of 16.32 months (range 6 months to 4 years). They observed 325 μ of residual bed thickness (RBT) to be the crucial figure rather than the conventionally accepted 250 μ. None of the eyes having

RBT >325 µ or attempted correction less than -8.0 D developed corneal ectasia, though some of the eyes with RBT 250-325 µ did show this complication[23].

As such about 37 cases of corneal ectasia following LASIK have been reported in the literature till April 2002[16, 19, 20, 22-26, 41], though many thousands of eyes have undergone this procedure. Two of the eyes had topographic changes of keratoconus preoperatively[26]. *This shows the rarity of this potentially vision threatening complication.*

In contrast to the occurrence of actual corneal ectasia, topographic changes, including *increase in anterior corneal curvature, forward shift (bulge) of the posterior corneal surface* not leading to ectasia and *increase in the central corneal thickness* are frequent observations after LASIK for higher degree of myopic corrections[18, 21, 27, 28].

Causes of Corneal Ectasia and Forward Shift of the Corneal Curvature

The following causes have been found to contribute to the pathogenesis of the decreased corneal integrity[18, 20, 24, 28] leading to corneal curvature change or ectasia as its severe manifestation after excimer laser refractive surgeries:

1. High to extreme myopia (-15 to -25 D) requiring *excessive ablation* resulting in *residual bed thickness* (RBT) < 325 µ (?< 250 µ).
2. Corneal flaps thicker than the intended cut.
3. Irregular corneal thickness (demonstrated by pachymetry maps).
4. Borderline cases of *thinning corneal disorders* without definite topographical evidence (keratoconus suspects, pellucid marginal degeneration).
5. Lower preoperative CCT vs. the amount of refractive correction required.
6. Higher preoperative intraocular pressure.
7. Inappropriate evaluation and selection of the cases.
8. Different ablation rate than expected: intra-operative dehydration leading to increased rate.
9. Predisposition to develop ectasia.

Predisposition to Develop Corneal Ectasia

This predisposition may probably be linked to the etiology of myopia. Corneal ectasia is mainly seen in the eyes belonging to the high and extreme (degenerative/pathological) myopia groups. These eyes are said to inherit a genetically weak sclera which cannot withstand the IOP. The sclera stretches under the 'normal intraocular pressure' and leads to globe enlargement, posterior staphyloma and other changes peculiar to this condition[38-40]. If the same pathology affects the collagen of the cornea, which is similar to that of the sclera (mainly type I), then possibility of such a predisposition for the corneal weakness also exists.

Evaluation of Central Corneal Thickness (CCT)

The above risk factors and the concept of RBT to avoid corneal ectasia as well as corneal curvature changes (which lead to regression of the refractive effect) calls for a *stringent evaluation of the preoperative central corneal thickness (CCT), pachymetry maps and anterior as well as posterior corneal topography* to detect and exclude cases which are at particular risk for developing this avoidable complication after LASIK.

Methods of Evaluating CCT: Optical vs. Ultrasonic

The method of evaluating corneal thickness also has great bearing on the outcome of the surgery as the results are directly related to the accuracy of preoperative data. Salz and Azen et al[29] compared the ultrasonic and optical methods of pachymetry and concluded that *ultrasonic pachymetry is a superior method of evaluating corneal thickness.* It showed great reproducibility, absence of interobserver and right-left eye readings variation as compared to the optical method which suffered from these drawbacks.

Olsen and Neilsen et al[30] discovered that the *optical principle of pachymetry gave lower than actual readings.*

Variables Affecting CCT Measurements

One also has to consider the *diurnal*[31] as well as *physiological variations in corneal thickness.*

In females, the corneal thickness increases on the 2nd, 14th and 21st day of the cycle due to estrogen (as assessed by the levels in urine). Moreover steepening of corneal curvature at the beginning of cycle and flattening after ovulation also has been found to occur[32].

The Orbscan, which also utilizes the optical principle, would also show variability and low reproducibility of readings and therefor would be *less reliable* method. Recently Genth et al[58], in May 2002 have reported that determination of corneal and flap thickness by 'optical low coherence reflectometry' (OLCR) was an appropriate alternative to U/S pachymetry.

Concern has been shown about the corneal thickness being less than average in Indian eyes, making them unsuitable for excimer laser surgery. Search of the international literature for the past three decades through internet-search did not reveal any such study on corneal thickness in Indian eyes, making this comment insignificant.

In fact only one report on *inter-racial difference in corneal thickness* could be found, which shows that cornea in Caucasians is about 60 µ thicker than in African Americans[33].

Moreover this concern about the unsuitability of the Indian eyes is without any supporting data. As stated above, the Orbscan uses the optical principle and needs long term evaluation and standardization to be comparable to the more reliable ultrasonic method. Hence the results from this source may not be so acceptable till studies on the predictability of this modality of CCT evaluation are made available.

Last but not the least, **a cornea does not become unsuitable for excimer laser surgery merely because it is little less in thickness than the average.** What is crucial is a critical evaluation of the required ablation visa vis the available tissue thickness, topographical analysis of the cornea and exclusion of the known contraindications and risk factors for the surgery.

RETINAL DETACHMENT

Another concern shown is about retinal detachment occurring after excimer laser procedures. Though a few case reports of RD after excimer laser refractive surgeries have appeared, *there seems to be no direct cause–effect relation between the two* and it is considered to be a consequence of myopia itself, due to the anatomical predisposition of the myopic eye[34]. As such the incidence of RD after photorefractive surgeries is very low whereas *34–79% cases of retinal detachments are caused by myopia itself*[35-37]. The incidence is even more in the high myopes.

The LASIK procedure raises the IOP to 60 mm Hg through the suction ring for a short time, thereby, theoretically stressing the intraocular structures.

Vakiti et al reported *one case* of *late onset retinal tear* in a patient who underwent LASIK. There was history of previous trauma and retinopexy. The tear was noticed at the margin of the previous treatment retinal scar. No causal relationship was attributed to LASIK[42].

Therefore one must carry a thorough retinal screening with the help of a competent retinal surgeon pre- and postoperatively as well as throughout the follow up for peripheral retinal degenerations and predispositions to retinal detachment.

Charteris DG et al[34] did not recommend prophylactic treatment of any *asymptomatic lattice* as they believed that 'there is no causal link between excimer laser surgeries and retinal detachment'. *However, it is prudent to treat all suspicious lesions judiciously, with minimum possible use of cryotherapy/laser photocoagulation to avoid excessive scar.*

Sakurai et al[43] reported one case of retinal detachment 7 months after LASIK surgery, who developed flap dehiscence at the time of scleral buckling. This case again stresses upon the fact that the adhesions of corneal flap are not strong enough for long period. The retinal surgeon has to be extra careful in handling cases of retinal detachment in post-LASIK patients because the *natural susceptibility of myopes to develop RD* would lend many of them for his intervention at any point of time.

DAMAGE TO CORNEA BY FREE-RADICALS

After excimer laser therapy, high influx of polymorphonuclear cells (PMNs) into the rabbit corneal stroma is detected. There is also increase in indicators of inflammation such as PGE_2 and leukotriene B4. This response is much more as compared to that found after mechanical keratectomy[44, 45].

The PMNs influx is reduced by local steroid application. But the use of inhibitors of inflammatory mediators such as diclofenac sodium, on the contrary, increases the actual number of PMNs during the early postoperative period. This increase of PMNs inspite of the inhibition of PGE_2 and leukotrienes is partly due to increase in oxidized lipids acting as chemotactic factors. These oxidized lipids increase by 87 to 198% in cornea ablated with 193 nm excimer laser. They are produced due to free radical damage to corneal tissue, which oxidize the lipids present in cell membrane, epithelium and stromal cells[46].

The toxic free radicals generated due to respiratory burst of the PMNs at the site of excimer laser ablation of bovine cornea can lead to peroxidative damage to the corneal tissue and might have some effect on the wound healing following excimer laser ablation. This might contribute to the corneal *haze* and *regression* after photorefractive surgery. The free radicals are transient products and are produced in cryogenic environment.

Use of topical steroids decrease influx of PMNs, which are responsible for free radical production after excimer laser ablation. They might minimize tissue free radical mediated damage to corneal tissue.

PHOTOKERATITIS

The measured threshold for photokeratitis with 193 nm excimer laser is 10 mJ/cm² of energy of UVB. Since only 0.001% of excimer energy is converted to UVB at the irradiance energy used for therapeutic purpose (see above), the accumulated UVB dose to cornea would be less than that necessary to produce photokeratitis[47].

MUTAGENESIS

A large number of experimental studies have shown that there is no risk of cytotoxicity to DNA or mutagenesis to the cornea with 193 nm ArF excimer laser irradiation.

Nuss and Puliafito studied the unscheduled DNA synthesis in rabbit cornea exposed to 193 nm ArF, 248 KrF and 254 nm excimer lasers. Excision repair through unscheduled DNA synthesis had been shown to be indicative of DNA damage by various cancer studies. They found that no significant increase in excision repair occurred in cornea exposed to 193 nm ArF laser in contrast to 248 nm and 254 nm wavelengths[48].

Green and Margolis et al[49] reported similar findings after ablation of the human skin, reiterating that 193 nm excimer laser had no significant risk of mutagenesis. They suggested that there may be formation of different DNA photoproducts which were not harmful.

Trentecoste et al[50] reported that more than 90% of 193 nm radiation is absorbed by each micron of protein constituents of the cell membrane and cytoplasm. The distance between the cell membrane and nucleus is about 1.5–3.0 μm. Thus, there is a *shielding effect of cytoplasm and membrane constituents* against any possible damage to the nucleus by the incident excimer laser.

Gebhardt and McDonald et al[51] studied the oncogenic potential of 193 nm excimer laser on mouse corneal tissue and keratocytes. They showed that keratocytes exposed to 193 nm laser and subsequently implanted subcutaneously in syngenic recipients showed no evidence of tumor growth after many months.

Kochever and Green et al reported that about 99% of incident energy of ArF laser is absorbed per micron of the cytoplasm, a finding similar to that of Trentecoste et al.

SHOCK WAVES AND SURFACE WAVES

These waves are reported by many researchers following *wide beam ablation.* No clinical study has shown any histopathological damage to cornea caused by these waves[51-54].

Acoustic Shock Waves

These waves are produced when the excimer laser beam strikes the corneal surface. These waves, recorded in animal studies under the cornea, using a piezoelectric transducer, traverse through the cornea at the speed of sound, i.e. at about 1.6 km/second and at pressure of about 100 atm.

Surface Waves

Surface waves of about 0.15–0.4 mm amplitude are produced by recoil forces of the 'ejection plume' of molecular fragments at the end of ablation. They travel at several meter/sec and have a high amplitude.

Earlier, during PRK procedures, they were thought to produce surface fluid from within the cornea during 'wide beam' ablation and lead to attenuation of corneal ablation centrally, thus causing **central steep island** formation[55, 56].

As mentioned earlier, the shock waves and surface waves are *mainly found during wide beam ablation.* All modern systems use the 'scanning spot' ablation where they are of no clinical significance.

SURFACE HEATING

This phenomenon is also a consequence of *wide beam ablation.* A temperature increase of about 10–20° C in the stroma adjacent to the area ablated with 193 nm ArF laser is detected using a thermal camera. It has been suggested that although these thermal spikes might not denature the lamellae, they might affect the keratocytes and corneal wound healing[57].

Other researchers have hypothesized that the leading edge of the large laser pulse creates a **surface plasma** which has a shielding effect for the laser light at the end of the pulse, thereby sequestering further energy at the surface and leading to surface heating. Shortening the pulse might eliminate this **plasma shielding effect** and minimize heating of corneal surface.

Suggested readings

1. Loertscher H et al: Preliminary repot on corneal incision created by a hydrogen fluoride laser. Am J Ophthalmol 1986; 102: 217-221.
2. Loree TR, Johnson TM et al: Fluorescence spectra of corneal tissue under excimer laser irradiation. Proc SPIE; 1988; 908: 65.
3. Muller Stolzenberg NW, Muller CZ et al: UV exposure of lens during]93nm excimer laser corneal surgery. Arch Ophthalmol 1990; (108): 915-916.
4. Tuft S, AI-Dhahir R, Dyer P et al: Characterization of the fluorescence spectra produced by excimer laser irradiation of the cornea. Invest Ophthal Vis Sci 1990; 31: 1512-1518.
5. Ediger MN: Excimer laser-induced fluorescence of rabbit cornea: radiometric measurement through the cornea. Laser Surg Med 1991; 11: 93-98.
6. Taylor HR, West SK et AL: Effect of ultraviolet radiations on cataract formation. New Eng J Med 1988; 319: 1429.
7. Pearlstein ES, Agapitos PJ et al: Ruptured globe after RK. Am J Ophthalmol 1988; 106: 755-756.
8. Bloom HR, Sands J et al: Corneal rupture after blunt trauma 22 months after radial keratotomy. Ref Corn Surg 1990; 6:197-198.
9. Campos M, Lee M, McDonnell PJ: Ocular integrity after refractive surgery: effects of photorefractive keratectomy, phototherapeutic keratectomy, and radial keratotomy. Ophthalmic Surg 1992; 23: 598-602.
10. Litwin KL, Moreira H, Ohadi C et al: Changes in corneal curvature at different excimer laser ablative depths. Am J Ophthalmol 1991; 111 : 382-384.
11. Bryant MR, Frederiks DJ, Campos M et al: Finite element analysis of corneal topographic change after excimer laser phototherapeutic keratectomy. Invest Ophthalmol Vis Sci 1993; 34 (Suppl): 804.
12. Miyata K, Kaimiya K, Takashahi T et al: Time course of change in corneal forward shifting after excimer laser PRK. Arch Ophthalmol 2002; 120(7): 896-900.
13. Shemesh G, Dotan G, Lipshitz I: Predictability of corneal flap thickness in LASIK using three different microkeratomes. J Ref Surg 2002; 18(3 suppl): S347-51.
14. Gokmen F, Jester JV et al: In vivo confocal microscopy through-focussing to measure corneal flap thickness after laser in situ keratomileusis. J Cataract Ref Surg 2002; 28: 962-970.
15. Spadea L, Palmieri G, Mosca L et al: Iatrogenic kreactesia following LASIK. J Ref Cataract Surg 2002; 18(4): 475-480.
16. Rumelt S, Cohen I, Skandarni P et al: Ultrastructure of the lamellar corneal wound after LASIK in human eye. J Ref Cataract Surg 2001; 27(8): 1323- 1327.
17. Probst LE, Machat JJ: Mathematics of laser in situ keratomileusis for high myopia. J Cataract Ref Surg 1998; 224(2): 190-195.
18. Wang Z, Chen J, Yang B: Posterior corneal surface topographic changes after LASIK are related to residual corneal bed thickness. Ophthalmology 1999; 106(2): 409-410.
19. Joo CK, Kim TG: Corneal ectasia detected after LASIK for correction of less than 12 diopters of myopia. J Ref Cataract Surg 2000; 26 (2): 292-295.
20. Vinciguerra P, Camesaska FI: Prevention of corneal ectasia after LASIK. J Ref Surg 2001; 17(3 suppl): S 187-189.
21. Seitz B, Torres F, Langenbucher A et al: Posterior corneal curvature changes after myopic LASIK. Ophthalmology 2001; 108 (4): 666-673.
22. Rao SN, Epstein RJ: Early onset ectasia following LASIK: case report and literature review. J Ref Surg 2002; 18(2): 177-184.
23. Pallikaris IG, Kymionis GD et al: Corneal ectasia induced by LASIK. J Ref Cataract Surg 2001; 27 (11): 1796-1802.
24. Argento C, Cosentino MJ, Tytiun A et al : Corneal ectasia after laser in situ keratomileusis. J Cataract Ref Surg 2001; 27 (9): 1440- 1498.
25. Magallanes R, Shah S, Zadok D et al: Stability after LASIK in moderately and extremely myopic eyes. J Cataract Ref Surg 2001; 27 (7): 1007-1112.
26. Schmitt-Bernard CF, Lesage C, Arnaud B: Keractesia induced by LASIK in keratoconus. J Ref Surg 2000; 16 (3): 368-370.
27. Chayet AS, Assil KK, Montes M et al: Regression and its mechanisms after LASIK in moderate and high myopes. Ophthalmology 1998; 105 (7): 1194-1199.
28. Baek T, Lee K, Kagaya F et al : Factors affecting forward shift of posterior corneal surface after LASIK. Ophthalmology 2001; 108 (2): 317-320. Comments in Ophthalmology 2002; 108 (3): 407-410.
29. Salz JJ, Azen SP, Berstein J et al: Evaluation and comparison of sources of variability in the measurement of corneal thickness with ultrasonic and optical pachymeters. Ophthalmic Surgery 1983; 14 (9): 750-754.
30. Olsen T, Neilsen CB, Ehlers N: On the optical measurement of corneal thickness : Optical principles and sources of error. Acta Ophthalmologica (Copenh) 1980; 58 (5): 760 766.
31. Harper CL, Boulton ME, Bennett D et al: Diurnal variation in human corneal thickness. Br J Ophthalmol 1996; 80 (12): 1068-1072. Erratum in Br J Ophthalmol 1997; 81 (2): 175.
32. Keily PM, Carney LG, Smith G: Menstrual cycle variation of corneal topography and thickness. Am J Optom Physiol Opt 1983; 60 (10) : 822-829.
33. La Rosa FA, Gross RL et al: Central corneal thickness of Caucasians and African Americans in glaucomatous and non- glaucomatous populations. Arch Ophthalmol 2001; 119 (1): 23-27.
34. Charteris DG, Cooling RJ et al: Retinal detachment following excimer laser. In J Ophthalmol 1997; 8: 759-761.

35. Schepens CL, Marilen D: Data on the natural history of retinal detachment: further characterization of some unilateral non0traumatic cases. Am J Ophthalmol 1966; 61: 213-226.
36. Ashrafadeh MT, Schepens CL et al: aphakic and phakic retinal detachments. Arch Ophthalmol 1973; 89 : 476.
37. Perkins ES : Morbidity from myopia. Sight Sav Rev 1979; 49 : 11-17.
38. Otsuka J: Research on the aetiology and treatment of myopia. Acta Soc Ophthalmol Jap 1976; 71: 13.
39. Balch RK : The nature of pathological myopia: A clinopathological study. Master's thesis, University of Cambridge 1964 : 47-58.
40. Curtin BJ: Physiologic vs. pathological myopia: genetics vs. environment. Ophthalmology1979; 86: 681-691.
41. Speicher L, Gottinger W: Progressive corneal ectasia after LASIK. Klin Monatsbl Augenheilkd 1998; 213 (4) 247-151.
42. Vakiti R, Taubu S, Lim ES: Successful management of retinal tear post LASIK retreatment case. Yale J Bio Med 2002; 75 (1) 55-57.
43. Sakurai E, Okuda M Nozaki M: Late onset LASIK flap dehiscence during retinal detachment surgery. Am J Ophthalmol 2002; 134 (2): 265-266.
44. Landry RJ, Pettit GH, Hahn DW et al: Preliminary evidence of free radical formation during argon fluoride excimer laser irradiation of corneal tissue. Laser and Light in Ophthalmol 1994; 6: 87-90.
45. Philips AF, Szerrenyi K, Campos M et al: Arachidonic acid metabolism after excimer laser corneal surgery. Arch Ophthalmol 1993; 111: 1273-1278.
46. Seizi Hayashi, Ishimoto S, Guey-Shuang W et al : Oxygen free radical damage in cornea after excimer laser therapy. Br J Ophthalmol 1997; 81: 141-144.
47. Krueger RR, Sliney DH, Trokel SL: Photokeratitis from sub-ablative 193- nanometer excimer laser radiation. Refract Corneal Surg 1992; 8: 274-279.
48. Nuss RC, Puliafito CA, Oehm E: Unscheduled DNA synthesis following excimer laser ablation of the cornea in vivo. Invest Ophthalmol Vis Sci 1987; 28: 287-294.
49. Green H, Margolis R et al: Unscheduled DNA synthesis in human skin after in vitro UV-excimer laser ablation. J Invest Dermatol 1987; 89: 201-204.
50. Gebhardt B, Salmeron B, McDonald M: Effect of excimer laser on energy growth potential of corneal keratocytes. Cornea 1990; 9: 250-210.
51. Trentacoste J, Thompson K, Parrish RK et al: Mutagenic potential of a 193-nm excimer laser on fibroblasts in tissue culture. Ophthalmology 1987; 94: 125-129.
52. Bor Z, Hopp B, Bacz B et at: Plume emission, shock wave and surface wave formation during excimer laser ablation of the cornea. Refract Corneal Surg 1983; 9 (suppl): S111-S115.
53. Bor Z, Hopp B, Bacz B et al: Physical problems of excimer laser corneal ablation. Opt Eng 1993; 32: 2481-2486.
54. Lubatschowski H, Kerman O et al: Characterization of acoustic effect in corneal photoablation and its possible use for on-line control of cutting depths (abstract), Refract Corneal Surg 1992; 18: 102.
55. Krueger RR, Saedy NF et al: Clinical analysis of steep central islands after excimer laser PRK. Arch Ophthalmol 1996; 114: 377-181.
56. Parker PJ, Klyce SO et al: Central topographic islands following photorefractive keratectomy. Invest Ophthalmol Vis Sci 1993: 34 (Suppl): 803.
57. Bende T, Seiler T et al: Side effects in excimer corneal surgery :corneal thermal gradients. Graefes Arch Clin Exp Ophthalmol 1988; 226: 277-280.
58. Genth U, Mrochen M, Walti R et al: Optical low coherence reflectometry for noncontact measurement of flap thickness during laser in situ keratomileusis. Ophthalmology 2002; 109(5): 973-978.

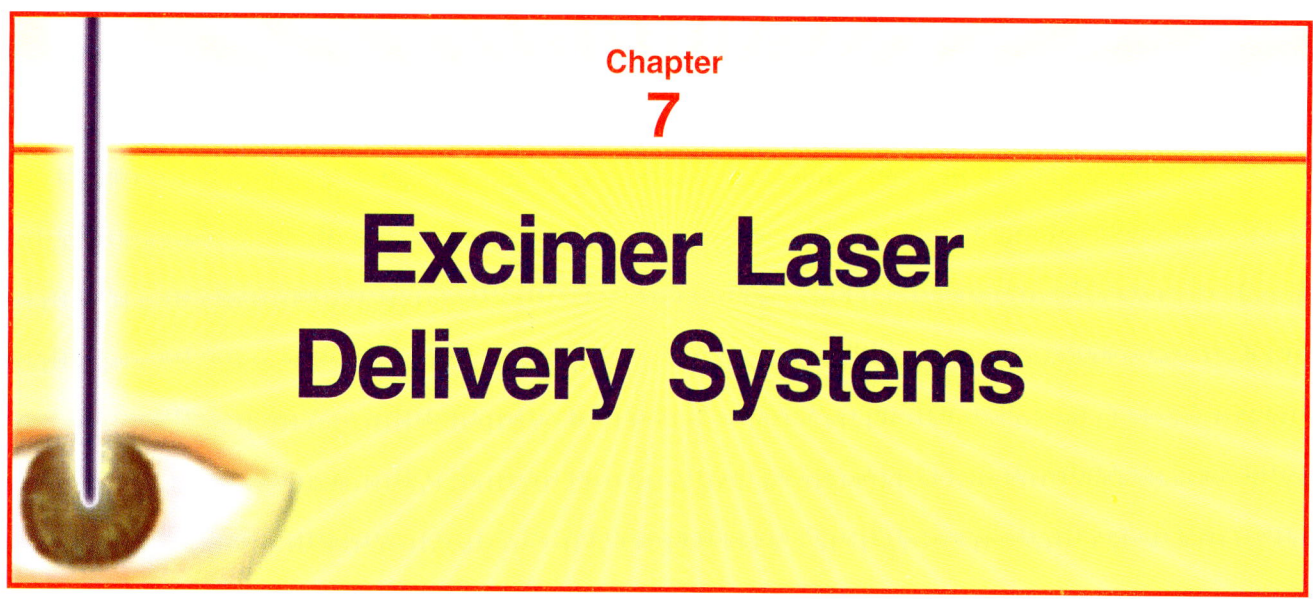

Chapter 7
Excimer Laser Delivery Systems

LASER DELIVERY SYSTEMS

Although extensive work is being done on *solid state excimer lasers,* all currently used excimer laser systems use *gas media* containing the noble gas *argon* and the halogen *fluorine.* The stimulated emissions is at 193 nm wavelength. The solid state excimer lasers are being developed in an attempt to make the system small, portable, cheaper and to enable one to use them for different type of surgical applications (vide supra).

A typical excimer laser system (Fig. 7.1) has the following components.

Laser Cavity

A typical excimer laser system consists of an elongated, large *aluminum protective housing* containing the *gas media* and surrounded by a *cooling system.* Two *metal electrodes* are placed inside this box, separated by 2 to 3 cm. An assembly of large number of *capacitors* is placed outside this box to supply very high charge, for initiating high electrical discharge, with voltage around 30,000 and current approximately 10,000 amp. A fan within the laser cavity circulates the gases across the electrodes.

Laser Pumping

A **thyraton** is a special switch based on *valve technology* to cope with the high current and fast switching, which is utilized for initiating the electrical discharge during excimer laser pumping. This device takes 5–10 minutes for *warming* due to its valve-like nature.

Thyraton failure used to be the commonest cause of *intraoperative laser failure*. This is prevented by use of improved technology using insaturable inductors, electrical pulse compression and better circuit designs which do not damage the thyraton.

The *linear accelerator* was used in the earlier excimer laser systems for pumping the high excitation energy.

Optical Arm

The long transmission arm contains many optical components, which vary depending on whether it is a wide beam system or a scanning system and also in different makes of the systems. Generally these components are the ones which are listed below.

1. Series of **mirrors** for redirecting the laser beam on to the patient's eye
2. The devices called **beam homogenizing system** such as the *image rotators* or the *optical integrators.* These are used for beam smoothening to remove any hot spots within the beam
3. Cylindrical **quartz lenses** for making the beam shape rectangular or square
4. A computer controlled **iris diaphragm,** used for making the laser beam circular and for varying the diameter of the beam in wide-beam systems.

46 Excimer Lasers in Corneal Diseases and Refractive Disorders

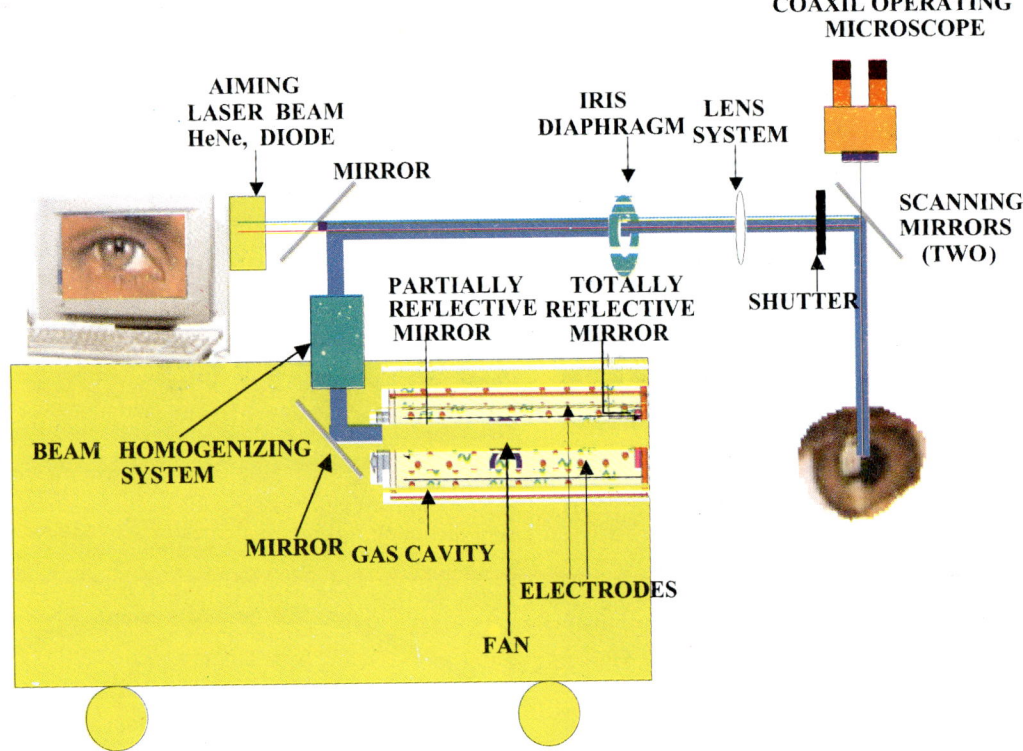

Fig. 7.1: Diagramatic representation of an excimer laser system showing its various parts.

5. Two **scanning mirrors,** which are computer controlled. They move the small beam of laser across the cornea in scanning beam systems.
6. A **shutter**, which is under computer control, is provided at the end of the arm. It opens at the time of the laser delivery.

Alignment System

It is attached to the optical arm and generates the aiming beam. The aiming beam consists of both Helium Neon green laser and the red diode laser.

Eye Tracking System

All modern excimer laser systems have the active eye-tracking system to make sure that it is the central optical zone which receives the ablation in a symmetrical pattern around the optical axis. This is crucial for avoiding a number of troublesome optical aberrations and undesirable refractive outcomes, including induced astigmatism.

This system consists of a high resolution S-VHS camera and an infra-red lighting system. The camera takes as much 50 frames per seconds and analyzes them with reference to the original co-ordinates of the pupil center with the help of the computer software. The camera is capable of a spatial resolution of 25 µ per pixel. The time taken for any change more than this is 20 milliseconds and the correction time for re-alignment is 40 ms. If there is a great displacement of the pupil (>2.5 mm) due to the eye movement, the camera loses the image and the ablation is automatically aborted.

Computer Unit

An attached computer software *controls all the laser operations* viz. the initiation of 'lasing action', the laser delivery, eye-tracking, ablation pattern, control of shutters and the operating microscope control, etc.

The following data is fed into the computer:

1. The patient's particulars
2. Type of ablation: myopic, hyperopic or plano (for PTK)
3. Central corneal thickness
4. The preoperative refractive error (for refractive correction)
5. The intended depth of ablation/depth of corneal pathology (for PTK).
6. Optical zone diameter.

The computer decides, utlizing the algorithm software provided by the manufacturer, the ablation pattern and the number of laser pulses to be delivered.

Operating Microscope

An operating microscope is integrated at the end of the optical arm. It has the eyepieces which are co-axial with the fixation target and the laser beam. It is a state of the art microscope with X-Y coupling.

MAINTENANCE OF THE LASING MEDIUM

The lasing medium (gases) are to be checked frequently to maintain a smooth laser output with appropriate energy level. This is ensured by using different methods for the laser calibration. Though, theoretically, it appears that the gases are not used up during the process of excitation and emission, but the following events do occur:

1. The fluorine gas, constituting about 0.1–0.2% of the gas mixture, is highly reactive and forms *by-products* by reacting with the material of the components of the laser cavity and with certain impurities, which might be present inside the cavity.
2. The electrical discharge forms hot plasma and UV rays, which further stimulate these reactions.
3. These reactions use up some of the gases, decreasing the lasing activity.
4. The by-products interfere with the energy transfer, absorb the laser energy or form coating on the optics of the cavity.
5. The result is a progressive decrease in the laser output on continued use, which may become inefficient at one time.

Therefore, maintenance of the lasing medium is crucial, which is done by the service engineers who perform calibration of the laser energy.

One of the following methods can be used for maintaining the purity of the gas medium:

1. **Frequent replacing** by flushing the cavity with fresh gases.
2. **Cryogenic purification** by 'liquid nitrogen cryogenic device' to maintain a stable laser output.
3. **Improved materials and laser cavity design** are used which emit less contaminants, decrease formation of the by-products and thereby reduce the need for frequent purification or exchange of the gas. Examples are the ceramic support for the electrodes and magnetic coupling for the fans.

CALIBRATION OF LASER ENERGY

The depth of ablation or *ablation rate* (tissue removed per pulse) is a function of the laser energy (mJ/cm^2, see chapter 4). The number of laser pulses to be delivered for a given ablation is decided by the computer, keeping a particular energy output into consideration. But if the energy level of the excimer laser is low, the desired ablation would not be achieved. Hence to achieve the *accuracy and precision* which is so characteristic of the excimer laser, the laser output must be frequently calibrated as per the guidelines of the manufacture. Two methods may be used for the laser calibration:

Direct Measurement This is difficult because meters give measurements within 20% accuracy limit.

Indirect Measurement This is done by measuring ablation on *plastic or PMMA* material, using one of the following devices recommended by the manufacture.

1. The depth of the material removed from a given disk.
2. The desired refraction produced by the lens formed by ablation of the material by the given laser pulses.
3. Whether the expected number of laser pulses are able to perforate the plastic 'Wratten filter' of a known thickness.

The ablated disk is also examined for any *hot-spots* and the *quality of the mire images* of the lens formed by the test ablation', using a lensometer. This ensures the homogeneity of laser beam energy and therefore the uniformity of the laser ablation.

EXCIMER LASER BEAM CHARACTERISTICS

The excimer lasers systems can be divided into the following two types depending on the mode of laser beam delivery.

1. Large beam laser systems
2. Scanning laser systems
   a. Slit scanning
   b. Spot scanning

Large/Wide Beam Laser System

In this system, a large circular beam, centered on the pupillary axis ablates the cornea in a *disc-like* manner with successive laser pulses. The laser beam is stationary although the diameter of the beam can be varied through computer controlled mechanical iris. The older excimer laser machines used this type of delivery system (Fig. 7.2).

For refractive ablation (PRK), the following two variations in this type of delivery can be made.

Transition Zone Ablation

In transition zone ablation, the iris diaphragm opens only once to create a single zone of ablation with successive pulses (Fig. 7.2 bottom).

Multizone/Overlapping Zones Ablation

Here the beam diameter is increased successively, many times, by computer controlled mechanical iris, to create several ablation zones of increasing diameter. After a certain amount of ablation of the corneal tissue, the iris opens again to ablate a more wider zone. With such successive ablations, the earlier central ablation zones also receive the laser and has deeper ablation than the latter zones, thus forming number of zones, which are successively less deep (Fig. 7.3).

Mechanical iris apertures are used to project myopic ablation pattern on to the cornea. A **contracting aperture** as well as an **expanding aperture** *produces stepped edges and discontinuities on the surface of the cornea.* Kruger and colleagues demonstrated that these steps could be minimized by **defocusing** the image of the aperture.

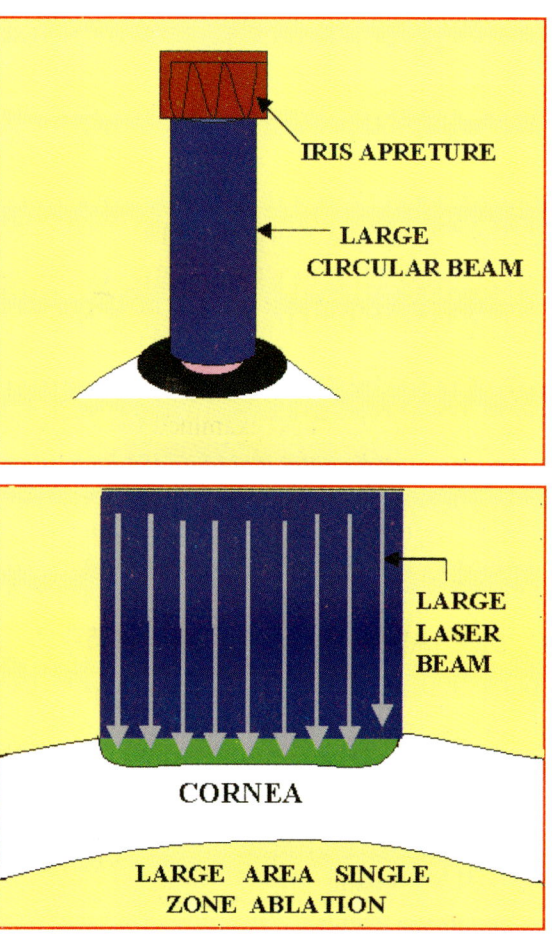

Fig. 7.2: Large (wide) beam ablation of cornea: 'Transition zone ablation' using only single diameter wide beam (the iris diaphragm opens once only)

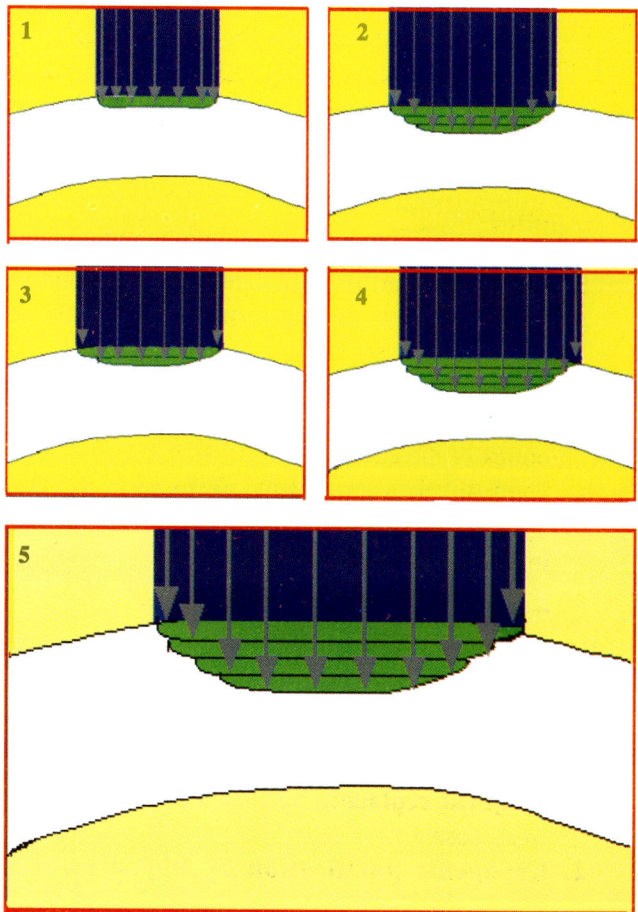

Fig. 7.3: 'Multizone ablation pattern' produced by large beam laser. Each time the 'iris diaphragm' diameter is increased, it removes tissue from the unablated surrounding area as well as from the already ablated central area thus causing central flattening of the cornea (myopic ablation pattern).

Disadvantages of Large Beam Laser Systems

1. The system requires high energy output per pulse, to be effective.
2. It requires 'homogenization' of the laser beam to avoid *hot-spots* within the wide/large beam.
3. It is therefore more complicated in design, larger in size and costlier in comparison to a scanning laser system.
4. Limited *refractive ablation patterns* are available with this system.
5. It produces more *shock* and *surface waves*.
6. It is more likely to produce *central steep islands*.

Advantages of Large Beam System

1. Ablation is quicker
2. Quicker ablation ensures better eye-fixation and less hydration changes (vide infra).
3. The ablated surface is smoother with a homogenized large beam than with a scanning beam.
4. The central steep islands can be avoided by making the beam *energy distribution* and *hydration* of the corneal surface *uniform*.

Energy Profile of the Laser Beams

The Shape of the laser beam can be of four types depending on the energy profile within the beam.

1. Derby shaped beam.
2. Flat top beam/top hat-shaped beam.
3. Laser beam with Gaussian distribution.
4. Trumcated Gaussian beam.

Both, the wide as well as the scanning laser beams can have the above types of energy profile.

Derby-Shaped Beam

Usually a large beam has more energy in the central part, which drops-off towards the periphery of the beam. Such a beam would lead to an *ablation pattern* in which the periphery is less ablated than the central area (the shape like a *derby*), hence the above name (Fig. 7.4). This ablation pattern results in hyperopic shift.

Flat Top /Hat-Shaped Beam

Energy profile within a *large beam demands a beam with uniform energy distribution*. This is an ideal beam for 'plano-ablation', such as for PTK. Such a laser bean would remove tissue uniformly over the entire area receiving the laser. The ablation pattern would have the top-hat configuration, hence this name (Fig. 7.5). To achieve *this ideal excimer laser beam*, with uniform energy distribution is not an easy process.

Gaussian Beam

It differs from the derby shaped beam because although the energy is lower towards the periphery, it decreases smoothly following a Gaussian distribution curve. This beam produces a smooth transitions zone in case of wide beam ablation. For scanning beams also, this distribution is of great advantage because a smoother ablation is produced at the overlapping sites of the flying spots. Use of the Gaussian beam has improved the results of photorefractive surgeries (see Chapter 25).

Truncated Gaussian Beam

The beam combines the energy profile of the flat top and the Gaussian beam. (Fig. 7.6). This beam gives a good corrective ablation like that of flat top beam and a smoother surface as produced by a Gaussian beam. This beam is specially being used for customized ablation.

Homogenization/Smoothening of Large Beam

The large beam excimer laser suffers from the inherent disadvantage of variance of energy across the laser beam. The areas with higher energy density are called **hot-spots** and the ones with less energy as **cold-spots**. The hot-spots produce more ablation. Therefore ablation with such laser beam results in *uneven surface* and *undesired refractive profile*.

A number of methods have been used to smoothen or homogenize the large laser beams, the detailed discussion of which is out of the scope of this book. Some beam homogenizing methods are:

Image Rotators

The laser beam is inverted by rotating it around its central axis by a mirror system or by prisms during successive pulses. The net effect at the end of the ablation is that of rotational symmetry.

Optical Integrators

This method uses an optical system which splits the beam into many segments. These segments of the beam are made to overlap at the time of ablation.

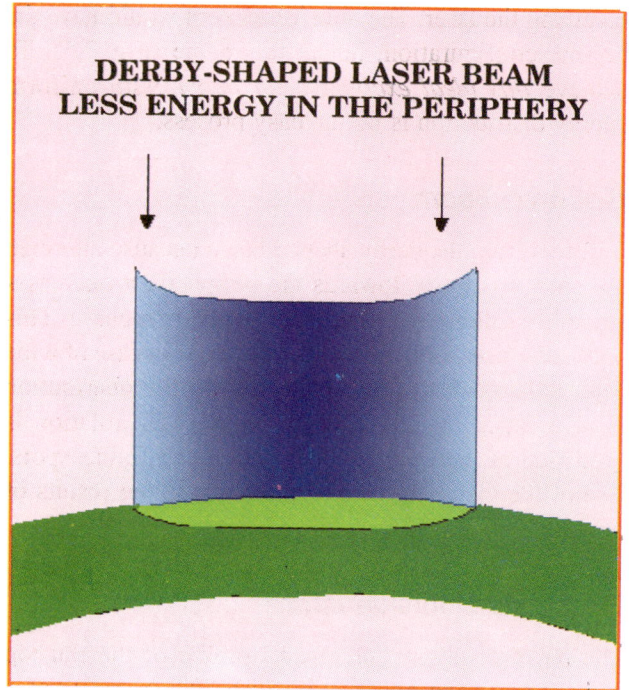

Fig. 7.4: Ablation pattern with a non-homogenized (derby-shaped) large laser beam

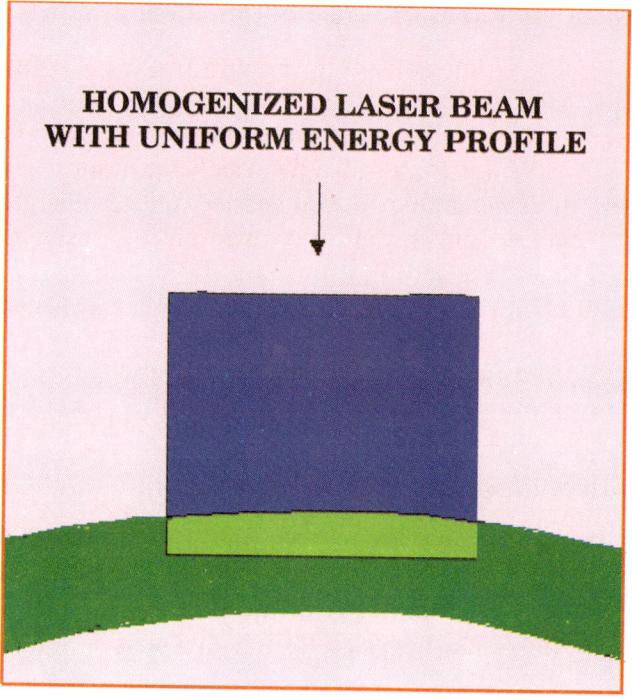

Fig. 7.5: Ablation pattern with a homogenized (flat top) large laser beam

Both of the above systems are ineffective in removing the hot-spots, which are merely rotated around rather than removed.

Wobbling Mirrors

This method is also not fully effective in providing a completely homogenous laser beam.

Spatial Filtering

This is more effective in removing the hot-spots but still there is no 100% guaranty of a perfectly uniform energy distribution.

Scanning Laser Systems

All modern excimer laser systems are scanning laser beam systems because algorithms can be easily developed for a varied type of '*refractive ablations*' using a scanning beam.

In this type of delivery the laser beam moves around or scans the corneal surface according to the ablation pattern decided by an algorithm *(myopic, hyperopic or plano)* under computer control. The number of pulses delivered depend upon the ablation depth/amount of refractive correction to be achieved. The irradiance of a scanning beam is much lower than that of a large beam laser because more laser pulses are used in the scanning mode of delivery.

Two modes of scanning beam ablations are available. The first one is most commonly used by many of the excimer laser systems.

1. Spot scanning/flying spot laser system
2. Slit scanning laser system

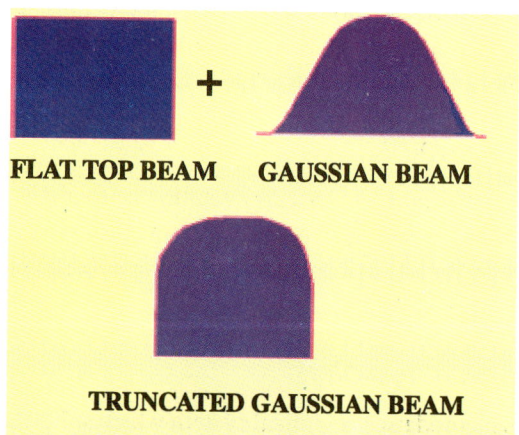

Fig. 7.6: Truncated gaussian laser beam

Spot Scanning/Flying Spot Ablation

The laser beam is a small, fixed diameter (1–2 mm) beam that scans the corneal surface rapidly as it 'flies' within the ablation zone (Fig. 7.7).

Slit Scanning Ablation

The laser beam is a narrow, rectangular slit-beam of fixed width which moves across the corneal surface back and forth and than rotates on its central axis to repeat the scanning. This process is repeated for 360 degrees (Fig. 7.7).

Advantages of Scanning Laser Systems

1. Different types of '*refractive ablations*' can be performed with the 'flying spot delivery'.
2. They are simple to design.
3. They are less demanding as for as beam smoothening is concerned.
4. The requirement for the complicated optics of a large beam system is avoided.
5. These systems are smaller in size.
6. They are cheaper in cost and easier to maintain in comparison to the wide beam laser systems.

Disadvantages of Scanning Laser Systems

1. During scanning, the beam edges overlap. Therefore the ablation is not as smooth as with a large beam.
2. The small beam takes *log time to scan* and to perform the ablation.
3. This makes eye-fixation difficult and the *active eye-tracking system becomes mandatory* for spot scanning.
4. Longer operative time also leads to corneal dehydration, requiring maintenance of intraoperative hydration to maintain smooth ablation.
5. Rapid pulse repetition rate is required to compensate for the time taken for slower scanning. Very high pulse frequency might result in thermal change (vide supra).

Some Large Beam Systems

1. The Summit Apex Plus Laser System (6.5 mm beam)
2. The VISX 2015 with 110-120 mJ/cm^2 (5.0–6.2 mm)
3. The VISX 2020 with 160 mJ/cm^2 (4, 5 and 6 mm)
4. The Chiron-Technolas Keracor 116 (6.0 mm beam)
5. The Coherent-Schwind Keratom (6.0 mm beam)

Some Scanning Laser Systems

1. The Nidek EC-500   rotating slit beam
2. The Meditek MEL 60   —do—
3. The Chiron-Technolas Keracor 117 and 217   spot
4. Kera Technology ISO beam   spot

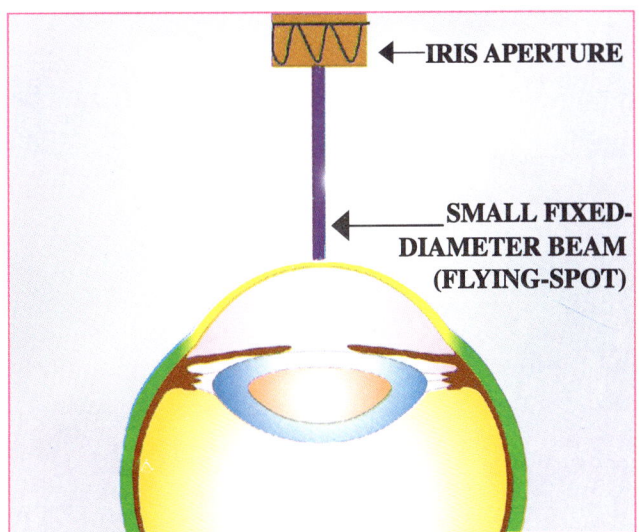

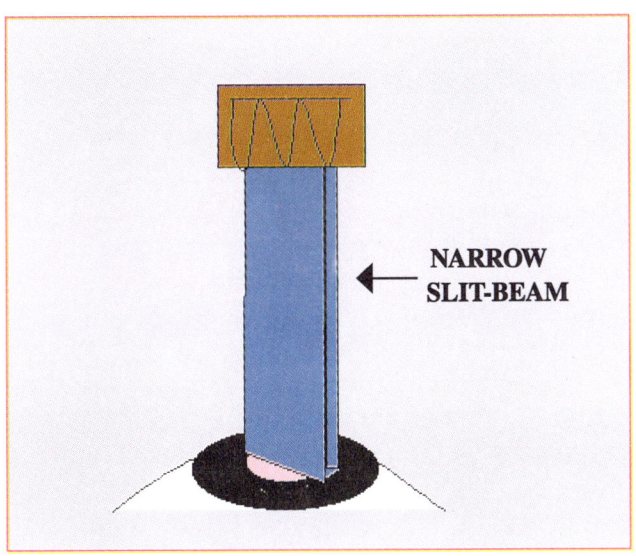

Fig. 7.7: Diagrammatic representations of spot-beam (top) and slit-beam laser delivery (bottom)

Suggested readings

1. Manns F, Shen J H: Söderberg P et al: Development of an algorithm for corneal reshaping with a scanning beam. Appl Optics 1995; 34: 4600–4608.
2. Manns F, Rol P, Parel J M et al: Optical profilmetry of poly (methylmethacrylate) surfaces after reshaping with a scanning photorefractive keratectomy (SPRK) system. Appl Optics 1996; 35: 3338–3346.
3. Ozdamar A, Aras C, Sener B, Bahcecioglu H: Two-year resuilts of photorefractive keratectomy with scanning spot ablation for myopia of less than –6.0 diopters. Ophthalmic Surg Lasers 1998; 29: 904–908.

Section III
Corneal Degenerations and Dystrophies

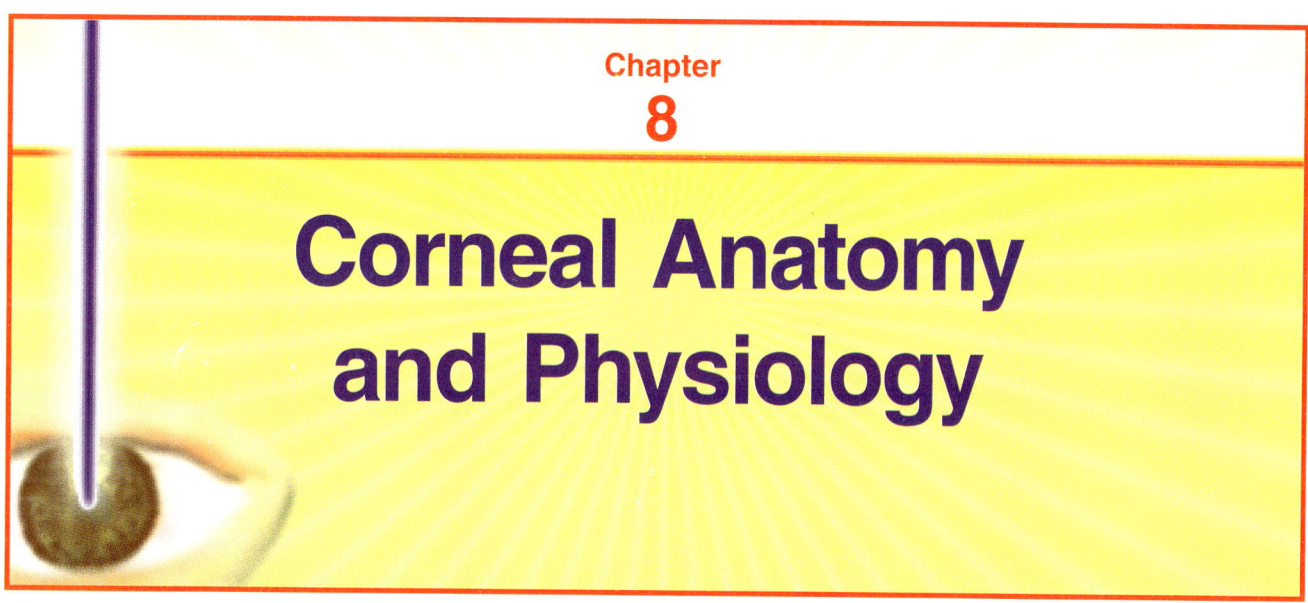

Chapter 8
Corneal Anatomy and Physiology

Cornea is a highly specialized, avascular, transparent structure forming the anterior most part of the eye-ball. Its anterior surface is elliptical horizontally due to greater overlap of sclera and conjunctiva superiorly and inferiorly while the posterior surface is circular. Its average dimensions in an adult are shown in Table 8.1.

Table 8.1: Corneal dimensions in adults

Anterior surface diameter:	Horizontal	11.7 mm
	Vertical	10.5 mm
Posterior surface diameter:		11.7 mm
Corneal thickness:	Central	540 μ
	Peripheral	670 μ

In the newborn the minimum corneal diameter is about 9.5 mm. If the corneal diameter is less than 11mm after the age of one year it is termed ***microcornea*** and if more than 13 mm then it is called ***megalocornea***. The cornea is clear in case of congenital megalocornea unlike that seen in buphathalmos.

CORNEAL CURVATURE

The dioptric power *(an average of 44 D, 2/3 of the total dioptric power of an adult eye)* of the cornea is determined by its curvature. The corneal curvature is a complex geometry. Simple profiles as ellipsoidal, parabolic, hyperbolic or spherical do not exactly represent it. The cornea is flatter in the periphery than in the center.

Regular Astigmatism

When the steep and the flat meridians of the corneal curvature are arranged at 90° from each other, i.e. they are orthogonal, it is termed regular astigmatism. Three types of regular astigmatism may occur:

1. **With-the-rule astigmatism**
   Generally the curvature is more in the vertical (or within ±15° of the vertical axis) than in the horizontal meridian.
2. **Against-the-rule astigmatism**
   When the corneal curvature is opposite of this, i.e. the greater curvature is horizontal or within ± 15° of this meridian, it is termed against-the-rule astigmatism.
3. **Oblique astigmatism**
   If the orientation of the most steep and flat axis is outside the ± 15° of the vertical or horizontal axis, it constitutes what is called an oblique astigmatism and is uncommon.

Though the newborn has a wide range of astigmatism, it changes to with-the-rule astigmatism that persists up to about 50 years of age after which an increasing incidence of against-the-rule astigmatism occurs. Decreasing lid pressure in the older individuals is thought to be responsible for this change. Lid pressure may modify the keratometry recordings also. Manipulations of lids during such procedure and while doing videokeratoscopy should be avoided.

Irregular Astigmatism

When the maximum and minimum curvature (and corneal power) meridians are not placed at 90° of each other, it constitutes an irregular astigmatism. There may be even absence of such meridians and axial symmetry. Irregular astigmatism is not *a feature of* the normal corneas but is associated with *scarred, traumatized, post-keratoplasty and pathological corneas.* It is difficult to correct it with glasses. Use of hard contact lenses may help such cases. *Excimer laser PTK* with the use of proper masking agent *is a promising alternative mode of treatment in this condition.*

APICAL/CORNEAL CAP OR APICAL ZONE

The central 4 mm zone of the cornea is taken to be spherical in curvature and is called the apical cap, corneal cap or the apical zone.

Radius of Curvature of the Apical Zone

Anterior surface ——— 7.8 ± 0.6 mm
Posterior surface ——— 6.5 mm

STRUCTURE OF THE CORNEA

The cornea has the following layers.

1. The epithelium (50-60 µ)
2. The stroma (constitutes 90% thickness)
3. The endothelium

Epithelium

The epithelium is stratified squamous epithelium having 5-7 layers. It is a transparent structure and has a smooth surface covered with the tear-film. This transparency is due to sparcity of the cytoplasmic organelles.

The epithelial cells are tightly adherent to each other by desmosomes, interdigitations, gap junctions and tight junctions. The epithelial cells are of the following three types.

1. **The squames**
   The outer three to four layers of flattened cells are called squames. The cells membranes of the most superficial layer have undulations or microplicae and microvilli, which are thought to have some binding role with the innermost mucin layer of the tear-film.
2. **Wing cells**
   These 1-3 layers of cells having thin wing-like extensions from the round cell bodies, are also called the *umbrella cells.*
3. **Basal cells**
   Basal cells are the innermost single layer of columnar cells. The basal cells are firmly attached to the underlying basement membrane and to the superficial part (1–2 µ) of the Bowman's layer by *adhesion complexes.* The adhesion complexes consist of *hemidesmosomes and anchoring fibrils (type VII collagen).*

Basement Membrane

The basement membrane or the *'basal lamina'* is secreted by the basal cells. It has two parts, the superficial *lamina lucida* and the deep *lamina densa.* These are seen by electron microscopy.

The adhesion complexes are poorly formed in cases of diabetes mellitus. In addition to the above abnormality found in diabetes, the basement membrane also is thickened and duplicated and the anchoring fibrils have decreased penetration. All these factors may account for the instability of the epithelium in advanced cases of diabetes mellitus.

Functions of the Epithelium

The epithelium serves the following functions.
1. **Barrier function**
   The superficial cells or the squames are tightly adherent to each other by *tight junctions or zonula occludens.* This acts as a barrier for fluids, pathogens and other factors which may otherwise find an access from the environment to the stroma.
2. **Binding with the tear-Film**
   The microvilli are covered with glycocalyx which has affinity with the innermost mucin layer of the tear-film.
3. **Smooth refractive surface**
   The epithelium forms an optically smooth refractive surface in association with tear-film.

Regeneration of Epithelial Cell

Older Concept of Epithelial Regeneration

The corneal epithelium is renewed every 5-7 days completely. There had been misconceptions about the origin of the cells replacing the older ones due to be shed away from the epithelial surface. It was thought that these are the basal cells which multiply and move upstream through the overlying layers. This concept has changed in the light of the following facts.

The XYZ Hypothesis (Thoft and Friend 1983)

The above researchers have advocated the following hypothesis for epithelial regeneration.

Stem Cells   All the cells in the basal layer do not have the germinative potential, as was believed earlier. The germinative region of the corneal epithelium lies at the basal layer of the limbus only, which contains the stem cells.

Transient Amplifying Cells or Transit Cells   The *stem cells undergo division once* and migrate centripetally in the basal region. This is a *slow process*. Their progeny is called transient amplifying cells or transit cells. These cells are the ones which undergo a number of cell divisions and differentiate to other corneal cell types while moving upwards towards the surface and are finally shed off (Fig. 8.1). The **transitional cells** identified just inside the limbal region by some other researchers are thought to be nothing but these transient amplifying cells of Thoft et al.

Corneal Stroma

The stroma forms little less than 90% of the corneal thickness. It is a transparent connective tissue due to the peculiar arrangement of the collagen fibrils constituting it. It consists of the following.

1. The collagen fibrils
2. The ground substance
3. The keratocytes (modified fibroblasts)
4. Occasional cells–lymphocytes, macrophages and rarely polymorphs

The stroma can be further divided into two parts.

1. The anterior part: *Bowman's layer*
2. The stroma proper or *Substantia propria*

Bowman's Layer or Anterior Limiting Lamina

The Bowman's layer is the anterior-most, 8–12 µ thick, modified acellular region of the stroma consisting of collagen fibrils and proteoglycans. It was earlier thought to be derived from the basal layer of the epithelium. Various functions like maintaining a regular refractive surface formed by the epithelium, formation of an acellular barrier between the epithelium and the stroma to avoid activation of the keratocytes that cause extracellular matrix formation inside the stroma, have been attributed to this layer.

Violation of this layer during surgical procedures was said to result in corneal opacity and poor refractive surface. The excimer laser has successfully removed this layer without disturbance in the refractive quality of the

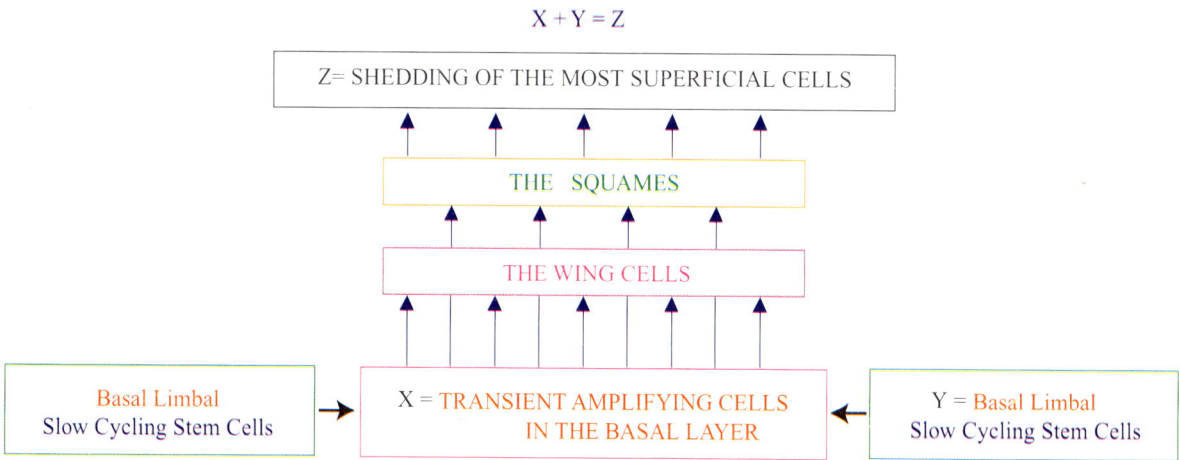

Fig. 8.1: Epithelial regeneration: The XYZ hypothesis

cornea. Moreover all other mammals, who lack this structure, do not suffer from any refractive or epithelial problem.

The Stroma Proper (Substantia Propria)

It consists of layers of 200-250 regularly arranged *lamellae of collagen bundles* which are parallel to each other and to the corneal surface. The lamellae generally run from limbus to limbus. Each lamella is about 2 μ thick, ribbon-like flattened layers of 9-250 μ width. The adjacent lamellae are oriented at about 90° angle to each other in the deeper layers of stroma. This arrangement is less precise in the more anterior stroma where some interweaving may be observed with some fibrils getting inserted obliquely into the Bowman's layer. The collagen bundles consists of fibrils of 27-35 nm diameter or 270-350 A° units (1 nm = 10 Å).

Keratocytes Keratocytes are flat, stellate cells. They are modified fibroblasts. Keratocytes are present between the lamellae of the stroma.

Their long processes attach to the tips of other cell processes by *gap junctions*. These cells thus form a network of interconnecting cell bodies within the stroma. The cell connections between the keratovytes are confined to the cells in the same horizontal plane and do not occur in antero-posterior direction between the cells of adjacent planes (lamellae).

The keratocytes are responsible for formation and maintenance of the stromal lamellae. After injury they transform into fibroblasts and lay down the scar tissue.

Ground substance The ground substance is secreted by the keratocytes. It consists of proteoglycans.

TRANSPARENCY OF THE CORNEA

Though the corneal stroma has similar structural constituents, yet it is 100% transparent to the light unlike the sclera. This transparency of the cornea is due to the special arrangement of the collagen fibrils within the stroma and the transparency of the epithelium as explained above. Following theories deal with the special arrangement of the collagen fibers resulting in transparency of the cornea.

The Lattice Arrangement Theory of Maurice (1957)

The collagen fibrils are of *equal diameter* and are arranged *equidistance* from each-other in a perfect lattice fashion. This arrangement along with small diameter of the fibrils is able to completely suppress the back-scatter of light by destructive interference resulting in complete transparency of the tissue.

The Modification by Goldman (1968)

The fibril diameter and the distance of their separation is more important for sufficient *destructive-interference* to occur and a perfect lattice periodicity is not must. The fibril separation and the diameter should be less then one-third of the wavelength of the incident light for total transparency to occur. This is what happens in a normal cornea.

Mechanisms of Loss of Transparency

Loss of transparency occurs when there is either:
1. Loss of the above regular arrangement of collagen fibrils as in the case of corneal scarring.
2. Increased separation of collagen fibrils due to pockets of fluid as in case of corneal edema.
3. Loss of glycosaminoglycans (GAGs) in corneal edema causing aggregations of collagen fibrils.

Endothelium

The innermost lining of single layer of low-cuboidal, hexagonal cells is the endothelial layer. The cells are rich in the cell energy-houses, the mitochondria, for their metabolic function. *This cell layer is neuroectodermal in origin.*

Specular microscopy is the method of visualizing and finding endothelial cell density. Table 8.2 shows the endothelial count at different ages.

Table 8.2: Endothelial cell count

At birth	:	about 6000 cells/cm^2
End of first year	:	26 % decrease in count
End of twelth year	:	another 26 % decrease
Young adult	:	3000-3500 cells/cm^2
Old age	:	2000-2500 cells/cm^2

The endothelial cells do not undergo mitosis to compensate for the cell loss due to chemical, mechanical or other trauma and inflammatory process. To fill up the space of cell loss they undergo sliding, rearrangement and increase in size. The enlargement of the endothelial cells is called **polymegathism.** This leads to *pleomor-*

phism of the cells which can be documented and followed up by specular microscopy.

Descemet's Membrane

It is a 8–12 μ thick basement membrane secreted by the endothelium which measures about 3 μ at birth. It has two parts in the adult.

1. **The fetal part** is the anterior one-third to half of the Descemet's membrane consisting of banded collagen. The is the oldest secreted layer whose thickness varies on the age of the individual.
2. **The inner amorphous part** is the posterior part of the Descemet's membrane.

Endothelial Pump

An active Na^+-K^+ ATPase dependant transport system, requiring energy, exists in the endothelium which moves Na^+ and bicarbonate ions from the stroma into the aqueous humor. This generates an *osmotic gradient* which draws water out of the stroma. This enzyme is inhibited by *ouabain* leading to corneal swelling. Another enzyme, *carbonic anhydrase*, in the endothelium generates carbonate ions from CO_2 and H_2O.

Carbonic anhydrase inhibitors, therefore, theoretically may inhibit this pump function and deturgescence of the stroma.

This pump function, which maintains the normal corneal hydration at about 78%, is dependent upon a certain level of active transport, which in turn is dependent upon a certain minimum number of *normally functioning* endothelial cells. The **critical number** of cell below which corneal edema must develop is a matter of speculation but certainly any drastic cell loss is a high risk factor. There are reports of clear cornea in certain cases of corneal grafting with a cell count as low as 400 cells/cm^2 and of corneal edema where the cell count is much higher than this. The areas of cell loss having large cells would give low readings of cell density. But if one happens to evaluate area where mostly normal cells are present, one would get better cell density readings despite an actual decrease in the total cell number. The physiological function of the cell itself is also of importance rather than the cell count only. Increased pump function occurs in early stage of Fuchs' dystrophy.

CORNEAL PHYSIOLOGY

Corneal Metabolism

The cornea is an avascular structure. Therefore it depends for its O_2 supply mainly on the diffusion from atmosphere and nutrient (glucose, amino acids, vitamins and minerals, etc.) supply from the aqueous by passive leak through the incomplete endothelial barrier. The peripheral cornea may derive these from the paralimbal vasculature.

The energy production from glucose is mainly by *anaerobic glycolysis,* but also through *MP shunt* and occasionally by *sorbitol-pathway.*

The partial O_2 pressure in the tears is 155 mm Hg when the eye is open. It falls to 55 mm Hg on closing the eye but is sufficient for maintaining the *aerobic metabolism of pyruvate* through Krebs cycle which otherwise would be converted to lactate under anaerobic conditions. Prolonged eye closure such as during sleep causes fall of partial O_2 pressure to still lower levels which leads to some lactate accumulation and mild corneal edema, which soon recovers during aerobic metabolism on awakening.

Corneal Hypoxia

Poorly fitted contact lenses or the ones having low oxygen permeability can cause corneal hypoxia. A critical fall in oxygen tension bringing it down to about 10-15 mm Hg, may occur after contact lens use during sleep or with therapeutic contact lens wear. Under such severe hypoxia, the following pathological changes take place in the cornea.

1. **Accumulation of lactate**
   Accumulation of lactate occurs, which cannot diffuse out due to the epithelial barrier. This increases the pH, causes epithelial edema and interferes with other essential cellular functions like cell division and repair.
2. **Na^+-K^+ ATPase inhibition**
   The arachidonic acid is metabolized to 12-(R)-hydroxy eicosatetraenoic acid [12-(R)-HETE] and 12-(R)-di-HETE due to hypoxia. The former [12-(R)-HETE] inhibits the Na^+-K^+ ATPase. This can be of significance in causing stromal edema.
3. **Corneal neovascularization**
   Formation of new vessels and growth into the cornea can be mediated by 12-(R)-di-HETE.

DETURGESCENCE

Maintenance of Corneal Thickness

The bulk of corneal thickness (up to 90%) is constituted by the stroma. The water content of this structure is about 78%. Any increase in the corneal thickness is due to increase in stromal thickness which is *mainly because of water retention* in the stroma (scar formation is other cause). Edema of the stoma causes number of pathological changes.

1. Absorption of water by the ground substance causes separation of the collagen fibrils.
2. There is loss of glycosaminoglycans (GAGs) due to edema which causes aggregations of collagen fibrils.
3. There is uneven spacing and distribution of the fibrils disturbing the *'lattice arrangement'*.
4. An amorphous material appears forming lakes between the lamellae.
5. Later epithelial edema appears which may leave behind subepithelial opacity.
6. Epithelial edema, if severe, can result in the formation of bullae within this layer of the cornea. Their rupture leads to pain, lacrimation and photophobia. Subsequent healing causes opacity in the subepithelial region resulting in the further loss of visual acuity, which is already compromized due to the corneal edema.

These changes hamper corneal transparency. Epithelial edema results in coloured halos, glare and reduced contrast sensitivity. Therefore hydration of stroma is to be maintained strictly.

Forces Causing Stromal Turgescence

1. **Corneal stromal swelling pressure**
   There is a tendency for the stroma to imbibe water and swell. This is due to presence of collagen, proteoglycans and salts which give the stroma a *hypertonic milieu in comparison to tears and the aqueous*. The corneal stromal swelling pressure is of the order of 60 mm Hg.
2. **Intraocular pressure**
   The intraocular pressure also works to move water in the stromal direction.

Forces Causing Stromal Deturgescence

1. **The epithelial barrier**
   The epithelial barrier is a complete one as described above. However a break in this barrier as by scraping, photoablation or large erosions can cause swelling up to 200 μ.
2. **The endothelial barrier**
   The endothelial barrier is an incomplete one as the apical tight junctions do not completely encircle the cells and the gap junction and cellular interdigitations on the lateral aspect do not offer total resistance to the movements of ions and small molecules.
3. **The endothelial metabolic pump**
   As has been described above, the metabolic pump, is an active process that removes water from the stroma, which moves in through the *leaky* endothelial barrier (*pump-leak–hypothesis*). It is the main factor that works to maintain the corneal hydration within normal limits.

Suggested readings

1. Azar DT et al: Decentred penetration of anchoring fibrils into the diabetic stroma: A morphometric analysis. Arch Ophthalmol 1989; 107: 1520.
2. Benedek BG: Theory of transparency of the eye. Applied Optics 1971; 10: 459.
3. Bonanno JA et al: Effect of rigid CL oxygen transmissibility on stromal pH in the living human eye. Ophthalmology 1987; 94: 1305.
4. Dikstein and Maurice et al: The metabolic basis of the fluid pump of the cornea. J Physio 1955; 221:29.
5. Friend J, Thoft RA: The diabetic cornea. Int Ophthalmol Cli 985; 24: 111.
6. Gipson IK: Adhesive mechanisms of the corneal epithelium. Acta Ophalmol suppl 1992; 202: 13.
7. Gipson IK: The epithelial basement membrane zone of the limbus. Eye1989; 3: 132.
8. Hall P, Watt FM: Stem cells: The generation and maintenance of cellular diversity. Development 1989; 106: 619.
9. Holden BA, Mertz DW: Critical oxygen levels to avoid corneal edema for daily and extended wear CL. Invest Ophthalmol Vis Sci 1984; 25: 1161.
10. Khodadoust A et al: Adhesion of regenerating corneal epithelium: The role of basement membrane. Am J Ophthalmol 1969; 65: 339.
11. Laule A et al: Endothelial cell population changes of human cornea during life. Arch Ophtha 1978; 96: 2031
12. Maurice DM: The cornea and the sclera. In H Davson (ed.), The Eye (3rd edition). Orlando: Academic 1985; 1b pp. 1-158.
13. Rozenman Y et al: Contact lens related deep stromal vascularization. Am J Ophthalmol 1989; 107: 27.
14. Thoft RA, Friend J: Corneal epithelial metabolism. Arch Ophthalmol 1971; 88: 58.

15. Thoft RA, Friend J: The XYZ hypothesis of corneal epithelial maintenance. Invest Ophthalmol Vis Sci 1983; 24: 1442.
16. Tsubota K, Laing RA : Metabolic changes in corneal epithelium resulting from hard contact lens wear. Cornea 1992; 121: 11.
17. Warwick R: (Ed) " Eugene Wolff's Anatomy of the Eye and Orbit", 8th Ed; 1997.
18. Zieske JD, Bukusoglu G et al: Characterization of a potential marker of corneal epithelial stem cells. Invest Ophthalmol Vis Sci 1992; 33: 143.

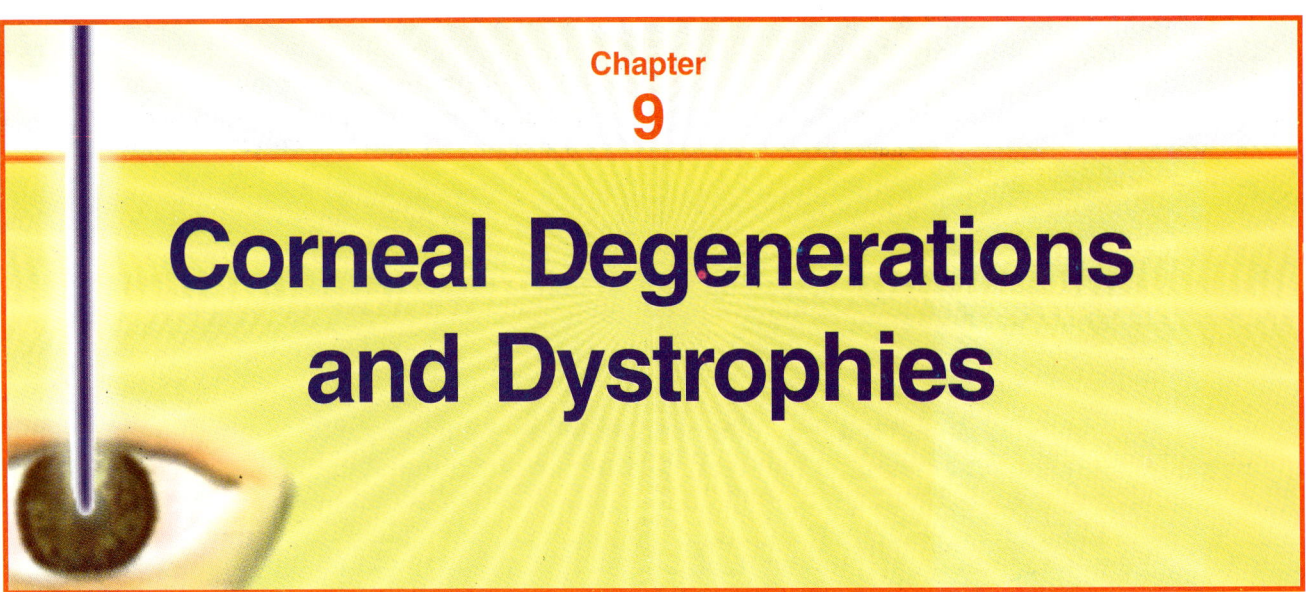

Chapter 9: Corneal Degenerations and Dystrophies

INTRODUCTION

The following overview deals with various corneal degenerations and dystrophies in a simplified manner with emphasis on conditions which are tackled with the excimer laser PTK. For a detailed description of other conditions the reader should refer to any standard text book on cornea.

Although there are numerous exceptions*, the points given in Table 9.1 differentiate dystrophies from degenerations in general.

Table 9.1: Differential features of corneal degenerations and dystrophies

Corneal Degenerations	Corneal Dystrophies
1. Usually unilateral	Usually bilateral
2. Asymmetric if bilateral	Symmetric
3. Lesions located peripherally	Located centrally
4. Accompanied by vascularization	Avascular
5. No inheritance pattern or genetic predisposition	Hereditary, usually *autosomal dominant* **Exception (recessive):** • Macular dystrophy type - III • Lattice dystrophy • Gelatinous drop-like dystrophy
6. Onset in middle or latter life	Usually early in onset, by second decade
7. Progressive	Very slowly progressive or stationary
8. Secondary to • aging • trauma • local or systemic disorders • environmental conditions. • inflammations etc	Usually unrelated to any such condition

CORNEAL DEGENERATIONS

The corneal degenerations are common conditions. These can be one of the following.

1. Age-related corneal degeneration
   a. Arcus senilis
   b. Vogt's limbal girdle
   c. Cornea farinata
   d. Hassal-Henle bodies
   e. Crocodile shagreen of Vogt
2. Band keratopathy
3. Salzmann's nodular degeneration

---

*Arcus Senilis and Hassal-Henle bodies are peripheral but bilateral degenerations. Eighty percent cases of Salzmann's degeneration are bilateral. Pellucid Terrien's marginal degenerations are bilateral. Degeneration where familial cases have been reported are band shaped keratopathy (BSK), cornea farinata, Salzmann's and spheroidal degenerations. Cornea farinata and mosaic shagreen of Vogt's are usually bilateral and centrally occurring degenerations.

4. Spheroidal degeneration
5. Pellucid marginal degeneration
6. Terrien's marginal degeneration
7. Arcus juveniles
8. Hyaline degeneration
9. Lipid degeneration
10. Pigmentary degenerations

AGE-RELATED DEGENERATIONS

These are changes occurring due to aging, presenting in specific patterns, hence described in distinction to physiological senile changes.

Arcus Senilis

Incidence

It is a bilateral, most common, asymptomatic, age-related degeneration seen in 60% of people between 40-60 years and universal in those above 80 years. It is common in black race and occurs 10 years earlier in men.

Appearance

It is seen as yellowish white deposits, first in the inferior, then in superior and eventually in the whole peripheral cornea.

There is a clear area, called *lucid interval of Vogt*, between the limbus and the arcus. The outer border has sharp and the inner border diffuse edge, sometimes with dark crisscross lines within.

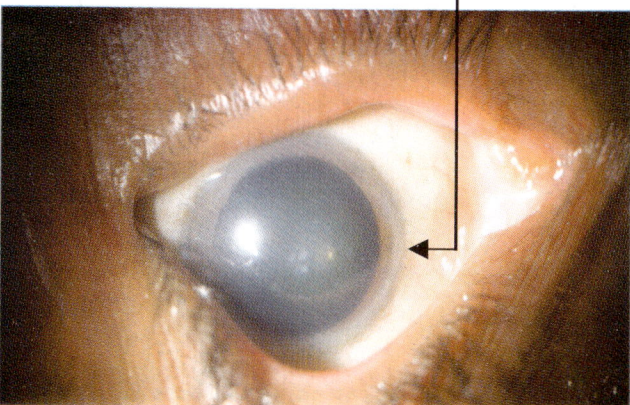

Fig. 9.1: Arcus senilis

Pathogenesis

With increasing age, the increased permeability of the highly vascularized limbal zone to low density lipoproteins, specially in the presence of hypercholestrolemia, leads to deposition of cholesterol, cholesterol esters, phospholipids and triglycerides into the peripheral cornea. The loss of proteins and formation of nonlabile lipids occurs later.

The arcus may occur in association with familial and non-familial dyslipoproteinemias, specially type II.

Arcus Juvenilis

This condition is not age-related. It occurs in individuals below 40 years of age. Arcus juvenilis can be found in the following conditions:

1. Familial dyslipoproteinemias
2. Atopic keratoconjunctivitis
3. Vernal keratoconjunctivitis
4. Megalocornea
5. Keratoconus
6. Osteogenesis imperfecta
7. Blue sclera

Unilateral Arcus

It is a rare entity, which may be seen in cases of *ocular hypotony* and *carotid obstructive disease*.

White Limbal Girdle of Vogt

Incidence

White limbal girdle of Vogt is found in almost 55% of general population between the age of 40–60 years. This condition is asymptomatic.

The type I and type II described in earlier literature are not accepted currently. The type I, which has a clear area separating it from the limbus is taken as early-stage band shaped keratopathy.

Appearance

It appears as chalky white crescent in the temporal and nasal palpabral area, with no clear zone between the limbus and the lesion.

Pathology

There is *elastotic degeneration* of subepithelial collagen probably related to sun–exposure.

Cornea Farinata

Occurrence

It is usually a bilateral, age-related condition though unilateral and familial cases have been reported.

Appearance

On slit-lamp examination, there is a speckling of dust like /flourlike opacities in the posterior, occasionally in the middle or anterior part of stroma.

Pathology

There is accumulation of a degenerative pigment *(lipofusin)* in the keratocytes of stroma. This condition is to be differentiated from pre-Descemet's dystrophy which clinically, resembles it and also shows accumulation of lipofusin.

Hassal-Henle Bodies (Descemet's Warts)

Incidence

More than 70% of the population over 40 years of age would show one or more of these bodies as incidental findings which increase in number as one grows older.

Appearance

Hassal-Henle bodies are seen by specular reflection as tiny dark spots disrupting regular mosaic pattern of the endothelium. The dark spots are caused by excrescencies or small nodular thickening on the Descemet's membrane facing the endothelium.

The location of these bodies is peripheral, in contrast to the identical findings of **cornea guttata** which occur in the central part of cornea.

They do not become pathological because the endothelial pump sites also increase in number to enhance the pump function as the their number increase.

Pathology

The thickenings on the inner surface of the Descemet's are due to overproduction of *hyaline* material by the endothelium.

Mosaic Shagreen of Vogt (Crocodile Shagreen)

Clinically this degeneration resembles *central cloudy corneal dystrophy* and is also to be differentiated from *corneal edema* (by the absence of thickening and Descemet's folds). The corneal sensation is reduced and corneal neovascularization may be present. Vision is rarely reduced.

Appearance

It is formed by asymptomatic polygonal, grayish white opacities located in the central cornea. There are two types, the anterior crocodile shagreen and posterior crocodile shagreen.

1. **Anterior crocodile shagreen**

   This is more frequent, in which the opacities involve the anterior two-thirds of stroma. The tension on the collagen lamellae of the anterior stroma that enter the Bowman's layer is relaxed due to aging, causing the mosaic pattern through formation of ridges that indent the epithelium. Calcium deposition, rupture in Bowman's membrane and subsequent fibrosis between the epithelium and Bowman's layer may occur. Other factors which can relax the normal tension are trauma and prolonged hypertension.

2. **Posterior crocodile shagreen**

   This is less common. Here the opacities are in the posterior stroma. Electron microscopy has demonstrated an irregular saw-tooth appearance of the corneal lamellae in which 100 nm–spaced collagen is interspersed.

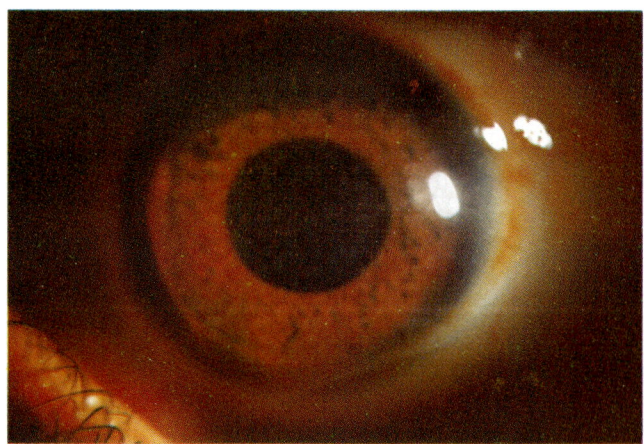

Fig. 9.2: Mosaic shagreen (crocodile shagreen) of Vogt

Juvenile form of Crocodile Shagreen

Juvenile form of crocodile shagreen is seen in the following conditions.

1. Megalocornea
2. Iris malformation
3. Peripheral calcific band keratopathy

CORNEAL DEGENERATION NOT CAUSED BY AGING

Band Shaped Keratopathy: BSK (Dixon 1848, Bowman 1849)

Appearance

A rough, whitish yellow area of calcium characteristically on interpalpebral region of the cornea, having a sharp margin separated from the limbus by a clear zone. Many holes are visualized on slit-lamp examination where corneal nerves penetrate the Bowman's layer.

1. Smooth band keratopathy

The surface is smooth and the epithelium is intact over the calcification. The calcific plaques in this case are limited in their extent. The lesions are located at the level of Bowman's layer only and do not penetrate further into the deeper level (Colour Plate 1, Photograph 7).

2. Rough band keratopathy

The band is thick, the epithelium unstable and the calcification extends deeper into the anterior stroma with breaks in the Bowman's layer. The eyes are severely symptomatic and vision is much affected (Colour Plate 1, Photograph 5 and 6).

Symptoms

Lesions of calcium deposition cause considerable ocular irritation, foreign body sensation, glare and photophobia, lacrimation and pain occurs when the surface epithelium is breached over the calcific lesions.

Pathogenesis

The band is formed by deposition of calcium (mainly hydroxyapatite), in the Bowman's layer, basement membrane and the most superficial part of stroma, starting in the periphery and extending to the central cornea. The calcified Bowman's layer may break forming plaques with transparent clefts.

The calcium present in the tears can be easily precipitated by rise in the pH, evaporation or increase in concentration of either calcium or phosphate, which are otherwise normally present in the body fluids and blood at levels that exceed their solubility. The localization in the palpebral fissure area is explained by increased evaporation of tears, loss of CO_2 causing rise in the pH and lack of blood vessels in the cornea which might have buffering effect through blood. Since the pH in the deeper stroma is low, calcium precipitation does not occur there.

The main causes associated with this condition are:

1. *Local degenerative diseases,* e.g. chronic uveitis, phthisis bulbi, absolute glaucoma, juvenile rheumatoid arthritis and interstitial keratitis
2. *Idiopathic* in the elderly
3. *Hypercalcemia,* e.g. Vitamin D intoxication, hyperparathyroidism, sarcoidosis and nephrocalcinosis,
4. Silicon filled eyes
5. *Chronic exposure to chemical irritants,* e.g. mercury fumes and calcium bichromate vapor.
6. *Skin disorders,* e.g. Icthyosis, DLE, tuberous sclerosis and Rothmund-Thomson syndrome.

Treatment

Chelating agents and *mechanical keratectomy* are often used for treatment of band keratopathy.

Chelation is done with 0.05 mol/L of 1.5% neutral and sterile solution of ethylenediamene tetra-acetic acid (EDTA). After good local anesthesia, the epithelium is scraped and a cellulose sponge saturated with the solution is applied for few minutes on the calcified area and calcium is removed with a cotton-tipped bud.

Repeated applications may be needed. Spilling–over of the chemical is to be avoided as it is very irritant to the eye. Some people use a water bath over the cornea to avoid spill-over of the medicine.

Superficial keratectomy is done in cases of thick, rough band keratopathy.

Calcareous Degeneration

This affects the deeper layers of the cornea also and is seen in severely injured eyes, phthisis bulbi and necrotic neoplasm. It is to be differentiated from band keratopathy.

Salzmann's Nodular Degeneration

Symptoms

Most patients are initially asymptomatic. Irritation, photophobia, lacrimation occur later due to breach in the single layered epithelium over the nodules.

Appearance

Grey or bluish-grey, elevated, nodular lesion in the superficial stroma, one to nine in number, on the central or peripheral cornea (Colour Plate 1, Photograph 1–4). They may be located in the previously scarred cornea or at the edge of the transparent cornea. A pigment line at the base of the nodule may be seen. Women are more often affected.

Pathogenesis

This degeneration develops as a *late sequelae* to a number of conditions suffered during childhood:

1. Phlyctenulosis
2. Trachoma
3. Keratitis sicca
4. Exposure keratopathy
5. Vernal keratoconjunctivitis
6. Measles and other viral diseases
7. Scarlet fever

The nodule shows hyaline degeneration of the superficial stroma, loss of the Bowman's layer and single layered epithelium.

Treatment

No treatment may be required in most cases unless symptoms become significant or there is loss of visual acuity due to the location of the lesion. *Superficial keratectomy* with or without *lamellar keratoplasty* may be used to shave off or excise a few lesions but the visual clarity may not be optimum. *Penetrating keratoplasty* is occasionally done to improve vision but recurrences have been reported after many years.

Spheroidal Degeneration (Labrador/Climatic droplet keratopathy)

This condition has the most number of eponyms including chronic actinic keratopathy, oil droplet keratopathy, corneal elastosis, elastoid degeneration, hyaline degeneration, Nama keratopathy, fisherman's keratopathy and proteinaceous keratopathy.

Appearance

Examination with a slit-lamp shows accumulation of clusters of tiny yellow or amber-coloured droplets or granules in the superficial stroma. These droplets form a band on the corneal surface of interpalpebral region.

It starts in the periphery, spreads to involve the center of the cornea and may vary in severity from localized oily granularity to large areas of bigger lesions (Colour Plate 2, Photograph 8).

Pathogenesis

Exposure to environmental factors, such as actinic radiations; dry, windy or sandy conditions, ice etc. are often implicated in the causation of this degeneration (therefore the above eponyms). It affects men more than women (spending more time outdoors). Aging, welding, extremes of temperature and corneal inflammations are supposed to enhance the progress of this degeneration.

There is **elastotic degeneration** of the collagen in the cornea and conjunctiva. Lipoprotein deposits are found beneath and at the level of the Bowman's layer. Three types or grades are described according to the severity:

Type I (Grade 1) It is a primary form which is *age-related* and not associated with any other factors. It is bilateral and affects only the periphery without affecting the vision.

Type II (Grade 2) In this type the pupillary area is also involved, reducing vision to 20/100 to 20/200. It occurs *secondary* to climatic factors or previous corneal conditions or both.

Type III (Grade 3) The vision is reduced to less than 20/200 in this extreme form due to the large opalescent, yellowish nodules. It occurs with pinguecula in most of the cases and is a severe form of conjunctival and corneal spheroidal degeneration.

Treatment

1. *Superficial keratectomy* can be done to excise the lesion. Recurrence is unusual.
2. *Lamellar or penetrating keratoplasty* are done for cases affecting vision.

Lipid Degeneration (Lipid Keratopathy)

Appearance

Dense opacities of yellowish white colour with feathery edges in the cornea. These consists of neutral fats with some cholesterol and phospholipids.

Pathogenesis

1. **Primary lipid degeneration**
   Bilateral, central lipid deposits occur without any vascularization and associated corneal diseases. This is a less common form.
2. **Secondary lipid degeneration**
   This is the more often seen type occurring secondary to chronic inflammatory diseases and trauma, which result in necrosis and vascularization of the cornea. Most common causes are herpes simplex and herpes zoster disciform keratitis and contact lens wear after cataract surgery. Increased permeability of the limbal vessels, increased production or decreased ability of corneal cells to metabolize the lipids are the possible reasons leading to the lipid degeneration.

Treatment

Argon laser photocoagulation of the feeder vessels has been employed for management of the secondary type. Control of the primary disease is must to avoid re-vascularization. Penetrating keratoplasty is done to improve the vision in both types.

Hyaline Degeneration

Appearance

A band of granular or nodular, yellowish brown opacities in the lower half of the cornea with a clear limbal zone. It resembles Salzmann's nodular degeneration, spheroidal degeneration as well granular dystrophy.

Pathogenesis

Climatic factors have been implicated in the causation of this condition as it occurs, like climatic droplet keratopathy, in some geographical locations only.

Treatment

Treatment is by lamellar keratoplasty, if required.

Pigmentary Degeneration

A number of disorders are associated with deposition of iron in the cornea as a ring, line or diffusely. The source of the iron is not exactly known except in case of injury with iron foreign bodies. It probably may be the perilimbal blood vessels from which the tear and corneal transferrin carry it to the site of its deposition.

1. **Coat's white ring:** A ring of iron deposition occurs at the level of Bowman's layer or superficial stroma. This is caused by injury with metallic foreign body.
2. **Fleischer ring:** It is found around the cone of keratoconus.
3. **Ferry line:** These lines occur near a filtering bleb.
4. **Stocker-Busaca line:** The iron deposition line seen in case of pterygium is called Stocker-Busaca line. This is found ahead of the advancing head of the pterygium.
5. **Hudson-Stahli line:** This may be seen in some cases of epithelial breakdown.

Pterygium

Pterygium is not a corneal but primarily conjunctival degeneration which affects the cornea. The term is derived from the Greek word 'pterygion' meaning a "wing".

Appearance

A triangular fibrovascular sheet extending from the conjunctiva onto the cornea, most often on the nasal side. It is firmly adherent to the underlying cornea throughout. Progressive growth may invade the central cornea (Colour Plate 2, Photograph 9). A pterygium has three parts: the body, the head and the cap.

The Body   It is pinkish red, flat sheet of highly vascular connective tissue.

The Head   It is the corneal part, firmly adherent to the superficial stroma, white in colour and slightly elevated from the surface.

The Cap   It is the grey coloured avascular area surrounding the head like a halo.

Stocker's Line   It is deposition of iron in the corneal epithelium that may be seen ahead of the advancing head of the pterygium.

The activity of a growing pterygium is reflected by the associated redness and inflammation.

Symptoms

Growth of white flesh, irritation and decreased vision due to astigmatism produced by the growth in the periphery or it directly covering the pupillary area in extreme of cases.

Pathogenesis

The interpalpebral location and geographical distribution of the patients affected by this condition point towards an environmental cause. It is found in people living in sunny, hot or dry climate and in welders in Japan. The histology of the excised lesion shows a vascular fibrous tissue base underlying degenerated elastic tissue. The cornea shows destruction of the Bowman's layer and superficial stroma. Invasive fibroblasts are found at the level of Bowman's layer which are responsible for recurrence of the pterygium after excision.

Treatment

Surgical excision is required in the following situations.

1. Cosmetic reasons
2. Decreased vision due to irregular astigmatism
3. Growth encroaching upon the visual axis

Excision Superficial keratectomy starting from clear cornea adjacent to the opaque head of the pterygium combined with excision of the bulbar conjunctiva, thus removing the tissue as one piece, is done. This may be done as '*bare sclera technique*' or with '*conjunctival autograft*' from the superior temporal area. A high recurrence (40%-60%), as early as four months, after the bare sclera technique but only 5% recurrence after 24 months of excision and conjunctival autograft has been reported.

Adjunctive Therapy Use of adjunctive therapy with beta radiation or mitomycin-C may further reduce the long term recurrence rate and help in the management of recurrent pterygium.

1. *Beta radiation*
   The dose is 900-3000 rads (9-30 Gy) given over a 3 weeks period. The main complications are scleral ulceration and cataract.
2. *Mitomycin C*
   This can be used in two ways.
   a. Topical Therapy: As 0.04% eye drops given four times daily for 2 weeks after the surgical removal.
   b. Intraoperative Use: In concentration of 0.02% or 0.04% applied for 5 minutes with a cellulose sponge on the exposed sclera while protecting the cornea. The recurrence rate is 8.3% with the use of 0.02% mitomycin-C and 2.9% with 0.04%. The main complications are persistent corneal and conjunctival defects, scleral thinning and corneal ulceration.

Pseudopterygium

It is a fibrovascular growth or a fold of the conjunctiva adherent to the cornea seen in corneal diseases like marginal keratitis, chemical burns and ocular cicatricial pemphigoid.

This growth is fixed to the globe only at its apex and is *not differentiated into the body, head and cap*, unlike a true pterygium.

Malignant growth like *squamous cell carcinoma* is also to be distinguished particularly from a recurrent pterygium.

Pellucid Marginal Degeneration

This is a rare, bilateral, slowly progressive, peripheral corneal degeneration occurring between the age of 20 and 50 years. Both sexes are equally affected and no hereditary predisposition is seen.

Appearance

A crescent shaped, 1-2 mm wide area of corneal thinning, extending from 4 to 8 O'clock, separated from the limbus by normal cornea. Scarring may be present underneath this thinned out band of cornea.

Symptoms

Presentation is with decrease in vision.

Pathogenesis

Protrusion of normal cornea occurs above the area of thinning leading to *high irregular astigmatism* (as much as 20 diopters) due to inferior steepening. This is in contrast to keratoconus where protrusion occur in the area of thinning. Moreover there is no Fleischer ring, no cone and no scarring in this area. Some workers consider it as a *corneal dystrophy* and a variant of keratoconus because of associated keratoconus in many cases, decreased levels of keratan sulfate and the histological similarity between these two.

Acute hydrops may develop due to breaks in the Descemet's membrane in the area of protrusion. Stromal edema and break in Bowman's layer are also seen.

Treatment

1. *Spectacle correction* may help in very early cases.
2. *Hard contact lens* are beneficial in some cases for correcting the irregular astigmatism but are liable to develop intolerance due to inferior decentration.

3. *Crescentic lamellar keratoplasty* or wedge resection with relaxing incisions are other procedure which may be needed in this situation.
4. *Hypertonic saline, eye patching or bandage contact lens* may be required if acute hydrops develop.
5. *Penetrating keratoplasty* is done if there is persistent corneal edema.

Terrien's Marginal Degeneration

This is a rare, bilateral asymmetrical, peripheral thinning of cornea, most often affecting men at any age.

Appearance

Initially there are fine, yellow-white, subepithelial opacities in the superonasal peripheral cornea separated from the limbus by a clear zone, which may resemble arcus senilis. Later, very slowly thinning of the cornea appears in that area. The overlying epithelium is intact, though a peripheral *gutter* is formed due to progressive thinning. This thinning and gutter formation may extend circumferentially. Superficial vascularization may be seen.

Pathogenesis

The cause of the corneal thinning is not known. In many, particularly young patients, there is inflammation, necrosis and neovascularization of the peripheral cornea and associated scleritis or episcleritis with episodes of pain. But this degeneration can be differentiated from Mooren's ulcer by normal level of immune complexes which are elevated in the later disease. Lipid deposition in the center of the gutter is seen in all cases of Terrien's degeneration.

Flattening of the thin cornea and ectasia of the normal cornea causes severe irregular astigmatism. Acute hydrops may develop or trivial trauma to the severely thinned cornea can cause perforation.

A pseudopterygium may form due to progressive vascularization.

Treatment

1. *Medical management*
   Acute hydrops and inflammatory episodes are treated medically with appropriate medications like hypertonic saline dropes, tear-drops and bandage soft contact lens.

2. *Surgical management*
   In severe cases excision of the thin cornea (gutter) with a lamellar or full thickness *corneoscleral graft* may be required. This procedure strengthens the cornea as well as reduces astigmatism caused by change in curvature due to corneal thinning. Re-thinning may occur after a decade.

CORNEAL DYSTROPHIES

As mentioned earlier, the corneal dystrophies are usually bilateral, centrally located, symmetric, hereditary (mainly autosomal dominant) conditions. The corneal dystrophies may be classified as shown in Table 9.2.

Table 9.2: Classification of corneal dystrophies

Epithelial Dystrophies
1. Meesman's dystrophy
2. Epithelial basement membrane dystrophy (microcystic dystrophy)

Bowman's Layer Dystrophy
1. Reis-Bucklers' dystrophy

Stromal Dystrophies
A. Anterior stromal
1. Granular dystrophy
2. Macular dystrophy
3. Lattice dystrophy
4. Central crystalline dystrophy (Schnyder's dystrophy)

B. Mid stromal (middle third of stroma)
1. Central cloudy dystrophy

C. Pan-stromal
1. Fleck dystrophy
2. Congenital hereditary stromal dystrophy

D. Posterior stromal
1. Posterior amorphous dystrophy
2. Pre-Descemet's dystrophy

Endothelial Dystrophies
1. Fuchs' endothelial dystrophy
2. Posterior polymorphous dystrophy
3. Congenital hereditary endothelial dystrophy

Ectatic Dystrophies
1. Keratoconus (anterior)
2. Posterior keratoconus
3. Keratoglobus

EPITHELIAL AND BOWMAN'S LAYER DYSTROPHIES

Epithelial Basement Membrane Dystrophy (EBMD)

It is the most common dystrophy that affects women over 30 years of age. The other eponyms are Cogan's microcystic dystrophy and *map-dot-fingerprint dystrophy*. Although it may show dominant inheritance pattern in some cases, no definite heredity pattern is known for the majority of cases.

Presentation

Presentation is with symptoms of recurrent corneal erosions but rarely as decreased vision.

Pathogenesis

Synthesis of abnormal basement membrane is the cause of this dystrophy. The basement membrane gets thickened and sends extensions into the epithelium. Hemidesmomes are not formed by the overlying epithelium which results in recurrent erosions.

Appearance

Slit-lamp examination shows three types of lesions found in a single location, either in the center or in the periphery of the cornea.

Maps This pattern formed by thickened basement membrane which extends into the epithelium. They appear as diffuse grey areas of varying size having clear areas within.

Dots The dots are intraepithelial cysts or blebs. They contain lipids, cytoplasmic and nuclear debris (Colour Plate 2, Photograph 12).

Fingerprints This pattern is formed by branching or intersecting refractile lines which appear in group. The lines are formed by deposition of fine fibrillar material and reduplication of the basement membrane.

Treatment

Treatment is for recurrent corneal erosion

Meesmann's Dystrophy

This autosomal dominant, bilateral dystrophy is also called juvenile hereditary epithelial dystrophy, which occurs during the first decade of life. It is a very rare condition and does not affect vision. Symptoms appear after fourth or fifth decade when the cysts break to cause pain, watering and photophobia or when irregular astigmatism is sufficient to cause decrease in vision.

Appearance

Tiny, round, clear vesicles are seen in the epithelium by direct as well as retroillumination mostly in the interpalpebral area. The cornea between the vesicles is clear.

Pathogenesis

The abnormality is probably in the cytoplasmic ground substance or filaments of the basal cells which undergo degeneration leading to accumulation of the intracytoplasmic fibrillo-granular material. The intra-epithelial vesicles contain this material.

Treatment

Meesmann's dystrophy remains asymptomatic for decades. Therefore, treatment is rarely required. Soft contact lens may help if the microcysts become symptomatic.

Reis-bucklers' Dystrophy/Bowman's Layer Dystrophy

This autosomal dominant dystrophy is relatively common. It presents early, during childhood with 3-4 episodes of recurrent corneal erosions every year.

The corneal erosions decrease or become infrequent by the fourth decade. This happens possibly due to the scarring of the Bowman's layer. Vision gets affected severely due to this scarring. Corneal sensation is decreased.

Grayson-wilbrandt dystrophy, honeycomb dystrophy and Wardenberg and Jonkers dystrophy are its clinical variants. These types do not affect the vision so severely and corneal sensation is normal.

Appearance

Initially there is a fine reticular opacification at the level of the Bowman's layer (Colour Plate 3, Photograph 14).

Established cases of Reis-Buckler's dystrophy show bluish white, ring or crescent-shaped opacities in the central part of the cornea. These opacities give the cornea a frosted glass or honeycomb appearance. The corneal surface is irregular and stains with fluorescein if erosions are present.

Pathogenesis

The Bowman's layer is replaced by fibrous tissue and filaments. The basement membrane is absent and no hemidesmosomes are formed in the affected region. these anatomical changes are responsible for the recurrent corneal erosions.

Treatment

The treatment is mainly for recurrent corneal erosions. Keratoplasty may be required for late cases with decreased vision due to subepithelial fibrosis.

ANTERIOR STROMAL DYSTROPHIES

Granular Dystrophy (Groenouw-I Dystrophy, Bread-crumb Dystrophy)

This anterior stromal dystrophy has an autosomal dominant inheritance pattern. It is asymptomatic or presents with photophobia or occasionally as recurrent erosions.

Appearance

The lesions appear as bilateral symmetrical, white, discrete, crumb like opacities in the superficial stroma of the central cornea with clear periphery. Over the years the opacities increase in size and number, coalesce and extend into deeper stroma. Three variants of this dystrophy are described.

Type I It presents during the first decade of life with asymptomatic opacities. The cornea between the opacities is clear. Vision is affected by the fourth decade when the opacities become bigger in size, more in number and ground glass haze develops between the lesions (Colour Plate 2, Photograph 11). Visual acuity may be as low as 6/60.

Type II It presents during the second decade with fewer, ring or disc shaped opacities (Colour Plate 2, Photograph 10). Progression is very slow by increase in size only not in number, recurrent erosions rare and the vision remains better than 6/18.

Type III It presents in infancy with painful recurrent erosions.

Pathogenesis

Abnormal keratocytes in the anterior layer of the stroma produce hyaline deposits consisting of proteins, sulfur-containing amino acids and phospolipids. These stain bright red with masson trichrome.

Treatment

Penetrating keratoplasty is done in late cases to improve vision. Recurrences are common in the graft.

Corneal Amyloidosis

Amyloid proteins may be deposited in the cornea as dots or as filaments. The tissue derived amyloid protein is labeled AA, serum derived as SAA and plasma component amyloid as AP. The amyloid material stains red-green with Congo red. This disorder is to be distinguished from lattice dystrophy.

Corneal amyloidosis can occur in a number of clinical settings; *some of which are considered dystrophies and other degenerations.* It is divided as follows:

1. Localized
   a. Primary
   b. Secondary
2. Diffuse/Systemic
   a. Primary systemic amyloidosis rarely involves the cornea
   b. Secondary systemic amyloidosis does not affect the cornea

Localized Corneal Amyloidosis

Primary Localized Corneal Amyloidosis

Gelatinous Drop-like Dystrophy (Nakaizumi)
This is a sporadic or recessively occurring dystrophy mainly reported in Japan. It presents in the first decade with foreign body sensation, photophobia and watering from eyes. Examination shows milky opacities in the central cornea of both eyes formed by amyloid material in the basal layer of a thin epithelium. Later the opacities form hemispherical, gelatinous, yellowish, raised masses on the corneal surface giving it a mulberry appearance. The periphery remains clear.

Treatment is by deep lamellar keratoplasty. Recurrence have been reported after years.

Polymorphic Amyloid Degeneration (Pillat) It is non-inherited disorder, occurring in older individuals, lack progression and does not cause vision loss. Both eyes are involved symmetrically. The punctate or filamentous opacities are produced by deposition of amyloid material in the stroma, more so in deeper part. These appear clear in retroillumination.

Treatment No treatment is required for this condition.

Secondary Localized Corneal Amyloidosis

A number of disorders like trachoma, trauma, neoplasms, leprosy, lipoidol degeneration, climatic droplet keratopathy, and phlyctenulosis can cause secondary localized amyloidosis. The amyloid deposits may be found in three locations: *sub-epithelial; in deep stroma* and *perivasvular*. Treatment is by penetrating keratoplasty if the vision is affected and the primary disorder permits the surgery.

Lattice Dystrophy (Biber-Haab-Dimmer Dystrophy)

Lattice dystrophy is an inherited disorder characterized by deposition of amyloid in the cornea in the form of refractile *lattice lines*.

Appearance

The characteristic *lattice lines* consist of a network of branching and interlacing, translucent and refractile lines formed by amyloid deposition in the anterior or mid stroma. There may be some dot-like, fluffy, anterior stromal and sub epithelial opacities. Initially the stroma between the opacities is clear but later becomes hazy. The corneal periphery remains clear.

Three clinical types have been recognized.

Type I The onset of this type is in the later part of first decade with recurrent corneal erosions. Inheritance is autosomal dominant. Progressive haze leads to diffuse opacification obscuring the lattice lines, dot-like opacities and causing profound loss of vision in later age. The corneal sensation also decrease.

Type II It is associated with systemic amyloidosis inherited in autosomal dominant manner. The systemic amyloidosis may manifest as mask-like facies, protruding lips, dry and itchy skin, cranial and peripheral nerve palsies and blepharochalasis. Onset is in the second decade. The lattice lines are thicker and less numerous. Vision is not affected much till old age. Recurrent erosions are also less frequent and occur late in life after fifth decade.

Type III The onset is still later, after 40 years. Recurrent erosions do not occur. The opacities are broad lattice-like lines and diffuse subepithelial deposits. Vision is not much affected till seventh decade. Inheritance is *autosomal recessive*.

Pathogenesis

The origin of the amyloid material is not known. Collagen degeneration or abnormal keratocyte synthesis could be responsible for its accumulation. In type I and II, the Bowman's layer may be abnormal/absent, the basement membrane fragmented and lacking hemidesmosomes; but it is intact in type III. This explains the absence of erosion in type III lattice dystrophy.

Treatment

Recurrent erosions are managed as described elsewhere. Penetrating keratoplasty is done when vision is affected significantly. Recurrences in the graft are common.

Macular Dystrophy (Groenouw-II Dystrophy)

This dystrophy differs from other stromal dystrophies in being *autosomal recessively* inherited, less common but affecting the vision early and involving the periphery of the cornea. Onset is in the second half of first decade. Recurrent corneal erosions are infrequent.

Appearance

Slit-lamp examination shows diffuse grayish-white irregular opacities with indistinct borders, in the anterior stroma. The intervening stroma has ground-glass appearance. Progression of the opacities leads to the involvement of the posterior stroma and the corneal periphery by third decade. Still later, the corneal surface become irregular due to its elevation by the subepithelial opacities.

Pathogenesis

The opacities are produced by accumulation of mucopolysaccharides in the endoplasmic reticulum of the cells. It stains blue with alcian-blue. Two types are recognized biochemically.

Type I In this type keratan sulfate is not synthesized. It is absent in the serum and very low in the cornea.

Type II Here the keratan sulfate is normal in serum as well as in the cornea.

Treatment

Treatment is by penetrating keratoplasty when vision decreases after the fourth decade.

Central Crystalline Dystrophy (Schnyder's)

Presentation

This dystrophy is autosomal dominant, associated with hyperlipidemia and xanthelasma or with genu valgum, which are also inherited disorders. Corneal arcus and limbal girdle develop in 80%. The opacities are due to deposition of fine, needle shaped crystals of cholesterol at the level of the Bowman's layer and anterior stroma. They form many morphological patterns like round, oval, discoid with ill-defined margins, discoid with garland like margin, annular with a clear center.

Progression

The dystrophy does not progress after second or third decade. Vision is not affected significantly and recurrent erosions are rare.

Treatment

Penetrating keratoplasty is occasionally needed. Hyperlipidemia is managed medically if present.

Peripheral Crystalline Dystrophy (Bietti's)

This dystrophy affects the corneal periphery. It may be inherited in autosomal recessive manner. Association with tapetoretinal degeneration or lipid disorder may be seen. The onset is in the third decade.

MID – STROMAL DYSTROPHIES

Central Cloudy Dystrophy (Francois)

The presentation of this autosomal dominant dystrophy is at any time after the first decade, though cloudy, gray, diffuse, ill defined lesions in the deep stroma of the central cornea occur early in life. It is bilateral symmetrical and non progressive dystrophy which does not affect the vision.

POSTERIOR STROMAL DYSTROPHY

Pre-Descemet's Dystrophy

This autosomal dominant dystrophy has poor penetrance. It appears late after fourth decade and is *asymptomatic*. Some consider it to be age-related degeneration. The opacities are in the pre-Descemet's membrane region, central, annular or diffuse and bilateral. Four clinical presentations are recognized.

1. The above type
2. The polymorphic stromal dystrophy
3. Associated with icthyosis or pseudoxanthoma elasticum,
4. Cornea farinata described previously

PAN- STROMAL DYSTROPHIES

Fleck Dystrophy (Speckled Dystrophy)

This autosomal dominant inherited dystrophy presents in the first decade or may be congenital. It may also occurs in association with keratoconus, limbal dermoid, central cloudy dystrophy or pseudoxanthoma elasticum. The pathogenesis of this dystrophy is not known. Characteristic small, gray-white, dandruff-like discrete specks are found in the stroma which are not progressive. The vision is not affected and no treatment is required.

Congenital Hereditary Stromal Dystrophy (CHSD)

This bilateral symmetrical, non-progressive, autosomal dominant dystrophy presents at birth with central corneal clouding caused by feathery and diffuse opacities, located in the anterior stroma which fade towards the periphery. The affected stroma consists of alternating layers of uniformly aligned and haphazardly placed collagen fibrils.

Visual impairment may leads to nystagmus and strabismus. Penetrating keratoplasty is to be done early to restore vision and prevent development of nystagmus and squint.

ENDOTHELIAL DYSTROPHIES

Cornea Guttata

It is a condition in which *excrescences* or **endothelial warts** appear on the inner surface of the Descemet's membrane which give the cornea a bronzed powdered appearance due to a golden hue on diffuse illumination. When viewed by retroillumination, the endothelial surface looks like beaten-metal with dispersed pigment on it. The excrescences appear as dark **guttate spots** on specular reflection.

Primary Cornea Guttata

It is *asymptomatic*, bilateral, symmetrical dystrophy which occurs between 20 to 30 years of age. The inheritance pattern is not clear. It is sometimes autosomal dominant. It, unlike Fuchs' dystrophy, remains stationary and the endothelial count, function and corneal thickness are within normal limit. Cornea farinata, a central degeneration, appears similar but occurs in old age while 'Hassal-Henle bodies' is a peripheral degeneration. The depth of the anterior chamber is normal. Posterior polar cataract has been reported in some familial cases. No treatment is required for this primary dystrophy.

Secondary Cornea Guttata

This condition may be seen in association with inflammations, corneal trauma, keratoconus and corneal degenerations.

Fuchs' Dystrophy (Epithelial-Endothelial Dystrophy)

Fuchs' endothelial dystrophy is sometimes inherited as autosomal dominant trait, is bilateral but asymmetrical disease, occurs in older individuals and is the most common endothelial dystrophy. It is 3–4 times more common in women and is more severe in them. An association with axial hypermetropia, shallow anterior chamber and angle-closure glaucoma has been reported in some patients.

Presentation

The disease presents in three phases affecting the central cornea of an elderly patient.

First Phase This phase may start early in young age, much before the second phase. There are no symptoms but the *abnormal endothelial cells* produce *new collagen* tissue which gives the Descemet's membrane a thickened and opaque appearance and also leads to the formation of *excrescences* (guttae) seen *as cornea guttata*. These excrescences may protrude into the anterior chamber, may be multilayered or may be buried within the new multilamellar collagen layer. Sometimes no guttae are seen. Dispersed pigment may also appears on the endothelial surface.

Second Phase Presents with hazy vision, worst on awakening, and glare, as the corneal edema develops due to gradual *failure of the endothelial pump* function. *Specular microscopy* shows large endothelial cells and loss of their hexagonal shape in addition to the guttae.
Progression of the edema involves the whole stromal thickness and the epithelium leading to first intracellular, then intercellular edema and eventually to painful bullous keratopathy when the stromal thickness exceeds 30%.

Third Phase The cornea becomes opaque and vascularized due to fibrosis in the stroma and subepithelial region prevents rupture of the bullae and loss of sensations. Vision is affected significantly, though the painful phase is gone. The intraocular pressure may be raised.

Treatment

Hypertonic Agents Hypertonic agents such as 5 % NaCl solution, are given to treat early cases of edema. Warm air applied to the cornea from distance with a hair-dryer particularly in the morning, when the edema and symptoms are worst, is also helpful.

Bandage Soft Contact Lens It is applied, along with the hypertonic agents, for painful bullous keratopathy for preventing rupture of the bullae. The intraocular pressure which further compromises the endothelial function should be lowered.

Penetrating Keratoplasty It is often needed to restore the severely affected vision. The graft should be larger than normal to provide more healthy endothelial cells as well as to prevent shallow anterior chamber and peripheral anterior synechia.

CHED: Congenital Hereditary Endothelial Dystrophy (Laurence)

This endothelial dystrophy is due to defective formation or degeneration of the endothelium *in utero*. The endothelium is absent or atrophic.

The posterior, non-banded layer of the Descemet's membrane, which is formed by the endothelium during the fifth month of gestation, is abnormal but guttate changes are not seen. The intraocular pressure and corneal size are normal which differentiate it from congenital glaucoma. Corneal changes similar to those of posterior polymorphous dystrophy may be seen in the asymptomatic relatives of the patient.

Congenital hereditary endothelial dystrophy is inherited in *both autosomal recessive as well as dominant* manner with variable expression.

Autosomal recessive

This type presents at birth as bilateral, cloudy or opaque cornea. In contrast to the 'congenital hereditary stromal dystrophy', the whole of the cornea up to the limbus is involved.

The corneal thickness is two to three times more than normal due to stromal edema. It is accompanied by nystagmus, occasionally associated with deafness and remains stationary.

Autosomal dominant

This type is less common, less severe and does not present at birth but during the first few years of life. It is a slowly progressive disorder and is not associated with nystagmus.

Treatment

Early penetrating keratoplasty is indicated in autosomal recessive type of this disorder to restore vision and amblyopia. The results of keratoplasty are highly variable.

Posterior Polymorphous Dystrophy (Koppe)

This rare, bilateral, dystrophy is present at birth or develops during the early life. The inheritance autosomal dominant or occasionally autosomal recessive. It also has been reported sometimes with Alport's syndrome.

Appearance

The posterior surface of the cornea gives *peau d'orange* appearance due to the presence of clusters of small vesicle like lesions, geographical areas of opacification and broad, sinuous bands.

Other abnormalities associated with this dystrophy are peripheral iridocorneal adhesions, anterior chamber cleavage syndrome, raised IOP, abnormal iris processes, corectopia, cornea guttata and posterior keratoconus.

Pathogenesis

The corneal changes are due to *mesenchymal dysgenesis* with presence of multilayered epithelium like cells on the posterior corneal surface and enlarged endothelial cells.

Presentation

Presentation may be with secondary glaucoma due to peripheral anterior synechia or with corneal edema due to the corneal abnormalities; associated with the above iris changes.

The *iridocorneal endothelial syndrome* appears similar but is not inherited, is unilateral, manifests at about 30-50 years of age and is seen more often in women.

Treatment

Many cases are asymptomatic and most have normal vision. Edema is treated medically, if present. Secondary glaucoma is managed medically/surgically. Penetrating keratoplasty is required for severe cases where opacity affects the vision. Results are better in the absence of the associated abnormalities.

Recurrent Corneal Erosion Syndrome (RCES)

Recurrent corneal erosion syndrome is a chronic relapsing disorder of epithelial instability.

Presentation

It presents as recurrent episodes of ocular pain, photophobia, lacrimation and blurring of vision characteristically on waking up. These symptoms decrease or subside over a few hours in mild cases but may persist and remain troublesome in severe chronic cases. Both eyes are affected in the case of dystrophies but those secondary to other causes, the erosions are unilateral.

Appearance

An eroded or loosely attached epithelium shows multiple, small corneal erosions which stain with fluorescein during the acute episode. In addition, slit-lamp examination would show the findings of primary dystrophy in both eyes.

Pathogenesis

Poor adhesions between the epithelium and the Bowman's layer are responsible for the recurrent erosions. All cases, irrespective of the etiology, show abnormality of the basement membrane and poor or absent adhesion complexes and hemidesmosomes. The causes are as follows.

Corneal Trauma Superficial *minor trauma* (scratch or minor surgical trauma, e.g. too vigorous epithelial debridement causing basement membrane abnormality) is the most common cause of recurrent corneal erosions. The presentation is unilateral and the abnormality does not involve the entire cornea (Colour Plate 3, Photograph 13 and 15).

Corneal Dystrophies The anterior dystrophies may be associated with the adhesion abnormality. Epithelial basement membrane dystrophy (EBMD/microcystic/Cogan's/map-dot fingerprint) is the commonest dystrophy associated with recurrent erosions. Other dystrophies, as described already, also may be associated with the erosions.

Superficial Minor Infection This may induce the same abnormality.

Spontaneous Cases Cases of recurrent corneal erosion have been reported to occur spontaneously.

Treatment

1. **Acute stage**
   a. *Pressure patching*
      In mild cases, pressure patch along with a cycloplegic and an antibiotic for 24 hours, gives relief from symptoms.
   b. *Epithelial debridement*
      To provide a smooth basement membrane for re-epithelization with a healthy epithelium, the devita- lized, loose epithelium is removed gently with a cellulose sponge and pressure patching is then done.

2. **Prevention**
   a. Lubricating agents such as artificial tear drops given at night time may help in preventing further episodes in mild cases.
   b. Bandage soft contact lenses (BSCL) may be effective in cases of severe recurrence. Bandage contact lens are to be used at least for 6 weeks or sometimes have to be continued for few months to allow time for formation of effective adhesion complexes.
   c. One study has shown effectiveness of oral tetracycline in prevention of recurrent erosions in cases associated with meibomian gland dysfunction.
   d. Anterior stromal puncture performed with a needle or with Nd: YAG laser may be an alternative for recalcitrant recurrent erosion cases. This form of treatment induces firm epithelial adhesions through the formation of microscars. On axis treatment is avoided.
   e. Newer microsurgical procedures
      i. *Diamond burr polishing of Bowman's membrane* is performed under the microscope.
      ii. *Peeling-off the hypertrophied basement membrane*
      These newer microsurgical procedures are performed under the operating microscope in recalcitrant cases under local anesthesia.

Table 9.3 shows the different conventional treatment methods for superficial corneal disorders.

Table 9.3: Available modes of treatment for superficial corneal disorders

Recurrent Erosions
1. Pressure patching
2. Epithelial debridement
3. BSCL
4. Lubricating agents
5. Anterior stromal puncture with needle or Nd:YAG laser
6. Newer micro-surgical procedures:
   a. Diamond burr polishing of Bowman's membrane
   b. Peeling-off the hypertrophied basement membrane

Degenerations and Dystrophies
1. Superficial keratectomy
2. Keratoplasty: lamellar, penetrating

Band keratopathy
Chelating agents: EDTA, sodium versanate

Corneal Scars
1. RGP contact lenses
2. Keratoplasty

DRAWBACKS OF PRESENT TREATMENT MODALITIES

Most of the surgical or non-surgical procedure utilized to treat the anterior corneal pathologies and the surgeries used for altering the corneal surface to bring a change in its refractive status are met with variable degree of scarring and surface irregularities.

These complications occur despite the *preciseness, skill* and *accuracy* utilized during the existing conventional procedures. The extent of corneal scarring depends on these variables as well on the amount of corneal tissue manipulation. *The end result is suboptimal corneal clarity and poor visual acuity because the altered cornea does not achieve the ideal optical properties.*

The corneal scarring and irregular surface were thought to result from the violation of Bowman's layer. Preservation of the Bowman's layer was considered to be indispensable for preservation of corneal clarity and uniform topography. This concept has been totally changed after the introduction of excimer laser corneal surgeries (vide supra).

The problems faced with the conventional modalities of management for different corneal disorders are innumerated in the following section.

Recurrent Corneal Erosions

1. Recurrent corneal erosions are not prevented in many cases despite prolonged use of conservative modes of treatment.
2. Use bandage contact lens for long period is associated with risk of infectious keratitis and corneal vascularization.
3. Anterior stromal puncture requires large number of punctures, multiple treatment sessions and carries the risk of perforation as well scars. This form of treatment is not appropriate for treatment in the optical zone.
4. The newer micro-surgeries are promising but are intensive and highly skilled procedures. These are again not free from the surgical risks and sub-epithelial corneal scarring.

Band Keratopathy

1. The efforts to remove the *calcific bands* are not always successful.
2. Calcium deposits may be resistant to removal with chelating agents and may require frequent use of the chelating agents.
3. Moreover, the surgical and chemical trauma leaves behind opaque and irregular corneal surface. Manual keratectomy is met with the same results.

Superficial Keratectomy

Superficial manual keratectomy, done in case of elevated lesions is associated with the following.

1. Rough and uneven corneal topography, not up to *optical standards.*
2. Damage to the underlying stroma resulting in some amount of scarring due to healing response.
3. Decreased corneal clarity.
4. Compromised visual function.

Penetrating and Lamellar Keratoplasty

1. Are more aggressive and *invasive surgeries.*
2. High rate of associated operative complications.
3. Scarcity of donor cornea in our subcontinent.
4. Longer rehabilitation time taken after these surgeries.
5. High incidence of graft failure.
6. Variable visual outcome due to high and irregular astigmatism and variable graft clarity.
7. Recurrence of dystrophy needs repeat surgery.

Suggested readings

1. Smolin Gilbert: In "The Cornea": Scientific foundation and clinical practice. Third edition, 1994, edi. Little Brown and company USA.
2. Severin, Krishhof B: Recurrent Salzmann's Corneal degeneration. Graefes Arch Cli Exp Ophthalmology 1990; 101: 228.
3. Freedman A: Climatic droplet keratopathy. Arch Ophthalmol 1973; 89: 193.
4. Grant WN: New treatment of calcific corneal opacities. Arch Ophthalmol 1952; 48: 681-685.
5. Brenin GM, DeVoe AG: Chelation of calcium with edathamil calcium di-sodium in band keratopathy and corneal calcium affections. Arch Ophthalmol 1954; 52: 846-851.
6. Wood TO, Walter CG: Treatment of band keratopathy. Am J Ophthalmol 1975; 80: 553.
7. Bokasky JE, Meyu RF, Suger : Surgical treatment of calcific band keratopathy. Ophthalmic Surgery 1985; 16: 645-647.
8. Freedman A: Climatic droplet keratopathy. Arch Ophthalmol 1973; 89: 193.
10. Smolin Gilbert: In 'The Cornea': Scientific foundation and clinical practice: Third Edition, 1994; (editorials) Little Brown and company USA.
11. Buxton JN, Buxton DF, Westphalen JA: Penetrating Keratoplasty: Indications and contra indications: in "Corneal Surgery: Theory, Techniques and Tissue; 2nd edition, 1984: (editorials) Brightbill FS: Mosby Publications.
12. Bokasky JE, Meyu RF, Suger A: Surgical treatment of calcific band keratopathy. Ophthalmic Surgery 1985; 16: 645-647.

13. Hykin DG, Foss AE, Pavesio C, Daor JKG: The natural history and management of recurrent corneal erosions: A prospective randomized trial. Eye 1994; 8: 35-40.
14. Hop-Ross MW, Chell PB, McDonnell ES et al: Recurrent corneal erosions: Clinical features. Eye 1994; 8: 373-377.
15. Foulks GN: Treatment of recurrent corneal erosions and corneal edema with topical osmotic colloidal solutions. Ophthalmology 1981; 88: 801-803.
16. Foulks GN: Treatment of recurrent corneal erosions and corneal edema with topical osmotic colloidal solutions. Ophthalmology 1981; 88: 801-803.
17. Mobilia EF, Foster CS: The management of recurrent corneal erosions with ultra thin lasers. Contact Intra ocular Lens Med J 1978; 4: 25-29.
18. McLean EN, McRae SM, Rich LF: Recurrent corneal erosions: Treatment by anterior stromal puncture. Ophthalmology 1986; 93: 784-787.
19. Geggel HS: Successful treatment of recurrent corneal erosions with Nd: YAG anterior stromal puncture. Am J Ophthalmol 1990; 110: 404-407.
20. Vegh M: Simplified microsurgical method of therapy for recurrent corneal erosions. German J Ophthalmol 1992; 1: 135-138 .
21. Freedman A: Climatic droplet keratopathy. Arch Ophthalmol 1973; 89: 193.
22. Rene Din, Christopher J, Rapuano CJ et al: Recurrence of corneal dystrophies after phototherapeutic keratectomy. Ophthalmology 1999; 106 (8): 1490-1497.

Section IV

Refractive Surgical Procedures

Chapter 10

Refractive Surgical Procedures

Although the problem of ammetropia might have existed with man since ever his evolution, serious efforts to achieve emmetropic state of the eye, by methods other than lenses, have been made only during the later half of the previous century. A number of factors including optical aberrations and other problems faced; temporary nature, cosmetic reasons etc. with spectacle use and the recurring cost, handling problems and complications arising from contact lens wear have led to the continued interest in invention, development and refinement of newer methods of refractive correction. Many methods for correcting refractive errors have been invented during the past few decades.

EMMETROPIA

The refractive apparatus of the eye consists of different optical components. These components are mainly cornea and the crystalline lens, though the refractive indexes of the aqueous and the vitreous humour also play some part.

In a normal eye, the *refractive powers of these various components* are in such a co-ordination or *harmony* that they bring about the bundle of parallel rays to a *sharp focus* on the retina, with *minimum circle of confusion,* so as to form an image with maximum clarity. This ideal condition of refractive state occurring in a normal eye at rest (without any accommodation) is termed emmetropia.

AMMETROPIA

Ammetropia is a pathological state of refraction of eye. Any deviation from the above mentioned ideal situation leads to ammetropia, in which the parallel rays of light are not brought to a sharp focus on the retina. The eye, then suffers from a refractive error.

The refractive errors may be one of the three types:

1. Myopia
2. Hypermetropia
3. Astigmatism

These abnormal states of refraction can result from certain pathological changes or deviation away from the above coordination, in any of the optical components of the eye. The following types of altered refractive states are recognized, based on *variations* in the *optical components* of *refractive apparatus* of a normal human eye.

1. **Axial refractive errors**
   The axial error occurs mainly due to variation in the axial length of the eye and less commonly due to forward or backward displacement of the lens.

2. **Curvature refractive errrors**
   The refractive error due to curvature variations occurs mainly because of deviation in the corneal curvature and less commonly because of deviation in the lens curvature.

3. Index refractive errors

This errors occurs due to change in the refractive index of the crystalline lens. While nuclear sclerosis causes a myopic shift, increase in the refractive index of the cortex in old age leads to hyperopic shift.

4. Absence the crystalline lens

This state of refractive error is called aphakia, which is either due to surgical removal or due to dislocation of the crystalline lens out of the visual axis.

5. Obliquity of the refractive components

Refractve errors also result from certain not so common, peculiar states of the refractive apparatus. For example a subluxated lens or an obliquely placed retina in case of posterior staphyloma would lead to an error of refraction.

Deviations in the corneal curvature and the axial length of the eye are the most commonly encountered causes observed for the refractive errors. Since the axial length of the eye cannot be manipulated and the cornea is easily accessible to the surgeon, the latter is exploited in particular to bring about the state of emmetropia by manipulating it in different ways.

Table 10.1a enlists various refractive surgical procedures that have been used by different surgeons or are being developed for correction of refractive errors.

Table 10.1a: Various procedures employed for achieving permanent refractive correction

I. CORNEAL SURGICAL PROCEDURES

A. THERMOKERATOPLASTY
  i. With heated probes and microwave heating
  ii. Laser thermokeratoplasty

B. LAMELLAR PROCEDURES
  1. Keratomileusis
     i. On corneal surface
     ii. On the under surface of a corneal flap
  2. Automated Lamellar Keratoplasty: ALK
  3. Keratophakia

C. INLAYS
  1. **Intrastromal Ring Segment** (PMMA): **ICRS**
  2. **Intracorneal Lenses** (hydrogel, polysulfone)

D. ONLAYS
  Epikeratophakia
  a. With donor lenticules
  b. With synthetic lenticules

E. INCISIONAL PROCEDURES
  1. **Radial Keratotomy: RK**
     i. Conventional
        a. The Russian or 'uphill method'
        b. The American or 'downhill method'
        c. The combined technique or the 'genesis method'
     ii. Minimum invasive or Mini-RK
  2. **Astigmatic Keratotomy**
     i. Transverse
     ii. Arcuvate transverse

  3. **Combined Radial and Astigmatic Keratotomies**
     i. Transverse incisions between radial incisions
     ii. Transverse incisions between semi-radial incisions (*Trapezoidal incisions*)
     iii. *Jump-T* or *flag incisions*: interrupted transverse incisions
     iv. *Jump Radial* incisions : interrupted radial incisions

  4. **Post-Keratoplasty Astigmatic Procedures**
     i. **Relaxing incisions** in the steep meridian
     ii. **Wedge-resection** in the flat meridian
     iii. **Relaxing incisions** in the steep meridian with **augmentation sutures** in the flat meridian
  5. **Hexagonal Keratotomy for Hyperopia**

F. EXCIMER AND OTHER LASER PROCEDURES
  1. Photorefractive keratectomy: PRK
  2. Photorefractive keratectomy for astigmatism: PARK
  3. Laser assisteds in-situ keratomileusis: LASIK
  4. Intrastromal refractive keratectomy: ISPRK with picosecond photo-disruptors
  5. Wavefront–guided or customized LASIK
  6. Laser thermokeratoplasty
  7. Excimer laser intrastromal keratomileusis: ELISK

II. INTRAOCULAR SURGICAL PROCEDURES

A. PHAKIC INTRAOCULAR LENSES
  1. **Anterior Chamber Lenses**
     a. Baikoff angle supported lenses
     b. Worst-Iris-Claw lenses
  2. **Intraocular Contact Lenses** between the iris and the anterior lens surface
     a. Collamer foldable hydrogel lenses
     b. Silicon lenses

B. CLEAR LENS EXTRACTION
  with or without intraocular lens

FACTORS THAT DECIDE THE FUTURE OF A REFRACTIVE SURGERY

Although many surgical procedures for correcting the refractive disorders have been developed, extensively used and refined during the later half of the twentieth century, not all of them have stood the test of time. These are continually being replaced by newer ones to achieve maximum *accuracy, precision, predictability, efficacy, safety, long-term stability of the results and optical clarity*. Though, clinically the above factors are the key determents for the success of the procedure, *patient's perception and acceptability, cost the surgery and surgeons familiarity and experience* with the procedure are other considerations that decide the future of a particular refractive surgical procedure.

Majority of refractive surgeries, whether mechanical or laser procedures, *revolve around changing of the corneal curvature.*

The concept behind all surgeries utlizing the corneal curvature as the main interventional area to alter the refractive state of the human eye is the fact that *cornea is the most powerful refracting component of the optical system* of an average eye.

Since the refractive index of the cornea is a constant factor, it is the anterior corneal curvature, which is main determinant of the refraction taking place due to this structure. In fact the contribution of the corneal curvature in the refractive power of a human eye is almost 70% of the the total diopteric power of the eye. Therefore any small change in its curvature would lead to substantial alteration in refraction of eye.

THERMOKERATOPLASTY

Thermokeratoplasty is a procedure that induces change in the corneal curvature by causing shrinkage of stromal collagen through heating of cornea. Collagen shrinkage causes flattening of cornea at the site of application. Historically a number of devices like *heated corneal probes, microwave heating,* insertion of *electrically heated wire*, etc. were used by different investigators.

Kaufman and others scientists used this procedure to flatten the cones in cases of keratoconus. But the resultant necrosis and thermal damage restricted its use for application to the central cornea for myopic correction.

The Thermomechanical Behaviour of Cornea

A crucial factor for understanding and *controlling the curvature change* of cornea through thermal shrinkage of its collagen fibers is '*the response of this tissue as a function of the induced temperature rise*'.

Laboratory experiments have shown that collagen shrinkage starts at 60° C, increases up to 90° C and then decreases after 100° C. This is because above this temperature the intermolecular bonds of collagen starts breaking[19]. Moreover destruction of the tissue begins above this temperature. The *maximum shrinkage rate*, 57 ± 12%, is found to occur between 75° C–80° C. Another study found maximum shrinkage force at 75° C and more refractive change after 60 seconds of irradiation with diode laser[16].

These *biomechanical properties* of corneal stromal collagen are crucial in *designing any laser system* for LTK, for developing a treatment *nomogram* for the refractive correction as well as for avoiding the tissue damage.

RADIAL THERMOKERATOPLASTY (TKP)

If the heating applications are made to the corneal periphery, the flattening effect of thermokeratoplasty would lead to steepening of the central corneal curvature *without causing any loss to clarity of optical zone.*

This fact was exploited by Fyodorov to treat hyperopia. In a study conducted on 117 eyes[1], he used electrically heated nichrome wire probes, deeply inserted into the stroma and applied in a *radial pattern* similar to the radial keratotomy incisions. He called it 'Radial Thermokeratoplasty' (Fig. 10.1). The temperature rise at the site of such applications is of the order of 600° C.

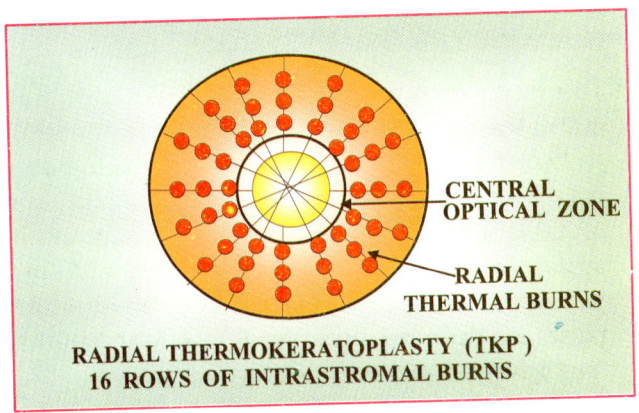

Fig. 10.1: Diagrammatic representation of radial thermokeratoplasty (TKP)

Results

Fyodorov obtained reduction in hyperopia by a mean of –3.84 D and post-operative visual acuity 6/12 using his method of radial thermokeratoplasty.

Drawbacks

1. Unpredictability of results
2. Instability of refraction on long follow up
3. Marked regression of effect[3]
4. Necrosis and scarring at the application site
5. Endothelial damage due to conductive effect of the very high temperature

Present Status of Radial Thermokeratoplasty

This procedure is no more in use.

LASER THERMOKERATOPLASTY: LTK

The lasers can also produce collagen shrinkage. This effect of lasers on cornea is called *photothermal tissue shrinkage*. It has been utilized for treating hyperopia and astigmatism by the procedure termed as *'laser thermal keratoplasty' (LTK)*.

Fyodorov used CO_2 laser thermokeratoplasty to correct hyperopia and opened the way for other lasers for similar application.

The cobalt-magnesium-fluoride, holmium: YAG (Ho: YAG) and the diode lasers cause the same effect. They can be used in a more controlled manner using the convenient fiber-probe or slit-lamp delivery systems[4-22].

Only the later two lasers have been used clinically in many studies during the last decade. The *continuous-wave infrared diode laser* is the most recent tool in the field of laser thermokeratoplasty[12-16].

Holmium: YAG (Ho: YAG) Laser

The Fiber Hand-piece Delivery System Seiler et al did the pioneering work in laser thermokeratoplasty.

Pulsed holmium: YAG laser at 2100 nm, with the pulse duration of 200 micriseconds and irradiance energy of 25–35 mJ was used by him. The technique involves application of 8 laser spots placed *concentrically* in the paracentral area with a fiber hand-piece. About 5–25 pulses are delivered at each spot. The temperature rise thus achieved is about 60° C.

The curvature change through this treatment was found to be inversely proportional to the distance of the applied laser spots from the corneal center.

The Non-Contact Slit-Lamp Delivery This mode of delivery was developed in 1994 and later used for phase IIa trial of FDA[13].

Two techniques were used for holmium YAG: laser thermokeratoplasty with the slit-lamp delivery system (Figs 10.2 and 10.3).

1. The single-ring technique
2. The two-ring technique

Subsequently many other clinical studies have been done on Ho: YAG thermokeratoplasty for low hypermetropia and cases of excimer laser overcorrections in myopia.

Advantage of Laser Thermokeratoplasty

It causes focal corneal shrinkage without the associated tissue necrosis, unlike that caused by CO_2 laser and radial TKP.

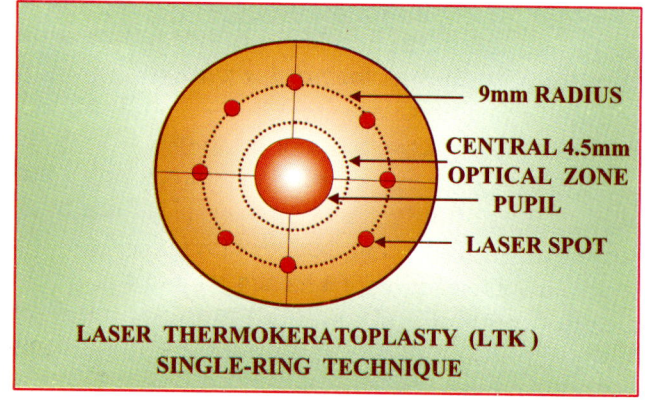

Fig. 10.2: Diagrammatic representation of the 'single-ring technique' of LTK

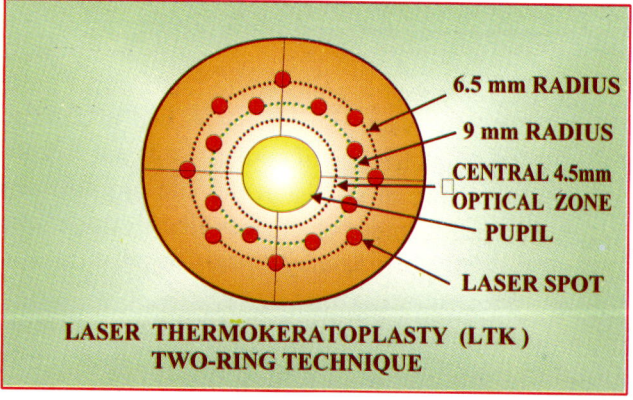

Fig. 10.3: Diagrammatic representation of the 'two-ring technique' of LTK

Drawbacks of Laser Thermokeratoplasty

1. Low predictability of the refractive outcome within a range of ±1.0 D of the desired correction.
2. Induced irregular astigmatism
3. Regression of the effect

Regression of the Refractive Effect

The regression of effect is the most disturbing problem of holmium: YAG LTK. Refraction may not stabilize for years.

1. The *regression* of refractive effect is found to be significantly *less with the two-ring technique* as compared to the one–ring technique.
2. It is found to be more in younger patients. This might be due to the higher water content of their cornea affecting the shrinkage effect on the stromal collagen.

Present Status of Holmium: YAG LTK

Its role is limited to the following conditions.

1. Low hypermetopes, particularly in the presbyopic age group.
2. Small group of overcorrected myopic patients after PRK procedure.

This is so because it has been observed that removal of the Bowman's layer by excimer laser improve the efficacy and stability of LTK. Nonetheless, this technique presently has no role in the treatment of myopia, myopic astigmatism and high hyperopia.

Diode Laser Thermokeratoplasty: DTK

Brinkmann and Greeling introduced diode laser thermokeratoplasty in 1998 using the continuous mode delivery at 1854 nm to 1870 nm wavelength, applied with a contact fiber-probe. The single-ring (8 spots) as well as double-ring (16 spots) techniques were used by them. The power used was 100–150 mW for 10 seconds[15].

Initial result on blind human eyes are as follows.

1. Maximum refractive change achieved with single-ring application was +4.9 D and +6.8 D with double-ring.
2. Refractive change produced with two–rings was more stable.
3. Refractive change increased linearly with decreasing *ring diameter* from 10 to 5 mm.
4. All eyes showed some amount of regression, mainly during first 6 months.
5. Regression continued up to second year in eyes with higher correction.
6. Eyes irradiated with 1854 nm wavelength showed *extensive endothelial damage*. Endothelial damage was limited with 1870 nm.
7. Refractive change up to +10 D could be achieved with 125–200 mW, but this energy would be more damaging to the endothelium.
8. Increase in irradiation time from 10 to 60 seconds showed approximately logarithmical relation with the refractive change in laboratory study on porcine eyes, but it was associated with more destructive changes.

Present Status of Diode LTK (DTK)

Refractive results of the diode LTK are promising but are haunted by the regression problem as well as concern for damage to the corneal endothelium[12].

Rad et al, in 2002, used LASIK with DTK (**LASIK-DTK bioptics**) to treat hyperopia from +5.0 to +10.0 D, to take care of the regression that follows the hyperopic LASIK. They were successful in preventing the regression. No comment on endothelial changes was made in this study with 9–12 months of follow[22].

Nonetheless, large prospective series spread over long period are needed to standardize the laser parameters and nomograms and to report on the effectivity, predictability and safety of this technique. *The appropriate irradiation parameters must also avoid or minimize the endothelial insult.*

LTK FOR HYPEROPIC ASTIGMATISM

Holmium: YAG laser thermokeratoplasty can be used for correction of astigmatism[18].

Laser spots given 'on the sides' of the *flat* meridian would cause steepening of that meridian. This refractive change is dependent on the following two factors.

1. *The coagulation angle,* i.e. the distance between the spots on the sides of the meridian being treated. Coagulation spots closer than 22.5° or more than 45° away did not show significant change in the refraction.
2. *The optical zone diameter* (OZD): The change in astigmatic error was found to be inversely proportional to the OZD kept clear of the treatment spots.

LAMELLAR CORNEAL SURGERIES

The following account deals with keratomileusis, keratophakia, epikeratophakia and automated lamellar keratoplasty, which are modified lamellar corneal surgeries to suit the refractive correction.

MECHANICAL KERATOMILEUSIS

Keratomileusis is a procedure by which the corneal power is altered by modifying its curvature using various *mechanical tools or lasers*. It literally means 'carving the cornea'. *Barraquer* did extensive work in this field and it is the result of those painstaking efforts by him over a period of 30 years that the concept of *excimer laser in-situ keratomileusis* came into being and later converted to reality by *Pallikaris*.

Surface Keratomileusis

Tissue can be removed from the corneal surface by a method similar to grinding. In this experimental study by Barraquer, all the animal eyes developed severe corneal scarring. Hence the procedure was abandoned.

Keratomileusis on the Undersurface of a Corneal Flap

This method involves the following steps:
1. Removing a cornel disc of uniform thickness with a microkeratome and freezing it.
2. Removing tissue from its undersurface by a special cryolathe (similar to the one used for making contact lenses) to shape a lenticules of desired power.
3. Re-suturing the lenticules back on to the patient's corneal bed (Figs 10.4 and 10.5).

Indications

Mechanical keratomileusis was indicated in cases of *very high* myopia, hyperopia and aphakia, in those who were intolerant to contact lenses or faced problems with spectacle correction. *The aim was to decrease the amount of refractive correction that these individuals needed.*

Exclusion Criteria

Patients with too flat or too steep corneas (< 39 D, > 52 D) are excluded because of problems with microkeratome sectioning and making a good tissue disk.

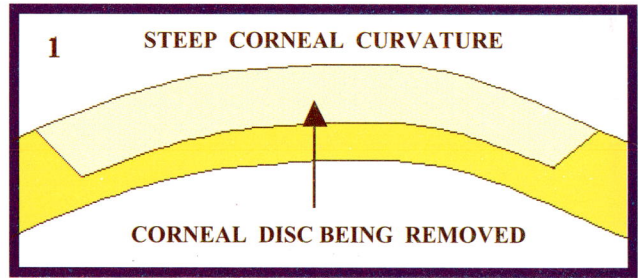
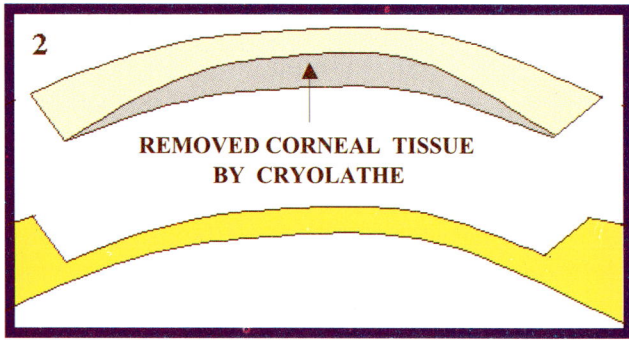
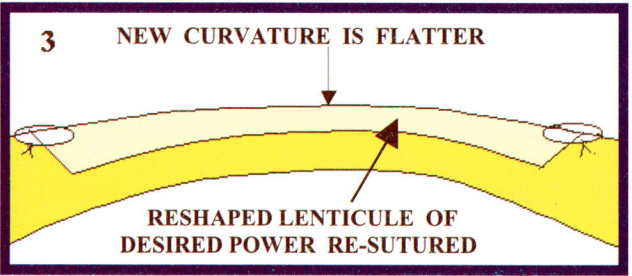

Fig. 10.4: Diagrammatic representation of myopic keratomileusis

Ocular surface problems, dry eye, glaucoma, small palpabral aperture and adenexal infections are also contraindications.

Drawbacks

1. *This is a highly complex surgery,* involving meticulous lathing and fashioning the corneal lenticules.
2. Microkeratome related problems, e.g. damage to the disk while lathing, even in inexperienced hands.
3. Decreased best corrected visual acuity due to loss of optical clarity because of:
   a. Interface scarring,
   b. Irregular astigmatism and
   c. Epithelial ingrowth.

SYNTHETIC IMPLANTS (INLAYS)

It was Barraquer, who conceived the idea of placing an intracorneal *flint glass* lens. Since then many types of intracorneal lenses have been studied experimentally and *some (hydrogel lenses) are undergoing clinical trials under FDA for correction of aphakia and myopia.*

When one is considering to implant any synthetic material inside the stroma, several important considerations are to be taken into account. These are:

The Long-term Biocompatibility of the lens material to the eye stroma.

Chemical Purity to avoid any toxicity to the corneal tissue.

Effect on Corneal Nutrition/Permeability to nutrients The supply of glucose and other nutrients to the epithelium and anterior stroma is from the aqueous. An implant that is impermeable to the nutrients would have damaging effects. An impermeable lens has to be smaller than 5 mm if it were to be physiologically non interfering.

Lens parameters and other characteristics

1. **Lens size:** A larger lens is more prone for extrusion and would be an obstacle for diffusion to nutrients while lens smaller than 5 mm would cause optical problems like monocular diplopia and glare.
2. **Lens Edge:** A lens with thinner edge is more likely to erode through the stroma while the one with a thick edge may create a gap in stroma.
3. **Lens Fenestrations:** The fenestrations made in the lens would make an otherwise impermeable lens permeable to the nutrients.
4. **Refractive Index:** A high refractive index, such as 1.633 for polysulfone lenses, would be beneficial for refractive correction over a wide range of refractive errors.
5. **Good optical quality**
6. **Imporosity to stromal tissue:** Keratocytes may migrate into the lens and cause opacity. Therefore, it must be imporous to stromal cells.
7. **Flexibility:** Inflexible lens may cause damage to the tissues, such the endothelium.

Lens position inside the stroma Deeper the implant inside the stroma, lesser is its effect on the anterior corneal curvature.

Based on the above consi... and lens designs are found t... of intracorneal implantatio...

1. Hydrogel intracornea...
2. Polysulfone intracorn...
3. Intrastromal corneal...

Hydrogel Intracorneal

These lenses have good lo... patibility), are permeable to... significant pathological... endothelium after 8 years of... except slight thinning of t... implant seen in most cases... reaction in the form of fibrob... extracellular material, docu... were attributed to chemica...

Polysulfone Non-Fenes...

The polysulfone intracorne... nutrients, hence are to be... (Fig. 10.7). Significant con... non-fenestrated polysulfo... ments using primate model... abandoned. These are:

1. Interface opacity in...
2. Anterior corneal ne...
3. Refractile particles...
4. Epithelial thinning...
5. Lens extrusion in 3...
6. Corneal vasculariza...

Polysulfone Fenestrate...

The problems of permea... cations has been taken ca... polysulfone lenses, which... to be free from the above c... lenses again are of two ty...

Earlier ones with 35 µ... These were optically uns... and hampered visualizatio... which implanted.

New Second Gener... lenses with 10 µ fenestrati... quality as well as all the saf... design. But the manufactu...

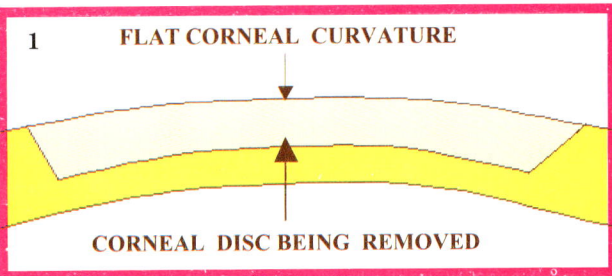

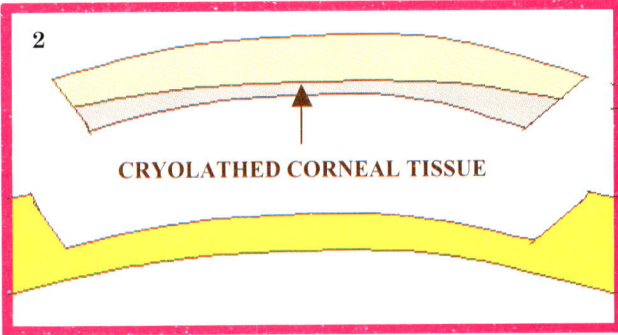

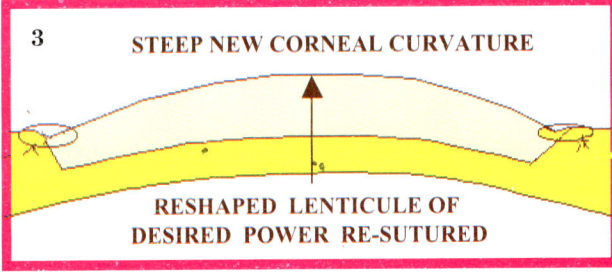

Fig. 10.5: Diagrammatic representation of hyperopic keratomileusis

4. Significant residual refractive error.
5. Prolonged recovery time,
6. Since the maximum and minimum keratometry which are found to be stable are 59 diopter and 37 D, it can correct up to 16 D of hyperopia and 10 D of myopia. This is so because in hyperopes, if average keratometry (K) reading is taken as 43 D, then it would change to 59 D. Similarly in mopes if average K is 47 D then it would flatten to 37 D after the surgery.

Present status of Mechanical Keratomileusis

This surgery is not being performed by many surgeons. It has been replaced by the much simpler 'epikeratophakia', if indicated.

AUTOMATED LAMELLAR KERATOPLASTY (ALK)

This technique involves *carving the curvature of the stromal bed* after removing *plano* superficial lenticule by using *automated, geared microkeratome*. This is in true sense, in-situ keratomileusis with mechanical means and is the forerunner of LASIK. In principle, this technique was introduced by Ruiz and Barraquer.

Indications

Automated lamellar keratoplasty has been used for correcting myopia ranging from –4.0 D to –16.0 D.

Results

Some studies have shown encouraging results using this technique.

Technical Problems

The procedure is highly complicated as it involves two keratectomies, which are machine dependent and hence are liable to be affected by mechanical failures malfunctioning.

1. There may be keratome failure due to loss of suction during activation.
2. The keratome might fail to complete full pass.
3. Decreased blade sharpness or warpage may lead to unpredictable results as well postoperative surprises.

Complications of ALK

The early studies have found significant complication rate, which include the following.

1. Significant under-corrections and over-corrections
2. Astigmatism, regular as well as irregular
3. Button-holing of the superficial plano lenticule
4. Decentration as well as loss of the lenticules
5. Interface particles
6. Corneal haze
7. Corneal ectasia
8. Anterior chamber perforation
9. Keratitis

Present status of ALK

Long–term studies and experience is needed for the automated lamellar procedure to have a role in future.

EPIKERATOPHAKIA (ONLAYS)

This method involves placement of a carved *donor corneal lenticule* of 8.5 mm or a *synthetic collagen lenticule*, on the surface of the cornea, after epithelial removal. It is sutured in place after making a peripheral, circular, 7.5 mm diameter and 0.2–0.3 mm deep groove with undermined edge, using a trephine and a spreader. This special cut is called **annular keratotomy**. This step prepares the site for the oversized lenticule to fit without buckling (Fig. 10.6).

Indications

The procedure is done in cases of adult and pediatric aphakia, myopia, keratoconus or other thinning of the cornea.

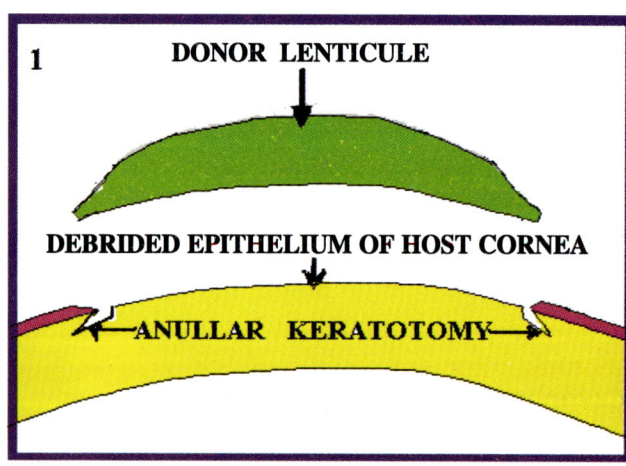

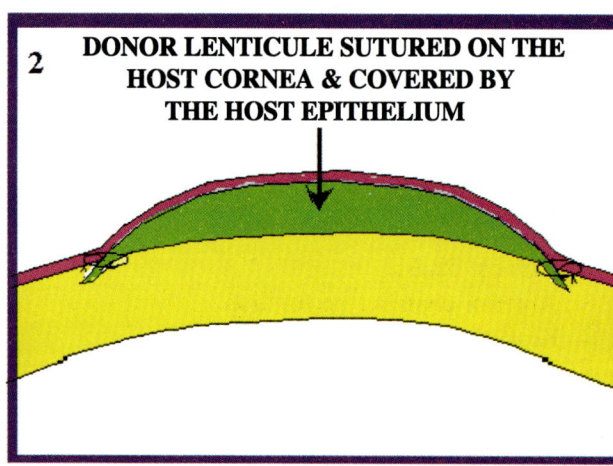

Fig. 10.6: Diagrammatic representation of epikeratophakia

Advantages

1. Simpler and widel
2. Can correct high d cularly aphakes, spectacle or conta IOL is not possibl
3. *Reversible* as well residua.
4. No risk of perforati cornea, unlike ker

Results

Improved uncorrected v epikeratophakia is indica

Drawbacks

1. In keratoconus, res keratoplasty in te rehabilitation peric
2. Results are poor in
3. Prolonged haze, poc infections, dehiscer

Present Status of Epik

Epikeratophakia is reserv

1. Patients with aphaki correction with lens
2. Patients with kerat central clear area, penetrating keratopl

KERATOPHAKIA

Keratophakia differs from that here the donor corneal within the stroma after rem cornea. The following ma tophakia.

Human Donor Cornec

These were used to correc from +10 D to +18 D. No

Synthetic Lenticules

These are discussed under

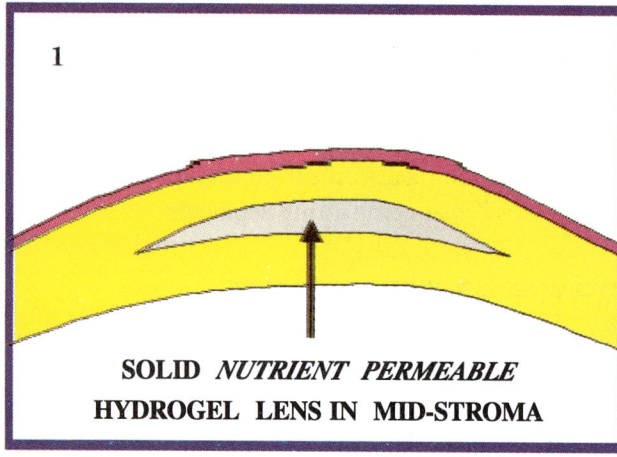

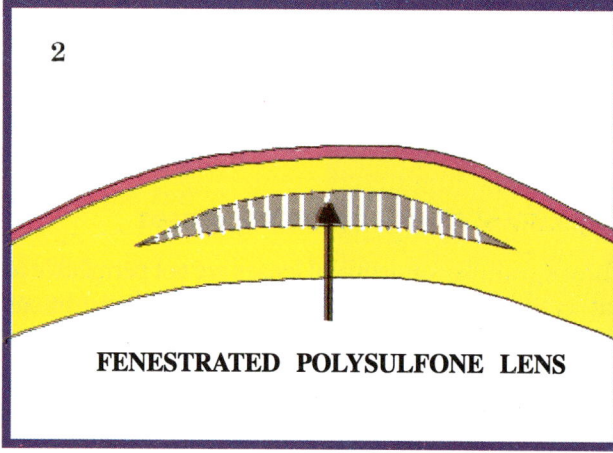

Fig. 10.7: Diagrammatic representation of synthetic keratophakia

INTRASTROMAL CORNEAL-RING SEGMENTS (INTACS)

They are also called intra-corneal ring segment (ICRS). They are specialized type of implants to treat low to moderate myopia and astigmatism. An INTAC consists of an optically transparent split-ring of PMMA (polymethylmethaacrylate). The split ring is inserted into the mid peripheral cornea at about 2/3 of its depth by making a tunnel with specialized corkscrew like dissector. New *microsurgical technique uses 1.2 mm* instead of 1.8 mm incision, *requiring no suture* (Fig. 10.8).

This device has undergone phase I and phase II trials and has *received the FDA approval in USA*.

Large number of clinical studies have agreed about the *safety, efficacy, predictability and stability* of ICRS/INTACS for mild (–1.0 to –3.5 D) myopia[47–56].

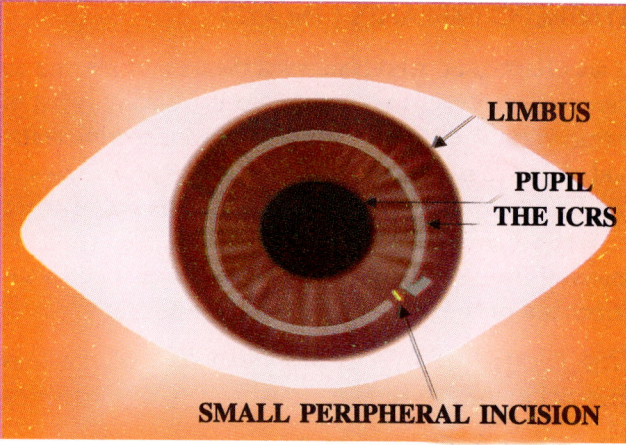

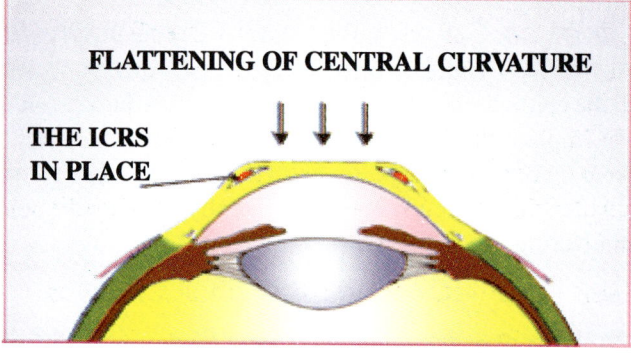

Fig. 10.8: Diagrammatic representation of ICRS in peripheral corneal stroma

Effect

When inserted into the above position, a 0.3 mm thick device leads to 2.7D of flattening of the central corneal curvature. An additional increase by each 0.27 mm in thickness causes 1.0 D flattening.

The *INTACS* are available in 6 insert thicknesses (0.21, 0.25, 0.3. 0.45, 0.4 and 0.45 mm). Phase II clinical trials have shown similar relationship using ICRS of 0.25–0.45mm thickness. Astigmatism may be tackled using modified ICR segments/INTACS.

Results

The European '**MECCA-trial**' presented clinical results in 1998 on 25 eyes after 12 months of follow up, as given below:

1. No case of visual loss, 60% eyes gained in BCVA.
2. Fifty six percent of the eyes gained one line in BCVA and 4% eyes gained two lines. In 40% eyes the best corrected visual acuity remained unchanged.

Corneal Changes

Some corneal changes occur, which are in the periphery and hence are *visually insignificant*. These are collagen/proteoglycans deposits on the ICRS and the tunnel and peripheral corneal haze.

Advantages

1. It is much cheaper than excimer laser procedures.
2. No intervention to the central optical zone, as compared to RK, PRK and LASIK.
3. Carries minimum risk as compared to the above keratorefractive surgeries.
4. One study reported better uncorrected visual acuity than LASIK after 1 month, which further improved over time.
5. Cases of corneal ectasia post-LASIK surgery can be effectively managed with this device.
6. Complete reversibility of the procedure.
7. LASIK can be safely done in case of removal.
8. The *INTACS* can be easily replaced, with improved refraction and uncorrected visual acuity.
9. Long-term results (up to 2 years) have found it to be safe, effective and predictable. No significant induced astigmatism or endothelial change have been seen.

Limitations of INTACS

1. Lengthy insertion technique taking up to an hour.
2. Application limited to myopia of only up to –4.0 D. This is because if higher correction is attempted then significant optical aberrations and visual impairment might occur.

INCISIONAL SURGERIES

Many types of incisional surgeries *used to be the mainstay* of refractive procedures before the advent of excimer lasers. *They are still preferred by some surgeons.* This could be because of one or more of the following reasons.

1. *Forced choice* due to high cost of excimer laser procedures.
2. More familiarity and experience with them.
3. Because of the special type of refractive problem faced in a particular case, which may be addressed to only by these procedures.

Table 10.1b gives an overview of the different incisional surgeries used.

Table 10.1b: Refractive incisional surgeries

Radial Keratotomy: RK
  1. Conventional
      a. The Russian or 'uphill method'
      b. The American or 'downhill method'
      c. The combined technique or the 'genesis method'
  2. Minimum invasive or Mini-RK

Astigmatic Keratotomy
  1. Transverse
  2. Arcuate transverse

Combined Radial and Astigmatic Keratotomies
  1. Transverse incisions between radial incisions
  2. Transverse incisions between semi-radial incisions (*trapezoidal incisions*)
  3. *Jump-T* or *flag incisions*: interrupted transverse incisions
  4. *Jump Radial* incisions: interrupted radial incisions

Post-Keratoplasty Astigmatic Procedures
  1. **Relaxing incisions** in the steep meridian
  2. **Wedge-resection** in the flat meridian
  3. **Relaxing incisions** in the steep meridian with **augmentation sutures** in the flat meridian

Hexagonal Keratotomy for Hyperopia

RADIAL KERATOTOMY (RK)

Radial keratotomy is an incisional surgery which is utilized to correct *myopia* by giving *radial, sub-total thickness* incisions into the cornea, avoiding the optical zone and extending to the limbus, thus leading to bulging of the weakened peripheral cornea by normal IOP.

This results in flattening of the central corneal curvature and therefore produces a hyperopic shift to correct myopia (Fig. 10. 9).

The idea of using incisions into the peripheral cornea originated with **Sato** in Japan, who used incisions given into the posterior surface of the cornea to induce corneal flattening effect, not being aware of the effect of endothelial damage, during those days (1930s). Most of the cses treated by Sato by this method developed corneal edema on long term follow up.

Yenaliev introduced and *Fyodorov* and coworkers popularized the modern technique of radial keratotomy using the anterior corneal surface in Russia.

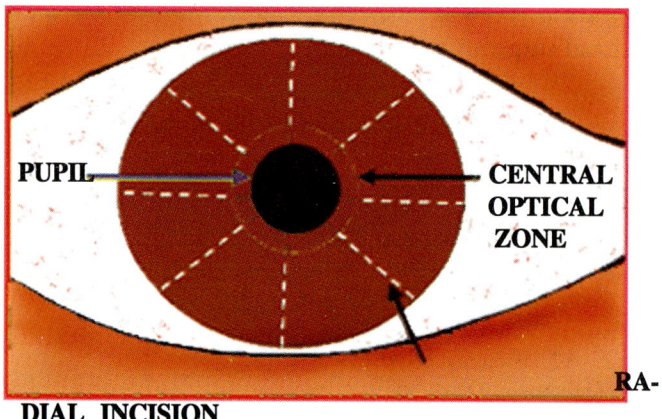

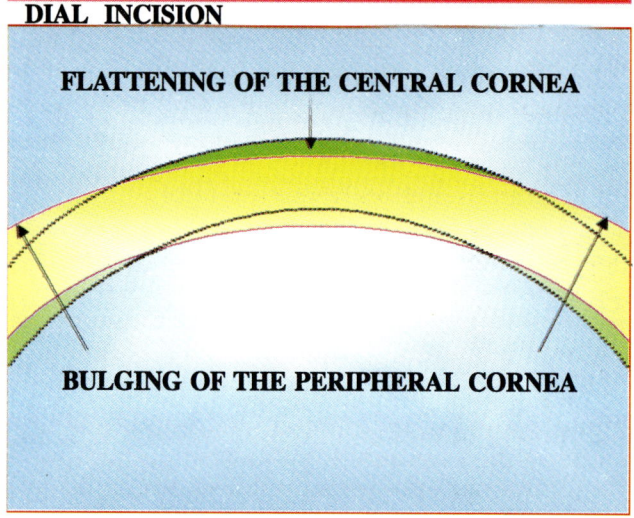

Fig. 10.9: Diagrammatic representation of surface and side-views to show the effect of radial keratotomy

FACTORS INFLUENCING THE OUTCOME AND PREDICTABILITY OF RK

These factors can be grouped under two major heads:

1. Surgical variables
2. Patient variables

Surgical Variables

1. Diameter of central clear zone
2. Incision numbers
3. Incision depth
4. The incision termination
5. Incision direction
6. Incision size

Diameter of the Optical Zone

The area of central cornea to be left uncut is of paramount importance for many reasons:

1. It is desirable to leave maximum area of central cornea, corresponding to different ambient light conditions, uncut and clear of any scarring that may occur as a result of the incisions.
2. It demands that this uncut optical zone be small if one is to achieve the maximum refractive change.
3. Smaller optical zones would have more risk of the associated 'edge effects' leading to various visual disturbances under different light conditions.

The PERK study group studied the effect of varying the diameter of the central uncut zone on refractive outcome, using this parameter as the only variable. It came out with the following results, summarized in Table 10.2.

Table 10.2: Effect of the central clear optical zone diameter on the refractive outcome

Baseline refraction (sphe. equivalent)	The central uncut zone diameter	Average 1 year refractive change
−2.00 to −3.20 D	4.0 mm zone	2.73 D
−3.25 to −4.37 D	3.5 mm zone	3.41 D
−4.50 to −8.00 D	3.0 mm zone	4.49 D

Incisions Numbers

Since the days of Yenaliev, the number of incisions have decreased from 32 to 16 during the Fyodorov era. The incision number was further decreased to 8 during the past years and recently to only 4 incisions (vide infra). This reduction in the number of the radial keratotomy incisions has been tried in an attempt to decrease the risk of corneal weakening visa vise the amount of refractive correction required.

When taking a decision as to how many radial incisions one should attempt in a particular case for the correction of myopia, it is of interest to take the following observations into consideration:

1. Four incisions give about 60% effect.
2. An additional 30% change is obtained by another 4 incisions
3. Eight incisions produce 88% to 91% effect in comparison of 16 incisions which bring about approximately 98% change in preoperative refraction.

Four Incision 'Staged Approach'

Lately, a four incision staged approach has been advocated by many researchers to correct myopia of less than −4.0 D (Bonham et al, 1965; Salz et al, 1986).

The four incision 'staged approach' needs specially formulated nomograms, which are different from those used for the 8- or16-incision radial keratotomy.

This approach is based on the fact that:

1. The initial 4 incisions produce the maximum effect.
2. Even if there is some undercorrection, later additional incisions can be given to augment the effect.
3. It induces less trauma and less structural weakening of the cornea.
4. It reduces the overcorrection rate as well as its degree.

Drawback of Four Incision RK

The major drawback of four incisions is that in an attempt to obtain the best effect, the diameter of the uncut optical zone is to be kept 3.0 to 3.5 mm. The reduction in the central clear optical zone to this level increases the chances of *glare* and *star pattern* during the postoperative months.

Glare may sometimes become disturbing and visually significant. Usually these are temporary symptoms and last for few months.

Incision Depth

Depth of the incision is the *second most important variable* affecting the refractive outcome. The refractive outcome varies depending on the incision depth. The following relationship has been observed between the two.

1. Incision depth less than 80% of the corneal thickness has no effect.
2. Incision depth 80–85% does not produce much effect and is associated with unpredictability and regression of results.
3. Incisions deeper than 90% of the thickness have greatest effect and can correct higher degrees of myopia but are associated with risk of perforations as well as **progressive hyperopic shift** (PHS) as a late complication.
4. 85–90% deep incisions are the *optimum* and reduce the risk of perforations and microperforations. With these incisions a larger optical zone may be left behind. This would *minimize the problems of glare and star pattern.*

Depth Control

The depth control of incisions has improved by pre-operative use of ultrasonic and Orbscan *pachymetry,* taking *multiple readings* and per-operative use of diamond *micrometer knives* with precise calibrations.

Optical pachymetry is found to be less reliable method due to inconsistency of the readings. Ultrasonic pachymeter was used in the PERK study. The readings are taken at least at four different peripheral positions of the central uncut zone from where the incisions are likely to begin.

The diamond knife settings are done keeping the thinnest pachymetry reading of this paracentral area in mind. **Usually the setting of the diamond blade is done at a level which is a little more than the minimum pachymetry reading.** This is because of the fact that the knife does not cut to its fullest setting.

The diamond knife has undergone many major improvisations in its design over the past decades, as have the *nomograms,* hand in hand with the refinements of the diamond blade. The techniques and the art of the complicated aspects of radial keratotomy are the subject matters of a full text book.

Incision Termination

Fyodorov postulated that it was dissection of the 'corneal circular ligament' through RK incisions, which was responsible for the bulging of the peripheral cornea. He extended the incisions past the limbus.

Experiences of other researchers in laboratory and clinical studies have not supported this concept. It has been concluded that:

1. *Incision, if terminated across the limbus,* may in fact result in less refractive change.
2. They may damage the trabecular meshwork.
3. Patients' eyes may develop scarring with neovascularization at the limbus.

Incision Direction

Depending on the direction of the RK incision with respect to the visual axis, the following three surgical methods exist.

The Russian or Uphill Method The incision is started at the outermost periphery of the cornea and carried out centripetally towards the optical zone. This method produces more refractive change because the incisions given in this manner are found to be deeper. But it has the risk of encroaching upon the visual zone and perforations.

The American or Downhill Method Here the incision is given in a centrifugal direction starting at the outer margin of the optical zone. The effect produced is less than that of the above method.

The combined or Genesis Method The incision starts as in the American method, at the margin of the OZ, but the direction is changed again after reaching the corneal periphery without removing the knife. Now the uphill incision is to gain the depth. Encroachment into the OZ is avoided as the termination is controlled by the initial incisions land mark. The diamond knife setting is done in relation to the pachymetry reading of the central zone. It, thus avoids perforations.

This method has the effectiveness of the Russian method as well as offers the safety of the American method.

Incision Size

Altgough, decreasing the length of the incisions reduces the effectiveness of RK procedure. Nonetheless the small radial incisions are useful for correcting low to moderate myopia.

Minimum Invasive RK or Mini-RK

It utilizes 4–8 incisions starting from the margin of the central 3 mm optical zone (OZ) and extending only up to a distance of 7 mm to 8 mm from the optical center of the eye (Fig.10.10).

Advantages of Mini-RK

1. Makes the surgery less invasive.
2. The long term instability of results is decreased.
3. Less diurnal fluctuations in vision.
4. Reduced incidence of hyperopic progression.

Patient Associated Variables Affecting the Outcome of RK

The PERK study (*Prospective Evaluation of Radial Keratotomy*) was a large prospective, collaborative study

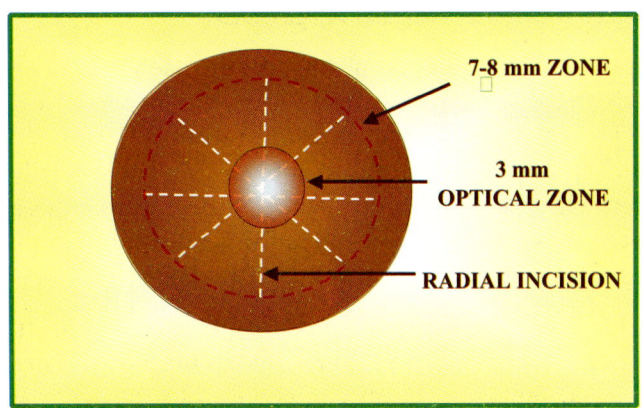

Fig. 10.10: Diagrammatic representation of Mini–RK

conducted in 9 different opthalmic centers in USA. It had a 10-year follow up. The aim of the study was to verify following variables independently, which were earliar supposed to affect the refractive outcome of radial keratotomy.

1. Age
2. Sex
3. Baseline refraction
4. Corneal curvature
5. Intraocular pressure
6. Ocular rigidity
7. Corneal thickness and its diameter

Age The patients were divided into third, fourth and fifth decade age groups. It was found that about 0.75 D additional increase in refractive change occurred in each successive age group.

Sex It was found that males with age above 40 years had more refractive change as compared to females, using the similar surgical parameters.

Preoperative Refraction A tendency was noticed that eyes with greater myopia had showed more change in refraction after RK.

Corneal Curvature No effect on the refractive outcome was noticed because of this variable.

Intraocular Pressure The association of IOP and refractive outcome was found to be weak.

Ocular Rigidity No effect of the ocular rigidity factor on the refractive results was noticed.

Corneal Diameter The baseline corneal diameter also showed no effect on the final refractive change after RK.

Corneal Thickness This variable also did not show any effect on the refractive outcome.

Side Effects and Complications of RK

Pain

Mild to moderate pain may last up to 48 hours. It might require use of oral analgesics.

Starburst Glare

This phenomena occurs after some months in most of the patients as a temporary effect lasting for one year or sometime even for longer periods. Visually disturbing glare is uncommon.

Epithelial Inclusion Cysts

These cysts may form sometimes but are not visually significant.

Endothelial Cell Loss

Endothelial cell loss up to 10% has been reported by some studies. This may be more if microperforations had occurred during the RK. The endothelial loss is *not progressive*.

Undercorrections

Undercorrection of refractive error is much more common than overcorrection. Undercorrection can be due to the following three reasons.

1. Failure to follow the parameters of *nomogram* properly.
2. The optical zone kept larger than normal.
3. Inadequate depth of the incisions.

The management of undecorrection requires to perform enhancement procedures, using specially designed '*enhancement diamond knives*' with strict adherence to various variables of the nomogram.

Overcorrections

Overcorrection of preoperative refractive error is again due to noncompliance to the nomogram. It is managed medically, *by not using the normally given topical steroids* and IOP lowering agents. Overcorrection of >1.5 D should be treated during the early postoperative period by applying *temporary* 10–0 nylon *sutures* to close the incisions.

Corneal Topographic Changes

The refraction at the optic zone of cornea behaves in a 'multifocal' manner. This occures due to increase in the *asphericity* of the central area. This change may result in an advantage to allow both near as well distance vision. But the following problems are also associated with the induced curvature changes of cornea.

1. Decrease in contrast sensitivity.
2. An increase in astigmatism.
3. The increased curvature in the periphery can interfere with contact lens fitting.

Decrease in BCVA

Best corrected vision may decrease in a minority of patients (up to 5% cases) probably due to the *corneal asphericity* of the central cornea caused by the surgery or occasionally due to trauma to the optic zone by inadvertent extension of incisions.

Instability of Refractive Effect

Regression of the Effect Regression of effect, i.e. the postoperative refraction becoming again myopic, is not common.

Hyperopic Shift This is a more common, long–term sequlae after RK. It occurs in two forms. In the simple form, which is common, the refraction changes to hyperopic side (1 to 3 D) after months of an uneventful RK. But it finally stabilizes, may be after years. Twenty two percent of the patients showed hyperopic shift in the PERK study after 6 months to 5 years.

In its severe form, called the **progressive hyperopic shift (PHS),** the corneal curvature continues to become more and more flatter with time.

1. The PERK study found that the hyperopic shift continued even up to 10 years of the follow up. The maximum change occurred during the first 2 years (mean change +0.2 D per year). The PHS was *more if higher degree of correction* was attempted which needed deeper and more number of incisions.
2. The PERTH study, after 5 years of follow up got similar observations. They *did not find* any case of *PHS in low myopes* (with –1 to –3 D).

Diurnal Fluctuation in Vision

On long term follow up, it is observed that many patients suffer from diurnal fluctuations in vision. This has been found to be a*ssociated with increase in the corneal thickness* in the morning (5.7% increase in corneal thickness after RK as compared to 1.7% in the controls). The incidence of this phenomenon in the PERK study was 52%.

Complications Causing Blindness

Rarely complications which are potentially blinding, can occur after RK (incidence 1–3%). They are:

1. Corneal perforation.
2. Cataract formation.
3. Endophthalmitis.
4. Bacterial keratitis.
5. Traumatic rupture of the globe is a rare complications that may also occur.

Vulnerability to Minor Trauma

Decreased strength of corneal tissue is a possibility due to multiple deep incisions of RK. Cases of rupture of the globe at the site of incision, after not so sever trauma, have been reported.

Present Status of RK

With the advent of *LASIK* and *wavefront guided LASIK*, radial keratotomy has a limited role in the present scenario. Its role is limited to cases of *low myopia*, if the cost of the excimer laser is a limitation and the surgeon has perfected in the technique of RK. Further improvements in the field of *surgical technique* and *instrumentation;* and *better nomograms* to improve the efficacy and predictability of results might keep its place in the future. A further comparison of RK and excimer laser refractive surgeries is given in the end of this chapter.

ASTIGMATIC KERATOTOMY

The correction of astigmatism requires giving the incisions in a *straight* or *arcuate manner*, placed in the *steep meridian*, perpendicular to it. These incisions are termed **transverse incisions** or **T-cuts**. They would *flatten* that meridian, thereby leading to steepening of the uncut meridian 90° away (Fig. 10.11).

1. The incisions should not be deeper than 80% of the corneal thickness in that area.

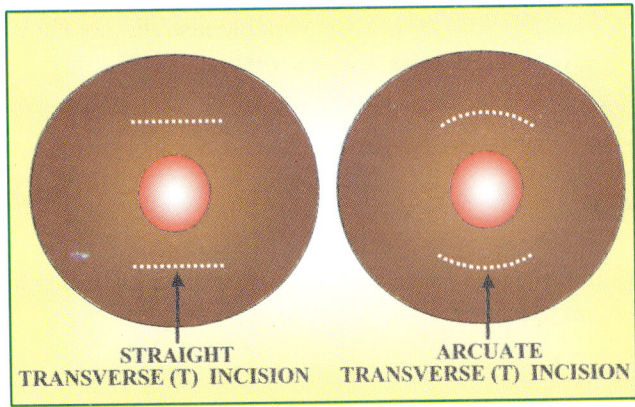

Fig. 10.11: Diagrammatic representation of astigmatic keratotomy

2. Incisions should be closer to the *optical center* to induce greater change in refraction but should not impinge upon the central OZ.
3. They may be single/multiple, parallel to each other but more than two pairs do not bring about further significant change in the effect.
4. Commonly 2 symmetrical arcuate incisions are used.
5. Arcuate incision induces more change because its actual length is 10-15% more with same chord length of a straight incision.

COMBINED RADIAL AND ASTIGMATIC KERATOTOMY

This combined approach addresses to the spherical myopia as well a large cylindrical component of refractive error in the same eye independent of each other. It utilizes the *radial* and the *transverse keratotomies* in *different combinations*. These combinations are complex patterns to suit the required refractive correction in a given case and are to be perfected after long term experience to master the right combination for achieving the desired change.

In general, two arcuate or straight incisions between, radial incisions are used commonly (Figs 10.12 and 10.13). *Intersection of the cuts is to be avoided to prevent wound gape, delayed healing and increased scarring.*

POST-SURGICAL ASTIGMATISM CORRECTION

Many surgical procedures have been used for correcting corneal astigmatism following cataract surgery and keratoplasty, *when spectacle or contact lens correction does not serve the purpose*. These are:

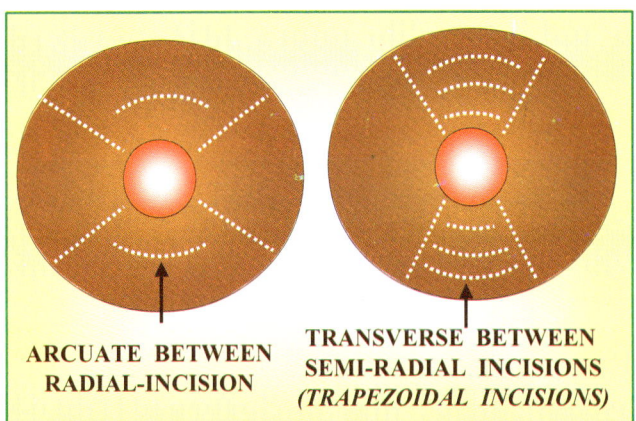

Fig. 10.12: Diagrammatic representation of combined radial and astigmatic keratotomy
Left - Spherical and astigmatic components are mild
Right - Astigmatic component is more severe

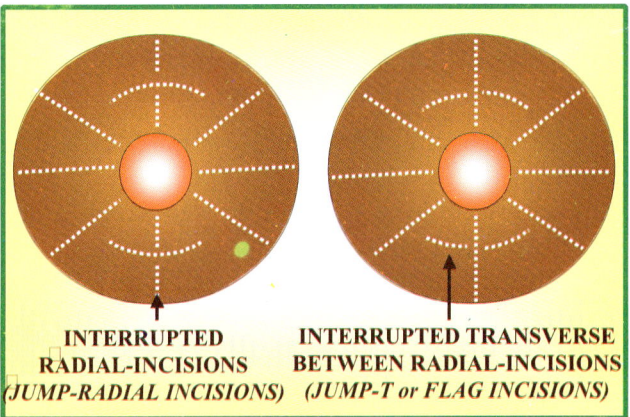

Fig. 10.13: Diagrammatic representation of combined radial and astigmatic keratotomy, when spherical component is more severe

1. Selected suture removal
2. Relaxing incisions
3. Relaxing incisions with augmentation sutures
4. Wedge resection
5. Holmium: YAG for hyperopic astigmatism
6. Photoastigmatic refractive keratectomy (PARK) and LASIK

Selected Suture Removal

Removing the sutures in the steep meridian is the simplest way of taking care of the post–surgical astigmatism. The effect of removing the tight sutures is maximum during the early months, once the wound is reasonably healed.

With large amount of astigmatism, this procedure may not necessarily take care of all of it, but then the residual error becomes easy to correct with cylinders.

Arcuate Transverse Keratotomy/Relaxing Incisions

For correcting high amount of astigmatism, once all the suture have been removed and the *wound has healed*, 'relaxing incisions' is the next procedure. It can be performed on the slit lamp under topical anesthesia (Fig. 10.14). Following are the steps used for this procedure.

1. The incisions are given at both the ends of the *steep* meridian, *directly into the healed wound* (the **classic technique).**
2. They also can be placed either on the donor side or the host side of the corneal tissue.
3. Though, the relaxing incisions given in the donor tissue have more effect, photophobia is a frequent sequelae.
4. Incision depth is 50–75% of the corneal thickness to avoid perforation.
5. They should extend at least 1 clock hour on either side of the steep meridian.
6. They are supposed to have maximum effect if made within 1–2 months of removing the sutures.
7. Maximum change in refraction is achieved at about 4–6 week after relaxing incisions.
8. Maximum change with relaxing incisions is of the order of about 2 D.
9. *Intra-operative use of the keratoscope helps to deepen or to enlarge the relaxing incisions to achieve the best effect.*

Relaxing Incisions with Augmentation (Compression) Sutures

When the above procedure is thought to be insufficient, in view of the magnitude of the astigmatism, it is supplemented by placing 2–6 sutures 90° away from the steep meridian on both the ends. This combined procedure can take care of about 6–7 D astigmatism (Fig. 10.14). They are left in place for many months but *removed early* in a gradual manner *only when the astigmatism remain still uncorrected.*

Wedge Resection

This procedure is carried out to steepen the *flat meridian.* This cannot be performed on the slit-lamp, unlike

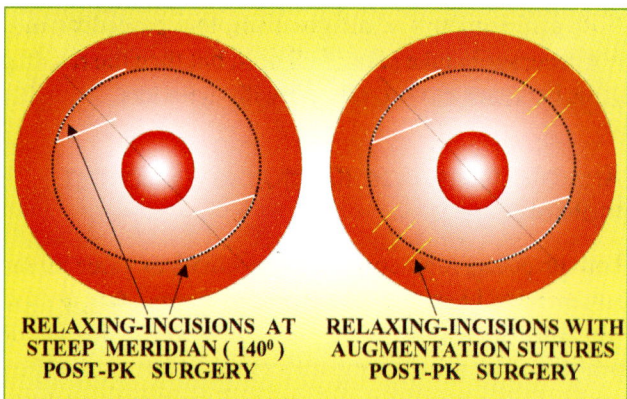

Fig. 10.14: Diagrammatic representation of relaxing incisions and combined relaxing incisions with augmentation sutures, post-PK

'relaxing incisions', but in the operating room with the usual anesthesia as for other intraocular surgeries (Fig. 10.15). The steps of wedge resection are:

1. A crescentic wedge, 1–2 mm wide and about 75% deep is dissected.
2. One of the incised margins of the crescent should be in the wound itself.
3. It is cut only at one end of the flatter meridian.
4. The wedge is preferably cut from the host tissue, if there is sufficient margin towards the limbus.
5. The extent of the wedge is about 1–1½ clock hour on either side of the flat meridian at that end.
6. The gap is approximated with about eight, interrupted 10–0 nylon sutures. A paracentesis is done to facilitate the closure.
7. Intraoperative use of the keratometer is of advantage in titrating the tightness of sutures.
8. Sutures are left in place for at least ½ months for the procedure to have its full effect.
9. Removal of the sutures is gradual in a phased manner.

Holmium: YAG Laser LTK for Hyperopic Astigmatism

The thermokeratoplasty spots are placed in the steep axis only. The effect is flattening in that axis due to collagen shrinkage (for more details on LTK, see in the beginning of this chapter).

HEXAGONOL KERATOTOMY FOR HYPERMETROPIA

Yamashita introduced incisional surgery for correcting hypermetropia, using 8 sided incisions surrounding the central OZ. Subsequently others modified the technique by using only 6 incisions and by decreasing the diameter of the area surrounded by these incisions (called **hex**) between 7.5 mm and 4.5 mm.

1. The incisions can be confluent, spiral, non-intersecting or non-intersecting supplemented by small transverse incisions placed at the corners of the '**hex**' (Fig. 10.16).
2. More the diameter approaches the central optic zone, greater is the refractive effect.
3. A 4.5 mm hex can correct up to 4.0 D of hyperopia.

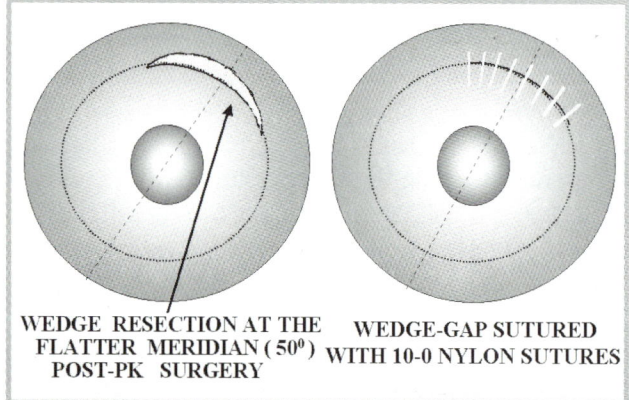

Fig. 10.15: Diagrammatic representation of wedge-resection for correcting post-PK surgery astigmatism

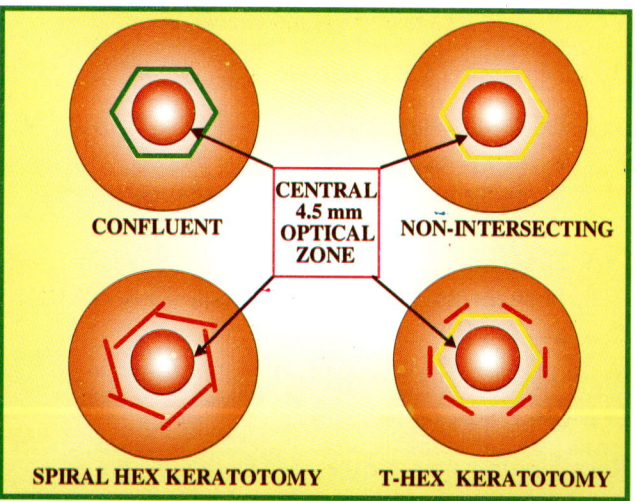

Fig. 10.16: Diagrammatic representation of hexagonal keratotomies for correcting hyperopia

Drawbacks and Complications

1. Results can be unpredictable.
2. Irregular astigmatism and loss of best corrected visual acuity can occur.
3. There may be excessive wound gaping and scarring after healing.

Present Status of Hexagonol Keratotomy

Since the refractive error corrected by this procedure is generally mild and can be easily taken care of by spectacles or by more predictable and safer *laser procedures* (vide infra), the role of hexagonal keratotomy in future is questionable.

INTRAOCULAR PROCEDURES

Various intraocular procedures were used for correcting refractive errors in the past. They have *again become popular in most severe cases of myopia, hypermetropia and astigmatism* because of limitations of other corneal refractive procedures, including excimer laser surgery, in these situations. But there are inherent complications associated with any intraocular surgery. These procedures may be divided into the following groups:

1. Clear lens extraction with or without an IOL
2. Phakic intraocular lenses (IOL)
    a. Anterior chamber lenses
        i. Baikoff angle-supported lens
        ii. Worst-Iris- Claw lenses
        iii. The Bakoff multiflex AC IOL
    b. Intraocular contact lenses between the iris and the anterior lens surface
        i. Collamer foldable hydrogel lenses
        ii. Silicon lenses

CLEAR LENS EXTRACTION

This is used to correct *high myopia* and *high hyperopia*. It was often used in the past but no prospective study with long term follow up is available. The following points must be considered:

1. The IOL power is calculated by one of the *third generation* formulas (SRK/T, Hoffer Q, Holladay).
2. The aim is postoperative emmetropia or slight myopia to compensate for the loss of accommodation. Whether or not to implant an IOL is based on this concept.
3. In unilateral case the eye is kept slightly myopic.
4. For bilateral surgery emmetropia is aimed.
5. Implantation of an *IOL even with zero power* with preservation of the posterior capsule is recommended to decrease the incidence of retinal detachment.

Surgical Technique

The latest technique of cataract surgery, *small incision phacoemulsification with foldable IOL* is to be preferred to give the best results with least complications. **The surgeon should have enough experience in this technique before venturing for clear lensectomy**.

Complications of Clear Lens Extraction

The major complications are:

1. Loss of best corrected visual acuity.
2. Loss of accommodation.
3. Endophthalmitis.
4. High posterior capsular opacification.
5. Retinal detachment.

The incidence of retinal detachment is found to be almost double of that seen in comparable high myopes, who do not undergo surgery. Preoperative treatment of holes, lattice, etc. and long term continuous surveillance of the operated cases is mandatory because this complication may develop even many years later.

PHAKIC INTRAOCULAR LENSES

Many researchers have worked for providing the desired refractive correction with intraocular implants without disturbing the natural lens, thus **maintaining the accommodation** as well as avoiding retinal detachment in the prone myopic eye.

Anterior Chamber Lenses

The anterior chamber IOLs are in common use for a long time. There have been ongoing efforts to improve the techniques of implantation and designs of anterior chamber IOLs and use of high density viscoelastics so that the associated corneal decompensation can be avoided.

The issue of corneal decompensation is of great concern because of the following facts:

1. The phakic anterior chamber is not as deep as in aphakia.

2. The lens is to be manipulated in this limited space while inserting it.
3. If the IOL is not well fitted in this limited space or not well immobilized away from the endothelium, it has the potential risk of rubbing against the endothelium.

Three types of anterior chamber (AC) IOLs have been used. These are:

1. **Baikoff Angle Supported AC IOL**
2. **Worst-Iris-Claw lens/Artisan Lens**
3. **The Bakioff multiflex AC IOL**

- Studies with the first two types have shown progressive endothelial cell loss of about 5–7% after 2 years. If this loss continues, it might result in corneal decompensation after many years.
- In addition the *Artisan or 'Iris-claw' lens* has the potential risk of causing chronic iritis, iris atrophy as well as dislocation. But it has the advantage of avoiding the UGH (uveitis, glaucoma and hyphema) syndrome, associated with the angle supported IOLs. These lenses are available in the power range of -3 to -23 D and +3 to +12 D.
- *Toric lenses* of up to 12 D of cylinder power have been used in post-PK high astigmatism in few case reports[119, 120].
- The third generation *Bakioff multiflex AC IOL* is found to be the safest regarding the above risks.
- Preoperative assessment of the AC depth and the endothelial count should help in deciding the feasibility of phakic AC IOL implantation.

Intraocular Contact Lenses

These are intraocular lenses implanted in the phakic eye, into the space between the iris and the anterior lens surface. The design of the lenses is such that they rest in the *prelenticular aqueous milieu* away from the anterior lens capsule.

Lens Design and Material

The lenses are specially designed. They consists of a *foldable material*. The dimension of the intraocular contact lens is 11.5–13.0 mm long with 6.5 mm width and 6.5 mm optic size. They have a *solid heptic* consisting of the same material (Fig. 10.17 and 10.18).

Presently two types of the intraocular lenses are available:

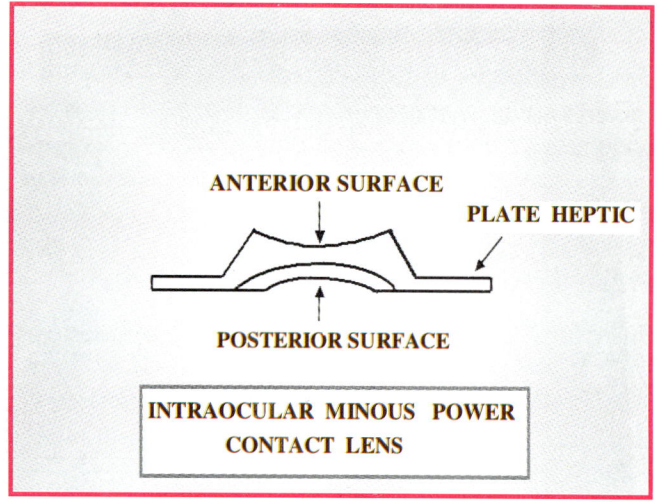

Fig. 10.17: Diagrammatic representation of an intraocular contact lens design.

The COLLAMAR Hydrophilic lens consists of collagen-silicone copolymer.

The Silicone Intraocular CL

Power Range

The power used ranged from −12.0 D to −19 D in one study and −8.0 D to −26.0 D in another.

Insertion Technique

The insertion is through a small *3 mm clear corneal incision* to cause minimal surgical damage to the

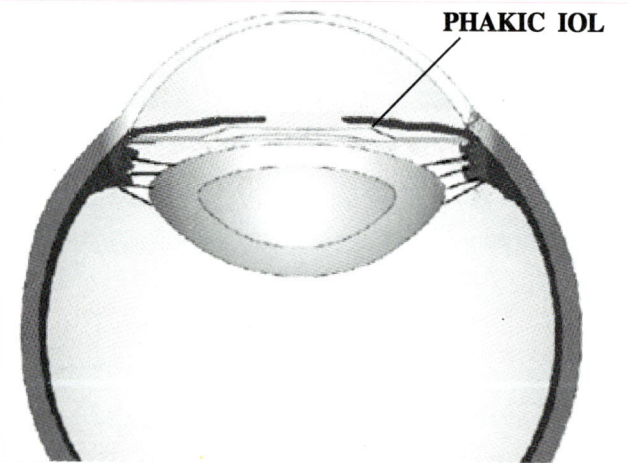

Fig. 10.18: Diagrammatic representation of an intraocular contact lens design and the same fixated in the sulcus

otherwise normal eye. Use of a high density viscoelastics substance is mandatory to keep the AC depth maintained for smooth transition of the IOL into the desired space without any significant touch to the crystalline lens and other intraocular structures. No suturing is required.

Complications of Phakic Intraocular IOL

Iris pigment dispersion, iritis, cataract due to inadvertent lens trauma during implantation, secondary pigment dispersion glaucoma and lens glare may occur. No case of endophthalmitis or retinal detachment was found after 7 years of follow up by one study[120].

Present Status

The technique is *easy* and *reversible* with good results. In cases of *very high/extreme myopia* not suitable for LASIK because of potential danger to the globe and retina due to very high suction pressure generated during the later, this procedure offers the correction without significantly disturbing the globe.

KERATOREFRACTIVE PROCEDURES WITH EXCIMER AND OTHER LASERS

The introduction of the excimer laser keratorefractive procedures have come as a new era in the field of refractive surgeries, heralding a major teccnological breakthrough.

Since the first clinical PRK series by McDonald and Kaufman in 1989, the *excimer laser refractive surgeries* have undergone many changes in the techniques to witness improvements in results and safety. Not only the *range* of refractive errors to be corrected has widely increased but also the *predictability and stability* of the outcome *continues to improve* with the newer techniques such as LASIK, wavefront-guided LASIK and LASEK. These techniques of refractive correction are described in the respective chapters with their results, advantages and safety/complications.

The only advantage of **RK** over the excimer laser procedures is that it is *relatively inexpensive*. But it has the major limitation that its application is **limited to low to moderate myopia and low degree of astigmatism.** Moreover it is associated with vision threatening complications like corneal perforations, endophthalmitis, retinal detachment, endothelial cell loss and cataracts as a result of frank or microperforations. Traumatic rupture of the globes at the site of incisions also have occurred. *Radial keratotomy is now very uncommon in clinical practice except* where the costly excimer laser surgery is not available and where RK is the surgeon's preference because of his long experience in this area. Nonetheless, it has played an important role at a time when the keratorefractive surgery was in its gestation period.

The excimer and other laser procedures have not been assosiated with sight-threatening complications in proper hands. Only PRK had its limitations due to the results being stable and predictable only in low to moderate myopia like RK. The outcome of newer techniques (LASIK, wavefront LASIK and LASEK) are promising in terms of range of corrections, predictability, stability and safety.

The other laser procedure, e.g. laser thermokeratoplasty and intrastromal PRK, are discussed elsewhere.

Suggested readings

1. Neumann AC, Fyodorov S et al: Radial thermokeratoplasty for the correction of hyperopia. Ref Corn Surg 1990; 6: 404-411.
2. Neumann AC, Sanders D, Raanan M et al: Hyperopic thermokeratoplasty: clinical evaluation. J Cataract Ref Surg 1991; 17: 830-838.
3. Feldman ET, Ellis W, Frucht-Perry J et al: Regression of effect following radial thermokeratoplasty in humans. Ref Corn Surg 1989; 5: 288-291.
4. Thompson VM, Seiler T, Durrie DS et al: Holmium: YAG laser thermokeratoplasty for hyperopia and astigmatism: an overview. Ref Corn Surg (suppl) 1993; 9: S134-S137.
5. Seiler T, Matallana M, Bende T: Laser thermokeratoplasty by means of a pulsed holmium: YAG laser for hyperopic correction. Ref Corn Surg 1990; 6: 99-102.
6. Seiler T, Matallana M, Bende T: Laser coagulation of the cornea with the holmium: YAG laser for the correction of hyperopia. Fortschritte der Ophthalmologie 1991; 88: 121-124.
7. Seiler T: Ho: YAG laser thermokeratoplasty for hyperopia. Ophthalmol Cli North Am 1993; 5: 773-780.
8. Durrie DS, Schumer DJ et al: Holmium:YAG LTK for hyperopia. Ref Corn Surg 1994; 10 (Suppl) S277-S280.
9. Tutton MK, Cherry PMH: H: YAG laser thermokeratoplasty to correct hyperopia: 2 years follow up. Ophthalmic Surg and Lasers 1996; 27 (Suppl): S521-S524.
10. Kohen T, Husain SE, Koch DD: Corneal topographic changes after Holmium: YAG laser thermokeratoplasty to correct hyperopia. J Cataract Ref Surg 1996; 22: 427-435.

11. Aker AB, Brown DC: Hyperion laser thermokeratoplasty for hyperopia. In Ophthalmom Cli 2000; 40 (3): 165-181.
12. Koop N, Wirbelauer C et al: Thermal damage to the cornea l endothelium in diode laser thermokeratoplasty. Ophthalmologe 1999; 96(6): 392-397.
13. Geerling G, Koop N, Tungler A, Laqua H et al : Diode laser thermokeratoplasty: initial clinical experiences. Ophthalmologe 1999; 96(5): 306-311.
14. Ismail MM, Perez-Santonja JJ et al: Laser thermokeratoplasty after lamellar corneal cutting. J Cataract Ref Surg 1999; 25(2): 212-215.
15. Geerling G, Koop N, Tungler A, Laqua H et al: Cintonuous wave diode laser thermokeratoplasty : first clinical experience in blind human eyes. J Cataract Ref Surg 1999; 25 (1):32-40.
16. Brinkmann R, Koop N, Geerling G et al: Diode laser thermokertoplasty: application strategy and dosimetry. J Cataract Ref Surg 1998; 24 (9): 1195-1207.
17. Ismail MM, Perez-Santonja JJ, Alio JL: Non contact thermokeratoplasty to correct hyperopia induced by LASIK. J Cataract Ref Surg 1998; 24 (9): 1191-1194.
18. Bende T, Jean B, Derse M et al: Ho: YAG thermokeratoplasty: treatment parameters for astigmatism induction based upon spherical enucleated human eye. Graefes Arch Clin Exp Ophthalmol 1998; 236 (6) : 405-409.
19. Sporl E, Genth U, Seiler T et al : Thermomechanical behaviour of the cornea. Gre J Ophthalmol 1996; 5 (6): 322-327.
20. Goggin M, Lavery F: Holmium laser thermokeratoplasty for the reversal of hyperopia after myopic PRK. Br J Ophthalmom 1997; 81 (7): 541-543.
21. Gezer A: The role of patient's age in regression of Ho: YAG laser thermokeratoplasty-induced correction of hyperopia. Eur J Ophthalmol 1997; 7 (2) : 139-143.
22. Rad AS, Jabbarvand M, Farahvash MM et al: LASIK and diode thermal keratoplasty for correction of hyperopia from +5.0 to +10.0 D. J Ref Surg 2002; 18 (3 Suppl): S318-S320.
23. Barraquer JI: Keratomileusis for myopia and aphakia. Ophthalmology 1981; 88: 701.
24. Barraquer JI: Queratomileusis para la correccion de la miopia. Arch Soc Am Oftalmol Optom 1964; 5: 27-48.
25. Barraquer JI: Long term results of myopic keratomileusis-1982. Arch Soc Am Oftalmol Optom 1983; 17: 137-142.
26. Barraquer JI: Refractive keratoplasty. Bogota: Instituto de America 1970.
27. Barraquer JI: Method for cutting lamellar grafts in frozen cornea: new orientation for refractive surgery. Oftalmol Optom 1958; 1: 1-271.
28. McDonald MB et al: On-lay lamellar keratoplasty for the tretment of keratoconus. Br J Ophthalmol 1983; 67: 615.
29. Kaufman HE, Werblin TP: Epikeratophakia for the treatment of keratoconus. Am J Ophthalmol 1982; 93: 342.
30. Troutman RC, Swinger CA et al: Keratophakia: a preliminary evaluation. Ophthalmology 1979; 86: 523.
31. Fouraker BD, Schanzlin DJ: Update on epikeratoplasty. Ref Corn Surg 1991; 7: 57.
32. Krumeich JH: Indications, techniques and complications of myopic keratomileusis. Int Ophthalmol Cli 1983; 23: 75.
33. McDonald MB et al: The nationwide study of epikeratophakia for myopia. Am J Ophth 1987; 103: 375.
34. Morgan KS et al: The nationwide study of epikeratophakia for aphakia in older children. Ophthalmology 1988; 95:526.
35. Morgan KS, Somers M: Update on epikeratophakia in children. In Ophthalmom Cli 1989; 29: 37.
36. Morgan KS, Stephenson GS: Epikeratophakia in children with corneal laceration. J Pediatr Ophthalmol 1984; 91:780.
37. Steinart RF, Grene RB: Postoperative management of epikeratoplasty. J Cataract Ref Surg 1988; 14: 255.
38. Panda A: Epikeratoplasty utilizing manually prepared plano lenticules from fresh M-K preserved cornea (a long term study). ISRK 1994; Oct: 75 Abstract.
39. Slade SD, Gordon JF, Dru RM: Aprospective multicenter clinical trial to evaluate automated lamellar keratoplasty for the correction of myopia. ISRK 1994; Oct :79 Abstract.
40. Neuman AC: ALK complications: avoidance and management. ISRK 1994; Oct: 80 Abstract.
41. McDonald MB, Mc Carey BE et al : Assessment of the long term corneal response to hydrogel intrastromal lenses implanted in monkey eyes for up to 5 years. J Cataract Ref Surg 1993; 19: 213-222.
42. Lane SS, Lingstrom RL et al: Polysulfone corneal lenses. J Cata Ref Surg 1986; 12: 50-60.
43. Lane SS, Lingstrom RL: One yer follow up on fenestrated intracorneal lenses: complications, reversibility and histopathology. Invest Ophthalmol 1988; 29 (Suppl): 311.
44. McCarey BE: Current status of refractive surgery with synthetic intracorneal lenses: Barraquer lecture, Ref Corn Surg 1990; 6: 40-46.
45. McCarey BE, Lane SS, Lingstrom RL: Alloplastic corneal lenses. Int Ophthalmol Cli 1988; 28: 155.
46. Climenhaga H, McDonald J et al: Effect of diameter and depth on the response to solid polysulfone intracorneal lenses in cats. Arch Ophthalmol 1988; 106: 818-824.
47. Chan SM, Khan HN: Reversibility and exchangeability of ICRS. J Cata Ref Surg 2002; 28(4): 676-681
48. Siganos CS, PallikarisI G et al: Management of corneal ectasia after laser in situ keratomileusis with INTACS. J Refract Surg 2002; Jan-Feb;18(1):43-46.
49. Suiter BG, Twa MD et al: A comparison of visual acuity, predictability, and visual function outcomes after intracorneal ring segments and laser in situ keratomileusis. Trans Am Ophthalmol Soc 2000; 98: 51-5; discussion 55-7.

50. Rapuano CJ, Sugar A, Koch DD et al: ICRS for low myopia: a report by the American Academy of Ophthalmology. Ophthalmology 2001 Oct; 108(10): 1922-8.
51. Gomez L, Chayet A: LASIK results after ICRS (Intacs). Ophthalmology 2001 Oct; 108(10): 1738-43.
52. Asbell PA, Ucakhan OO: Long-term follow-up of Intacs from a single center. J Cata Ref Surg 2001; 27(9): 1456-68.
53. Schanzlin DJ, Abbott RL et al: Two-year outcomes of ICRS for the correction of myopia. Ophthalmology 2001; 108(9):1688-94.
54. Tham VM, Hwang DG: The ICRS: Intacs. Ophthalmol Clin North Am 2001 Jun; 14(2): 295-9.
55. Asbell PA, Ucakhan OO, Abbott RL et al: ICRS: reversibility of refractive effect. J Refract Surg 2001 Jan-Feb; 17(1): 25-3.1
56. Ruckhofer J, Stoiber J et al: One year results of European Multicenter Study of ICRS. Part 2: complications, visual symptoms, and patient satisfaction. J Cataract Refract Surg 2001 Feb; 27(2): 287-96.
57. Sato T: Treatment of conical cornea (incision of Descemet's membrane). Acta Soc Ophthalmol Jpn 1939; 43: 544.
58. Sato T, Akiyama K et al: A new surgical approach to myopia. Am J Ophthalmol Jpn 1953; 36: 823.
59. Akiyama K: Study of surgical treatment of myopia (II report). Animal experment. Acta Soc Ophthalmol Jpn 1955; 59: 294.
60. Akiyama K: The surgical treatment for myopia (III report). Anterior and posterior incisions. Acta Soc Ophthalmol Jpn 1955; 59: 797.
61. Yamaguchi T et al: Bullous keratopathy after anterior-posterior radial keratotomies for myopia and myopic astigmatism. Am J Ophthalmol 1982; 93: 600.
62. Yenaliev FS: Experience in the surgical treatment of myopia. Vestn Oftalmol 1978; 3: 52.
63. Fyodorov SN, Durnev VV: Anterior keratotomy method application with the purpose of surgical correction of myopia. In Pressing Problems of Ophthalmosurgery. Moscow 1977; pp. 47-48.
64. Fyodorov SN, Durnev VV: Operation of dosaged dissection of corneal circular ligament in cases of myopia of a mild degree. Ann Ophthalmol 1979; 11: 1885.
65. Hecht SD, Jamara RJ: Prospective evaluation of radial keratotomy using the Fyodorove formula: preliminary report.Ann Ophthalmol 1982; 14: 319.
66. Assil KK, Schanzlin DJ: Radial keratotomy surgical techniques and protocols. In: Assil KK, Schanzlin DJ, eds. Radial and astigmatic keratotomies: A Complete handbook for the succesful practice of incisional keratotomy using the combined technique, (Slack: Thorofare; 1994); 87-110.
67. Bores LD, Myers W et al: Radial keratotomy: analysis of the American experience. Ann Ophthalmol 1981; 13:941.
68. Lynn MJ, Waring GO et al: The PARK study group: Factor affecting outcome an predictability of RK. Arch Ophthalmol 1987; 105: 42.
69. Waring GO, Lynn MJ, McDonnell PJ et al : Results of the prospective evaluation of RK study(PERK) 10 years after surgery. Arch Ophthalmol 1994; 112:1298-1308.
70. O' Donnell FE : Short incision RK: A comparative study in rabbits. J Ref Surg 1987; 3: 22.
71. Sanders DR, Diitz MR et al: Factors affecting the predictability of RK. Ophthalmology 1985; 92: 1237.
72. Salz JJ et al: A study of optical zone size and incision redeepening in experimental RK. Arch Ophthlmol 1985; 103: 590.
73. Salz JJ et al: Four incision RK for low to moderate myopia. Ophthalmology 1986; 93: 727.
74. Salz JJ, Salz MS: Results of 4 and 8 incision RK for 6 to 12 diopters of myopia. J Ref Surg 1988; 4: 46.
75. Salz JJ et al: Ten years experience with a conservative approach to RK. Res Corn Surg 1991; 7: 12.
76. Lindstrom RL: Minomally invasive radial keratotomy: Mini- RK. J Cataract Ref Surg 1995; 21: 27-34.
77. Chen V, Lindstrom RL: Oblique orientation of incisions in four-incision RK. Ophthalmic Surg 1992; 23: 359.
78. Hoffman RF: Reoperations after radial and astigmatic keratotomy. J Ref Surg 1987; 3: 119.
79. Gelender H, Flynn HW et al: Bacterial endophthalmitis resulting from RK. Am J Ophthalmol 1982; 93: 323.
80. Gelender H, Gelber HC: Cataract following RK. Arch Ophthlmol 1983; 101: 1229.
81. Stark WJ, Martin NF et al: Radial keratotomy II. A risky procedure of unproven long term success. Surv Ophthalmol 1983; 28: 106.
82. McRae SM, Matsuda M, Rich LF: The effect of radial keratotomy on the corneal endothelium. Am J Ophthalmol 1985; 100: 538.
83. Shivitz IA, Arrowsmith PN: Delayed keratitis after radial keratotomy. Arch Ophthalmol 1986; 104: 1153.
84. Bourque LB et al : Reported patient satisfaction, fluctuation of vision and glare among patients one year after surgery in the PERK study. Arch Ophthalmol 1986; 104: 356.
85. D'Day DM, Feman SS et al: Visual impairment following RK: A cluster of cases . Ophthalmology 1986; 93: 319.
86. Schanzlin DJ, Santos VR, Waring GO et al: Diurnal change in refraction, corneal curvature, visual acuity and IOP after RK in the PERK study. Ophthalmology 1986; 93:167.
87. MacRae S, Rich L et al: Diurnal variation in vision after RK. Am J Ophthalmol 1989; 107: 262.
88. Deitz MR, Sanders DR: Progressive hyperopia with long term follow up of RK. Arch Ophthalmol 1985; 103: 782.
89. Deitz MR, Sanders DR, Raanan MG: Progressive hyperopia in RK: Long term follow up of diamond knife and metal blade series. Ophthalmology 1986; 93: 1284.
90. Deg JK, Zavala EY, Binder PS: Delayed corneal wound healing following RK. Ophthalmology 1985; 92: 743.

91. John ME Jr, Schmitt TE: Traumatic hyphema after RK. Ann Ophthalmol 1983; 15: 930.
92. Pearlstein ES, Agapitos PJ et al: Ruptured globe after RK. Am J Ophthalmol 1988; 106: 755.
93. Bloom HR, Sands J, Schneider D: Corneal rupture from blunt trauma 22 months after RK. Ref Corn Surg 1990; 6:197.
94. Binder PS, Waring GO: Keratotomy for astigmatism, in: Waring GO, Refractive Keratotomy for Myopia and Astigmatism, (Mosby-Year Book : St Louis, 1992): 1087.
95. Thornton S: Astigmatic keratotomy: A review of basic concepts with case reports. J Cata Ref Surg 1990; 16: 430.
96. Thornton S: Inverse arcuate incisions, a new approach to the correction of astigmatism. J Cataract Corn Surg 1994; 10 : 27-30.
97. Gilbert ML, Friedlander M et al: Hexagonol keratotomy in human cadaver eyes. J Ref Surg 1988; 4: 12-14.
98. Neuman AC, McCarty GR: Hexagonol keratotomy for correction of low hyperopia: preliminary results from a prospective study. J Cata Ref Surg 1988; 14: 265-269.
100. Jensen R: Hexagonol keratotomy: clinical experience with 483 eyes. Int Ophthalmol Cli 1991; 31: 69-73.
101. Grandon SC, Sandera DR et al: Clinical evaluation of hexagonol keratotomy for the treatment of promary hyperopia. J Cata Ref Surg 1995; 21: 40-49.
102. Franks JB, Binder PS: Keratotomy procedures for the correction of astigmatism. J Ref Surg 1985; 1: 11.
103. Hall GW et al: Reduction of corneal astigmatism at cataract surgery. J Cata Ref Surg 1991; 17; 407.
104. Lindstrom R: The surgical correction of astigmatism: A clinician's perspective. Ref Corn Surg 1990; 6; 437.
105. Lindstrom R, Lindquist TD: Surgical correction of postoperative astigmatism. Cornea 1988; 7: 138.
106. Mandel MR, Shapiro MB et al: Relaxing incisions with augmentations sutures for the correction of post- keratoplasty astigmatism. Am J Ophthalmol 1987; 103: 441.
107. Van Rij G , Waring GO: Changes in corneal curveture induced by sutures and incisions. Am J Ophthalmol 1984; 98: 773.
108a. Rowsey JJ, Morley WA: Surgical correction of moderate myopia: Which method to use? RK will always have a place. Survey of Ophthalmol 1998; 43 (2): 147-156.
108b. Steinert RF, Bafna S: Surgical correction of moderate myopia: Which method to use? PRK and LASIK are the treatment of choice. Survey of Ophthalmol 1998; 43 (2): 177-179.
109. Lyle WA, Jin JC : Clear lens extraction for the correction of high refractive errors. J Cataract Ref Surg 1994; 20: 273-276.
110. Colin J, Robonet A: Clera lensectomy and implantation of low power posterior chamber intraocular lens for the correction of high myopia. Ophthalmology 1994; 101: 107-112.
111. Menejo JL, Cisneros AL et al: Iris claw phakic lens-intermediate and long term corneal endothelial changes. Eur J Implant Ref Surg 1994; 6: 195-9.
112. Mimouni F, Colin J, Koffi V et al: Damage to corneal endothelium from anterior chamber IOLs in phakic myopia. Ref Corneal Surg 1991; 7 : 277-81.
113. Saragoussi JJ, Cotinas J, Renard G et al: Damage to corneal endothelium by minus power anterior chamber lenses. Ref Corneal Surg 1991; 7: 282-90.
114. El Danasoury MA, El Maghraby, Gamali TO : Comparison of iris-fixed Artisan lens implantation with excimer laser in situ keratomileusis in correcting myopia between -9.00 and -19.50 diopters: a randomized study. Ophthalmology 2002; 109 (5): 955-64.
115. Grabow HB: Discussion section-management of patients with high ametropia who seek refractive surgical correction. Eur J Implant Ref Surg 1994; 6: 302-4.
116. Allemann N, Chamon W, Campos M: Saftey prediction in Baikoff lenses for high myopia correction using ultrasound biomicroscopy. ISRS 1995; 59-60 (Abstracts).
117. Marinho AA, Neves M et al: Posterior chamber IOLs (Silicone) in myopic phakic eyes: 2 years experience. ISRS 1995; 58 (Abstracts).
118. Zaldivar R: Hypernegative IOLs in the posterior chamber of phakic eyes for the correction of high myopia. SRS 1995; 58 (Abstracts).
119. Tehrani M, Dick HB: Implantation of an ARTISAN trade mark toric phakic intraocular lens to correct high astigmatism after penetrating keratoplasty. Klin Monatsbl Augenheilkd 2002 Mar; 219(3):159-63
120. Uusitalo RJ, Aine E, Sen NH, Laatikainen L: Implantable contact lens for high myopia. J Cataract Refract Surg 2002 Jan; 28(1): 29-36.
121. O'Brien TP, Awwad ST: Phakic IOLs and refractory lensectomy for myopia. Curr Opin Ophthalmol 2002 Aug; 13(4): 264-70.
122. Colin J, Robinet A, Cochener B: Retinal detachment after clear lens extraction for high myopia: seven-year follow-up. Am J Ophthalmol 2000 Feb;129(2):144-50.
123. Werblin TP, Patel AS, Barraquer JI: Initial human experiance with permalens myopic hydrogel intracorneal lens implant. Ref Corneal Surg 1992; 8: 23-26.

Section V

Excimer Laser Corneal Surgeries

Chapter 11

Phototherapeutic Keratectomy: Advantages and Indications

INTRODUCTION

PTK is a newer technique of laser keratectomy for treating various anterior corneal disorders which uses 193 nm ArF excimer laser. The corneal tissue from surface is removed by a photochemical reaction 'ablative photo-decomposition', in which the 6.4 eV photons of excimer laser cause disruption of covalent bonds of molecules leading to the tissue ablation. The ablated tissue is ejected out with a great velocity by the remaining energy of the photons being used as kinetic energy.

The physical qualities of 193 nm ArF excimer laser interaction with the corneal tissue have endowed it with a magical surgical action capable of *controlled removal* of corneal tissue in desired shapes and patterns with *submicron precision* without significant collateral damage; and *predictability* in terms of intended depth, length and reproducibility of cuts. It has been suitably termed as *laser scalpel* that can be used to create a new corneal curvature or to reconstruct the surface of the cornea, *thereby successfully replacing keratectomy, keratotomy and keratoplasty.*

Preservation of the Bowman's membrane during corneal surgeries has been proven to be a *myth*, which can be violated by the excimer laser without producing any opacity or irregularity. This is possible because the tissue removal with the excimer laser is so smooth and precise with minimum damage to the adjacent tissue.

ADVANTAGES OF EXCIMER LASER SURGERIES

1. Minimal collateral damage as compared to other laser and manual surgeries, < 100 nm.
2. High absorption by cornea (3-4 µ penetration per pulse), no intraocular penetrance.
3. Risk of cataractogenesis, mutagenesis, endothelial damage and photokeratitis non-existent.
4. Risk of corneal ectasia only if remaining cornea thickness is < 250 µ.
5. Easier, **non-invasive surgery** for correction of refractive errors and superficial corneal disorders.
6. Avoids the inherent complications associated with an intraocular procedure such as endophthalmitis and retinal detachment to name the serious ones.
7. *Early visual rehabilitation* and *very effective in restoring vision* in comparison to the other available keratorefractive surgeries and keratoplasty.
8. *Correction of refractive errors over a wide range* in comparison to the other available keratorefractive surgeries.
9. *High safety and predictability* of results and low variability of refractive outcome as compared to other keratorefractive surgeries.
10. Low in complication rate as compared to contact lens wear, (e.g. keratitis, allergy and giant papillary conjunctivitis, etc.)
11. Less demanding and cumbersome modality as compared to CL wear.

12. *Far superior visual and anatomical results* in case of corneal disorders *vs. keratoplasties*.
13. Much faster visual recovery in a matter of days rather than months, unlike keratoplasty procedures (lamellar and penetrating).
14. Recurrence rate of dystrophies is much less as compared to penetrating keratoplasty.
15. Most patients with dystrophies need repeat *keratoplasty* in their lifetime. Repeat *invasive* procedures are fraught with *high potential for risks*. Repeat PTK can be performed with least surgical risk as long as the residual cornea remains > 250 µ.
16. No problems like scarcity of donor corneas, prolonged waiting time and 'graft failure'.
17. Prevention of recurrent corneal erosions is achieved in majority of cases (70-100%).

LIMITATION OF EXCIMER LASER SURGERIES

The main drawback of excimer laser surgeries is that the laser system is highly expensive. Therefore the accessibility is limited to the population at large. These surgeries are not easily and freely available, particularlly in the developing countries. Other limitations are the complications associated with these surgeries. These are discussed in Chapter 26.

PHOTOTHERAPEUTIC KERATECTOMY (PTK)

REVIEW OF PTK LITERATURE

In 1985, *Oliva Serdarevic* and fellow researchers were the first to perform a series of successful excimer laser phototherapeutic keratectomies using rabbit model, to treat experimentally created fungal (candidial) ulcers of about 3 mm size. The results were clear healed corneas. They supported the observation of Marshall and Trokel that corneal transparency could be achieved in spite of removing the Bowman's layer.

In 1986, *Seiler, Bende* and colleagues were the first to use 193 nm excimer laser clinically for corneal resurfacing by removing diseased superficial corneal tissue in *blind human eyes*.

The following account reviews the indications and results of PTK for different corneal diseases.

Band Keratopathy

In the year 1988, *David Gartry* et al were the first to perform PTK on 25 *sighted human eyes* in patients of superficial corneal pathologies in UK, after the first ethics committee's approval for PTK. There patients were divided into groups of various *band types–rough and irregular* to *even and fine*, caused by Lattice degeneration, Salzmann's degeneration, Cogan's dystrophy, granular dystrophy, increased calcium, trauma, viral keratitis, uveitis and idiopathic, etc.

They reported that all patients of rough band keratopathy who had pain and glare disability had marked improvement after PTK. Sixteen of 25 patients (64%) had improved vision. One patients who had *overlapping ablation* had decreased visual acuity due to irregular astigmatism. Eight patients (32%) who had extensive pathological conditions of the eyes did not improve visually. They also reported a mean hyperopic shift of +2.5 D sph. equi. (spherical equivalent).

O'Brart and Gartry et al in 1993 treated 122 eyes with band keratopathy by PTK. They reported that 88% of cases had good BCVA. All of the patients had hyperopic shift with a mean of +1.4 D sph. equi. Forty four of the patients (95%), who had pain and glare disability experienced relief following PTK.

Claoue et al in 1995 reported 21 cases of band keratopathy treated with PTK. They had 100% success in pain relief, 53% cases with improvement in BCVA, and a mean of +2.4 D sph. equi. hyperopic shift.

Recurrent Corneal Erosions

Daush and colleagues had treated the first patient of recalcitrant corneal erosion in 1988 using excimer laser PTK. During the subsequent years, they reported their success in treating this condition with PTK in 74 eyes.

Many other researchers had successful experience in treating corneal erosions with 193 nm excimer cases PTK. The recurrence of erosions was reported from 0% to 25% in these studies (75–100% success). All these studies reported healing of epithelium in 4–6 days in a vast majority of cases.

Kremer et al in 1997 reported treatment of myopic patients with recalcitrant corneal erosions with excimer laser PTK, combined with PRK. with the technique called **pancorneal photoablation.** They demonstrated complete alleviation of erosions in all 16 treated eyes. A final myopic spherical equivalent was less than or equal to –1.0 D in 14 of 16 eyes.

Bullous Keratopathy

Thomann et al in 1985 reported results of PTK on 13 cases of bullous keratopathy with no visual potential, to relieve pain and reduce risk of secondary infectious keratitis. Bullae rarely persisted after 1–2 months following PTK.

Corneal Dystrophies and Degenerations

Fagerholm et al in 1993 treated 27 patients of corneal dystrophies such as granular, Meesman's, Schnyder's and epithelial basement membrane dystrophy (EBMD) with PTK. But the cases were not analyzed separately. They reported that 77.8% of the patients achieved the goal of improved visual acuity, reduction of pain and stabilization of refraction.

Nassaralla et al reported four cases of granular and lattice dystrophy, treated with PTK in 1996. Corrected visual acuity improved in all patients. There was a hyperopic shift in three eyes. Mean follow up was 47.8 months.

Rapuano in 1997 reported results of PTK treatment on six eyes with superficial granular dystrophy, five eyes with Salzmann's degeneration, three eyes with recurrent erosions, two eyes with keratoconus nodule and six eyes with other dystrophies and corneal scars.

The corneal smoothness and clarity improved in all eyes. There was improvement in visual acuity. Mean hyperopia was + 2.13 D sph. equi. with range of +7.25 D to 6.5 D. The overall success rate was 78.5% with moderate to significant recurrence of pathology in five eyes (17.8%). There was worsening in one eye.

Forster and associates treated 252 eyes of 216 patients with PTK in 1997. One hundred three eyes had recurrent corneal erosions, 86 eyes had previous surgery for pterygium, 29 eyes had band keratopathy and 4 eyes had scars, superficial stromal dystrophies, anterior corneal dystrophies, superficial infection and amyloidosis.

They reported 91% eye with recurrent erosions were recurrence free. All the patients with band-like keratopathy were pain free. In 88% of eyes the treatment goal was achieved. Loss of visual acuity occurred in only one patient with bullous keratopathy. Hyperopic shift was seen in all patients. It was suggested that the use of large area ablation could reduce this side effect.

Orndahl et al in 1998 treated 28 eyes with PTK which were having recurrent corneal erosions (8 eyes), map-dot finger print (nine eye), lattice type I (5 eyes), lattice type II (2 eyes), Meesman's (2 eyes), central crystalline (4 eyes), granular (5 eyes) and Fuchs' endothelial dystrophy (one eye).

They reported 84.6% of eyes had improvement in corrected vision. Two cases of lattice type II and one case of granular dystrophy recurred. In the case of Fuchs' dystrophy, there was recurrence of subepithelial fibrosis. None of the eyes with recurrent erosions had recurrence. Mean hyperopic shift was + 2.25 D sph. equi.

Meier and colleagues reported two cases of Schnyder's crystalline dystrophy with disabling visual acuity being successfully treated with excimer laser PTK in 1998. The best corrected visual acuity improved from 20/70 to 20/25 in one and 20/30 in other patient.

PTK for Scars

Neil Sher and colleagues, in 1991, were the first to perform PTK for superficial scarring due to various causes such as post-infective, post traumatic, recurrent corneal erosions and different corneal dystrophies, in 33 sighted eyes. A majority of their patients had reduction in the corneal scarring and about 50% had improved visual acuity. Epithelial healing was reported to occur after 4–5 days. A hyperopic shift was noticed in 50% of cases. They recommended immediate hyperopic steepening of cornea with excimer laser following PTK to avoid this complication.

McDonnell et al in 1992 reported a case of long standing post traumatic superficial scar that proved resistant to excimer laser ablation.

Herpes Simplex Keratitis Scars

Fagerholm et al in 1993 treated 30 eyes with post infectious scars. They achieved 73.3% success in scar removal and 80% improvement in visual acuity. One patient out of 15 with post herpes simplex scarring had recurrence of herpetic keratitis following PTK.

Compos and associates treated 6 patients of post-infective scarring in 1993. They obtained improved visual acuity in 50%. No recurrence of herpetic keratitis was reported during 15 months follow-up when they used acyclovir orally, 200 mg four times daily for 10 days, starting one day preoperatively. Old scars and calcific areas were found to be resistant to removal even with 140μm deep ablation.

Trachomatous Scarring

Goldstein et al in 1994 treated three patients with trachomatous superficial corneal scarring. Such patients had scarring of the conjunctiva and lids associated with corneal vascularization and would be highly unsuitable for penetrating keratoplasty. They reported significant improvement in visual acuity in 2 of the 3 patients.

PTK for Pterygium

Seiler and coworkers treated 31 eyes having post-excisional scarring and 24 eyes with recurrence of pterygium in which excimer laser PTK ablation was used to smoothen the wound bed immediately following surgical re-excision, followed by topical 0.04% Mitomycin-C. In the primary group there was no recurrence. In the second group there was 12.5% recurrence of pterygia. Overall 16.4% cases gained at least 2 lines of visual acuity by the first year.

Fagerholm et al reported satisfactory results of PTK in patients with post-pterygium excision scars.

Tuunanen et at in 1995 treated 11 eyes with primary or recurrent pterygium with PTK with an aim of preventing recurrence. However recurrence occurred in 36% (4eyes) of the cases.

Forster et al in 1997 used PTK on 86 eyes for smoothening the corneal surface after pterygium surgery. The reported that 42% of the eyes had recurrence of pterygium if the *bare sclera technique* was used and 33% recurrence if *free conjunctival graft* was used as procedure for primary pterygium surgery.

Superficial Infectious Keratitis

Therapeutic excimer laser has been used successfully for sterilization of micro-organism cultures, experimental microbial keratitis, infectious superficial keratitis resistant to medical treatment, etc.

Oliva Serdarevic and co-workers, in 1984 were the first to use excimer laser PTK to successfully treat experimentally induced fungal corneal ulcer in rabbit model.

Keats et al in 1988 used excimer laser for sterilization of microbial cultures.

Gottsch et al in 1991 used excimer laser for treating infectious superficial keratitis not responding to medical treatment.

Eiferman et al reported successful use of excimer laser PTK in case of infectious crystalline keratopathy.

Drawback of PTK for Keratitis

Pepose and co-workers in 1992 reported that since 193 nm excimer laser had poor penetration, less than 4 micron, deep stromal infiltration with the infectious process might limit the effectiveness of PTK for such cases. There could be risk of possible spread of micro-organisms. They also reported reactivation of latent herpes simplex virus following excimer laser PTK.

Miscellaneous Conditions

Keratoconus

Moodaley and colleagues used excimer laser PTK for proud-nodulae in keratoconus giving rise to contact lens intolerance. *Mortensen et al* in 1994 and 1998 used excimer laser for treatment of keratoconus nodules. No increased risk to cornea or any interference with subsequent corneal transplantation surgery was found and there was an improvement in vision as well as ability to wear contact lenses. *Rapuano* reported successful treatment of two cases of keratoconus nodules with PTK.

Vernal Keratoconjunctivitis

In 1994, *Cameron et al* reported there success in treatment of shield ulcers and corneal plaques in vernal keratoconjunctivitis, with excimer laser PTK.

Epithelial Melanosis

Kim and colleagues, in 1993, used PTK for treating conjunctival epithelial melanosis.

Cryoglobulin Deposits

Kremer et al reported in 1997, a case of paraproteinemia with subepithelial cryoglobulin deposits, successfully treated with PTK. They found marked improvement in visual acuity and reading capacity. The hyperopia induced by these deposits regressed by 5.75 D spherical equvalient.

Recurrent Numulli after Epidemic Keratoconjunctivitis (EKC)

Quentin et al had success in significantly decreasing the recurrence of the numulli.

PTK after other Corneal Surgeries

Fong et al successfully treated 4 cases of superficial corneal fibrosis after previous RK and *Lazzaro* et al one case of epikeratophakia lenticule scarring with partial success with PTK.

PTK after PRK, LASIK and LASEK

Edward et al reported success of PTK in treating '*central steep islands*' developing after PRK and LASIK, in 1998.

Vinciguerra et al in 2002, treated 45 eyes which had developed whitish *corneal scars* following LASIK in cases of hyperopia. The treatment was also aimed to at correcting the corneal *eccentricity (asphericity)* caused after LASIK and 'LASEK'. The ablation *profile* for this therapy was a *wider optical zone of 6.7 mm with transition zone of 9.5 –10.0* mm delivered with the Nidek EC–5000 excimer laser system. All cases of the corneal scars were treated successfully and the corneal eccentricity corrected substantially.

FDA APPROVED INDICATIONS

FDA Indications:1994

In early nineties, the first FDA (Food and Drugs Administration, USA) trial was done on 271 consecutive eye with VISX laser.

The following groups were included:

1. Visual impairment due to opacities in the anterior third of cornea.
2. Visual impairment due to fine corneal irregularities.
3. Superficial infectious keratitis.
4. Visual impairment due to pathological or post surgical refractive abnormalities.

Fifty five percent of the patients had corneal scars, 39% dystrophies and 5% surface irregularities. BCVA improved by two or more lines in 45% and worsened in 10% of the patients agter PTK.

FDA Indications:1995

The second FDA trial using Summit laser studied 67 eyes with the following groups of pathologies of cornea:

1. Opacity group
2. Surface irregularity group
3. Recurrent epithelial breakdown group.

The UCVA improved in 64–69%, BCVA in 77% in the *opacity group*, 70% in *irregularity group* and 30% in *erosion group*. Nine percent in the erosion group and 20% in the other two groups had worsening in visual acuity. The most important finding was a myopic shift in the opacity group which needed peripheral ablation.

Following success of these trials, FDA gave *conditional approval* for PTK in 1994.

Thus, the extensive work by a large number of researchers, as is evident from the above review, speaks of the success of this technique as a new modality of treating superficial corneal disorders.

Table 11.1 gives the current indications and goals of treatment of PTK.

Table 11.1: Current indications for PTK

Condition	Goal of Treatment

1. **Superficial Corneal Opacities**
  * Scars-Post-infectious
     Post-traumatic
  * Anterior dystrophies
     Granular dystrophy
     Lattice dystrophy
     Schnyder's dystrophy
  * Spheroidal degeneration
     of the central cornea
	Improve visual acuity
	Relieve symptom of glare, haloes
	Relieve **monocular secondary images**

2. **Irregular Surface**
  * Degenerative nodules:
  * Salzmann's nodules
  * Keratoconus nodules
  * Band keratopathy
	Improve visual acuity by improving optical quality of the cornea
	Allow contact lens wear
	Relieve symptoms of discomfort, pain, glare and photophobia

3. **Epithelial Instability**
  * Recurrent corneal erosions
  * Epithelial basement membrane dystrophy (EBMD)
  * Meesman's dystrophy
  * Vernal keratoconjunctivitis
	Re-establishment of an intact, healthy surface
	Relief of discomfort pain, glare, photophobia

4. Aids in the Surgical Removal of **Pt erygium**	Smoothen the corneal surface

5. **Iatrogenically Produced**
  *R*efractive errors*:
  Astigmatism following:
     Penetrating keratoplasty
     Cataract surgery
     Epikeratophakia
  **Central Steep Islands*
	Improve visual acuity

6. **Bullous Keratopathy**	Relief of pain

Suggested readings

1. Azar DT, Jain S, Woods K, et al: Phototherapeutic keratectomy: The VISX Experience. In: Salz JJ, ed., Corneal Laser Surgery (Mosby: St Louis, 1995).
2. Algawi K, Goggin M, O'Keefe M: 193 nm excimer laser phototherapeutic keratectomy for recurrent corneal erosions. Eur J Implant Ref Surg 1995; 7: 1-13.
3. Berlin M, Bende T, Seller T: Corneal resurfacing by excimer laser photoablation. ARVO abstracts, Invest Ophthal Vis Sci 1988; 29(Supp): 310.
4. Brancatto R, Sciadone A, Carones F et al: Excimer laser ablation of a corneal protuberances. J Cataract Refract Surg 1992; 18: 111.
5. Campos M, Hertzog I et al: PTK for severe post keratoplasty astigmatism. Am J Ophthalmol 1992; 114: 429-436.
6. Cameron JA, Antonios SR, Badr IA: Excimer laser phototherapeutic keratectomy for shield ulcers and corneal plaques in vernal keratoconjunctivitis. J Refract Surg 1995; 11: 31-35.
7. Claoue C, Stevens J, Steele A: Band keratopathy and excimer laser phototherapeutic keratectomy. European J Implant Ref Surg 1995; 7: 260-5.
8. Campos M, Nietsen S, Szerenyi K et al: Clinical follow-up of phototherapeutic keratectomy for treatment of corneal opacities. Am J Ophthalmol 1993; 15: 433-440.
9. Chamon W, Azar DT, Stark JW et at: Phototherapeutic keratectomy. Ophthalmol Clin North Am 1993; 6: 399-413.
10. Campos M, Nielsen S, Szerenyi K et al: Clinical follow-up of phototherapeutic keratectomy for treatment of corneal opacities. Am J Ophthalmol 1993; 115: 443-440.
11. Edward E, Manche MD et al: Treatment of topographic central islands following refractive surgery. J Cata Ref Surg 1998; 24 : 464- 470.
12. Eggink FA, Beekhuis WH: Granular dystrophy of the cornea: Contact lens fitting after phototherapeutic keratectomy. Cornea 1995; 14: 217-22.
13. Eiferman RA, Forgey DR, Cook YD: Excimer laser ablation of infectious crystalline keratopathy. Arch Ophthalmol 1992; 110: 18.
14. Fagerholm P, Fitzsimmons TD, Orndahl M et al: Phototherapeutic keratectomy for corneal diseases: A follow-up study CLAO Journal 1995; 21.
15. Fong VC, Chuck RS, et at: PTK for superficial corneal fibrosis after radial keratotomy. J Cata Ref Surg 2000; 26: 616- 9.
16. Forster W, Atzler U, Rakkay I et at: Therapeutic use of 193 nm excimer laser in corneal pathologies. Graefe's Arch Clin Exp Ophthalmol 1997; 235 (5): 296-305.
17. Forster W, Grewe S, Atzter U, Lunecke C, Busse II: Phototherapeutic keratectomy in corneal diseases. Refract Corneal Surg 1993; 9: S90-S95.
18. Goldstein M, Loewenstein A, Rosner M, et al: Phototherapeutic keratectomy following penetrating keratoplasty. J Refract Corneal Surg 1994; 10: S290- S292.
19. Gartry D, Kerr Muir M, Marshall J: Excimer laser treatment of corneal surface pathology a laboratory and clinical study. Br J Ophthal 1991; 75: 258-69.
20. Gartry DS, Kerr Muir M, Marshall J: Excimer laser photorefractive keratectomy: 18 month follow-up. Ophthalmology 1992; 8: 1209-1219.
21. Cottsch .JO, Gilbert ML, Goodman OF, et al: Excimer laser ablative treatment of microbial keratitis. Ophthalmology 1991; 98: 146-149.
22. Hersh PS, Spinak A, Carrana R, Mayer M, PTK: strategies and results in 12 eyes. Ref Corneal. Surg 1993; 9: 890-895.
23. John ME, Van der Karr MA, Noblitt RL, Boleyn KL: Excimer laser phototherapeutic keratectomy for treatment of recurrent corneal erosion. J Cataract Refract Surg 1994; 20: 179-81.
24. Kyle C et al: PTK in recurrent corneal erosions refractory to other forms of treatment. Eye 1997; 11 (4): 570-5.
25. Ketates RH, Drago PC, Rothchild EJ: Effect of excimer laser on microbiological organisms. Ophthalmic Surg 1998; 19: 715-718.
26. Loewenstien A, Lipshitz I et al: PTK for the treatment of myopia after epi-keratoplasty. J Ref Cata Surg 1994; 10: 8285- 8286.
27. Maloney RK, Thompson V et al: A prospective multicenter trial of phototherapeutic keratectomy for corneal vision loss. Am. J. Ophthalmol.1996; 60: 149-160.
28. Mc Donnell JM, Garbus JJ, Mc Donnell PJ: Unsuccessful PTK: Clinico-pathological correlations. Arch Ophthalmol 1992; 110: 977-979.
29. Mortensen J, Obstrom A: Excimer laser photorefractive keratectomy for the treatment of keratoconus. J Ref Corneal Surg 1994; 10: 368-72.
30. Moodaley L, Liu, C, Woodward EG, et al: Excimer laser superficial keratectomy for proud nodule in keratoconus. Br J Ophthalmol 1994; 78: 454-7.
31. McDonnell PJ, Seiler T et al: Phototherapeutic keratectomy with excimer laser for Reis-Buckler's corneal dystrophy. Ref corneal Surg 1992; 8: 306-10.
32. O'Brart OP, Muir MG, Marshall J: Phototherapeutic keratectomy recurrent corneal erosions. Eye 1994; 8: 378-83.
33. O'Brart OP, Gartry OS, Lohmann CP, et at: Treatment of band keratopathy by excimer laser phototherapeutic keratectomy: surgical techniques and long term follow up. Br J Ophthalmol 1993; 77: 702-8.
34. Pepose JS, Laycock KA, Miller JK et al: Reactivation of latent herpes simplex virus by excimer laser photokeratectomy Am J Ophthalmol 1992; 114: 45-50.
35. Rapuano CJ, Laibson PR: Excimer laser phototherapeutic keratectomy. CLAO Journal 1993; 19: 235-240.

36. Rao SK, Fogia RS et al: Excimer laser PTK indication, results and its role in the Indian scenario. Indian J Ophthalmol 1999; 47: 167-1.72.
37. Rene Din, Christopher J, Rapuano CJ et al: Recurrence of corneal dystrophies after phototherapeutic keratectomy. Ophthalmology 1999; 106 (8): 1490-1497.
38. Rapuano CJ, Laibson PR: Excimer laser phototherapeutic keratectomy for anterior corneal pathology. CLAO Journal 1994; 20: 253-7.
39. Seiler T, Kahle G, Kriegerowski M: Excimer laser (193 nm) keratomileusis in sighted and blind human eyes. Refract Corneal surgery 1990; 9: 165-173.
40. Seiler T, Schnelle B, Wollensak J: Pterygium excision using excimer laser smoothing and topical mitomycin C. German Journal of Ophthalmology 1992; 1: 429-31.
41. Sher NA, Bowers RA, Zabel RW, et al: Clinical use of 193-nm excimer laser in the treatment of corneal scars. Arch Ophthalmol 1991; 109: 491-498.
42. Stark WJ, Chamon W, Kamp MT, et al: Clinical follow-up of 193-nm, ArF excimer laser photokeratectomy. Ophthalmology 1992; 99: 805-811.
43. Stark WJ Chamon W, Azar DT, et al: Phototherapeutic keratectomy. Ophthalmol Clin North Am 1993; 399-413.
44. Steinert RF, Puliafito CA: Excimer laser phototherapeutic keratectomy for a corneal nodule. Refract Corneal Surg 1990; 6: 352.
45. Thomann U, Meier-Gibbons F, Schipper I: Phototherapeutic keratectomy for bullous keratopathy. Br J Ophthalmol 1995; 79: 335-8.
46. Tunnanen TH, Tervo TM: Excimer laser phototherapeutic keratectomy for corneal diseases. Refract Corneal Surg 1993; 9: S85-S90.
47. Wang GO: FDA panel recommends conditional approval of excimer laser phototherapeutic keratectomy. J Ref Cata Surg 1994; 10: 74-78.
48. Kasetsuwan N, Puangsricharern V et al: Excimer laser PTK for corneal diseases. J Med Assoc Thai 2000; 83(5): 475- 482.
49. Paparo LG, Rapuano CJ et al: PTK for Schnyder's Crystalline corneal dystrophy. Cornea 2000; 19(3): 343-347.
50. Dighiero P, Boudraa R et al : Therapeutic photokeratectomy for the treatment of band keratopathy. J France Ophthal 2000; 23(4): 345-9.
51. Fong YC, Chuck RS et al: PTK for superficial corneal fibrosis after RK. J Cata Ref Surg 2000; 26 (4): 616-619.
52. Faschinger CW: PTK for a corneal scar due to presumed infection after PRK. J Cata Ref. Surg 2000; 26 (2): 296-300.
53. Lazzaro DR, Starr MB et al: PTK For anterior scarring in an epikeratophakia lenticule. CLAO J 2000; 26(1): 52-53.
54. Amano S, Oshika T et al: Long term follow up of excimer laser PTK. Jap J Ophthalmol 1999; 43(6): 513-516.
55. Ho CL, Tan DT, Chan WK: Excimer laser PTK for recurrent corneal erosions. Ann Acad Med Singapore 1999; 28 (6): 787-790.
56. Stahl J, Fulcher S et al: Corneal subepithelial nodular scarring treated with PTK in a child with Rothmund-Thomson Syndrome. Cornea 2000; 19(1): 110-115.
57. Jain S, Austin DJ: PTK for treatment of recurrent corneal erosions. J Cata Ref. Surg 1999; 25(12): 1610-1614.
58. Cavanaugh TB, Lind DM et al: PTK for recurrent erosions syndrome in anterior basement dystrophy. Ophthalmology 1999; 106 (5): 971-976.
59. Quentin CD, Tondrow M, Vogel M: PTK after epidemic keratoconjunctivitis. Ophthalmologe 1999; 96(2): 92-96.
60. Talu H, Tasindi E et al: Excimer laser PTK for recurrent pterygium. J Cataract Ref Surg 1998; 24(10) 1326–1332.

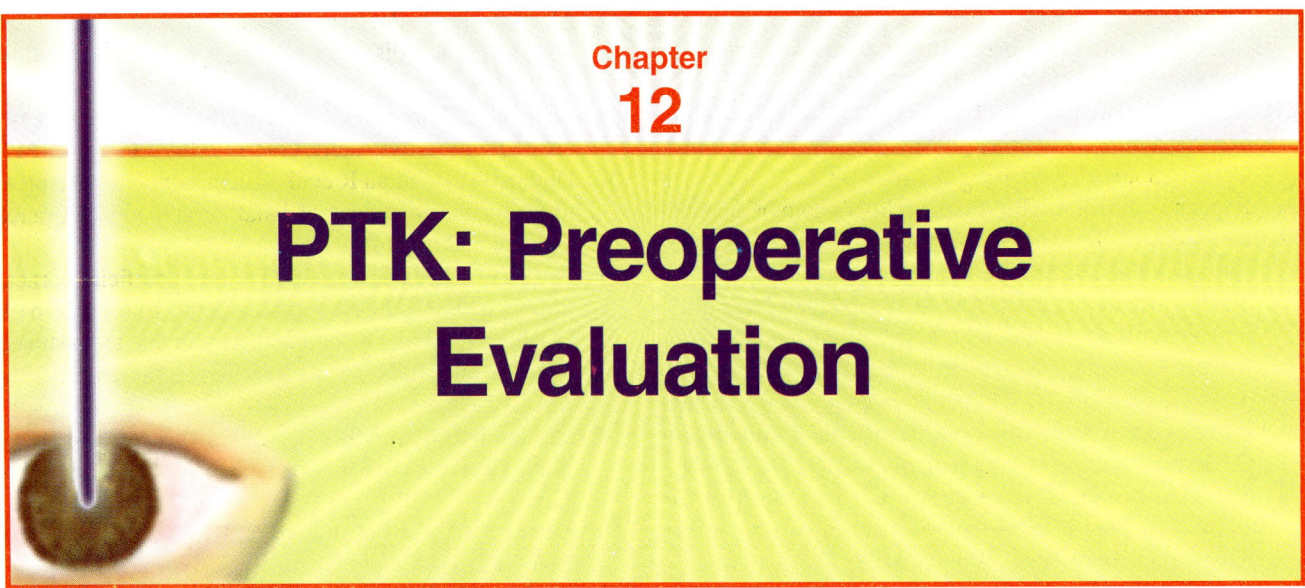

Chapter 12

PTK: Preoperative Evaluation

A careful preoperative selection of the patients is the first key to success for PTK. This evaluation involves several aspects, which are:

1. Assessment of the corneal pathology
2. Recognition of absolute and relative contraindications
3. Understanding of the functional needs and expectations of the patient
4. Evaluation of the risks and benefits
5. Preoperative refractive error of the patient.

ASSESSMENT OF THE CORNEAL PATHOLOGY

The corneal lesion is evaluated in terms of the following.
1. Depth
2. Horizontal distribution (extent, location)
3. Corneal sensations
4. Type of lesion.
5. Associated corneal vascularization
6. Associated corneal thinning, if any

This helps in deciding wheather PTK would be *beneficial* and if it is so then what should be the *treatment strategy*.

Depth of the Lesion: Vertical Distribution

The more *superficial* the lesion is, more is the success of phototherapeutic keratectomy. This is because of the following reasons:

1. Superficial pathologies are easier to remove.
2. Less ablation is required and less corneal tissue removed. Therefore, it has the following advantages.
   a. Less *refractive change* is induced after ablation (hyperopic shift, irregular astigmatism).
   b. Less *corneal haze*, better corneal clarity.
3. Less amount of laser used.
4. Re-treatment can be planned for residual lesions without causing significant corneal thinning.
5. No risk of corneal ectasia after PTK.
6. Deep ablation results in excessive thinning, more aggressive healing response leading to undesirable corneal haze and dramatic changes in refraction.

Most surgeons feel that less than 100 μ deep lesions are the ideal candidates. Lately many others have become more confident of removing more deeper lesions with new improved techniques to avoid the hyperopic shift, as long as the central corneal thickness is >250 μ.

Elevated lesions are better candidates than the ones located below the surface, if these are paracentral in location, because off-axis ablation can cause severe irregular astigmatism.

An approximate assessment of the depth is done by slit-lamp examination, which also confirms vertical location of the lesion from the corneal surface. *Optical pachymetry* by the Haag-Striet pachymeter assesses the depth of the lesion objectively. The procedure is performed in the same manner as for assessing the corneal thickness. But here the alignment of anterior surface of one half of the corneal section is done with the most posterior aspect of the lesion in the other half of the section. This is read on the scale to give the thickness of the lesion in micrometers.

No lesion, however thin, located in deeper stroma is a candidate for PTK.

Horizontal Distribution of the Lesions

The horizontal distribution of the corneal lesions may be considered regarding two aspects:

1. Horizontal distribution in relation to the visual axis.
2. Horizontal distribution according to the distribution pattern of the pathology.

Horizontal Distribution in Relation to Visual Axis

Horizontal distribution of the corneal lesion can be one of the following three types:

Central Involving the central 4 mm optic zone

Para-central Located in the 4 mm to 8 mm middle zone of the cornea

Peripheral Outside the 8 mm zone

- Lesions located in the central zone affect the vision most and are the ideal indications for PTK.
- Para-central lesions affect the vision and peripheral lesions usually do not affect it directly. They may do so by producing astigmatism.
- PTK may be done for a para-central lesions, combined with ablation of the central zone to avoid irregular astigmatism, which results from ablation in the para-central zone alone.
- PTK is not indicated for peripheral pathologies.

Horizontal Distribution According to the Distribution Pattern of the Pathology

Nodular Discrete nodule, one or more in number, elevated above the corneal surface and surrounded by the normal corneal tissue. These lesions are best treated by shaving off the elevated bulk of the lesion **(manual keratectomy)** followed by smoothening of the surface by excimer laser, while protecting the normal cornea with a masking agent, e.g. Salzmann's nodules, a small localized scar.

Segmental These are larger lesions than the above but occupy only a part of the optic zone, e.g. post-pterygium removal scarring, early band keratopathy. The treatment strategy is same as for a nodular lesion.

Diffuse Lesions are distributed throughout the optic zone but there are areas of uninvolved cornea within, e.g. Meesman's dystrophy, map-dot-fingerprint dystrophy and granular dystrophy. These are treated with a *large area PTK*. Frequent use of a suitable masking agent is required to achieve smooth surface while ablating the cornea because the lesion and the normal cornea may have different ablation rates.

Complete Here the lesion is distributed throughout the optical zone in a continuous manner without any area of normal cornea, e.g. advanced band shaped keratopathy and large corneal opacity.

Corneal Sensation

It is very important to test the corneal sensations in all cases undergoing excimer laser ablation. In cases of corneal opacity /scar, loss of corneal sensation would indicate towards a herpetic cause. They need adjuvant use of oral acyclovir to prevent reactivation of herpetic keratitis.

Type of Pathology

The pathologies may be divided into the following groups for the purpose of PTK.

1. **Superficial Opacities,** for example granular and lattice dystrophies, nebulomacular corneal opacities.
2. **Epithelial Instability,** for example recurrent corneal erosion syndrome, vernal keratoconjunctivitis.
3. **Surface Irregularity,** for example Salzmann's nodules, post-pterygium surgery irregular surface.
4. **Scars and band shaped keratopathy (BSK).**

Different sub-groups of disorders have been found to give different results after PTK. The superficial opacity and surface irregularity subgroups, which do not have significant corneal thinning, are found to be the best candidates by most researchers. Our own study on 48 eyes achieved best results in eyes with *nebulomacular corneal opacities* (post-herpes and others) and *post-pterygium surgery irregular surface* subgroups. In the later condition the PTK is combined with the manual removal of pterygium. *Old post-pterygium scars* do not do as well when PTK is done later.

The *scarred corneal tissue* and *calcium deposits* are found to be the worst candidates and even sometimes resistant to excimer laser ablation. Other coexisting ocular pathologies in case of band shaped keratopathy are also responsible for sub-optimal visual results.

Corneal Vascularization

Eyes with associated corneal vascularization are not good candidates for PTK. The blood absorbs laser energy and hampers smooth ablation, resulting in poor refraction or even irregular astigmatism postoperatively.

Corneal Thinning

Eyes with significant corneal thinning are also poor candidates for PTK. But if one is sure that the post-PTK corneal thickness would be > 250 microns, one may decide to go ahead with the laser ablation.

RECOGNITION OF ABSOLUTE AND RELATIVE CONTRAINDICATIONS

Phototherapeutic keratectomy is not to be performed in certain situations, either because of the potential complications or poor visual results in such cases. These are grouped under the following heads:

1. Conditions that would hamper corneal re-epithelization
   a. Systemic autoimmune disease
   b. Advanced diabetes mellitus
   c. History of abnormal wound healing
   d. Keloid formation
   e. Severe dry eye/keratoconjunctivitis sicca
   f. Significant lagophthalmos
2. Conditions that would preclude good vision
   a. Uncontrolled uveitis
   b. Posterior segment disorders causing loss of vision
      i. Retinopathies
      ii. Macular disorders
      iii. Retinal detachments
      iv. Vascular occlusions, etc.
   c. Uncontrolled glaucoma
   d. Posterior segment inflammations
3. Conditions that may predispose to infectious keratitis
   a. Uncontrolled blepharitis
   b. Lacrimal sac infection
   c. Conjunctivitis
4. Heavy corneal vascularization
5. Significant thinning of the cornea < 400 microns
6. Corneal lesion > 100 microns deep
7. Unwilling patients

It is to be understood that some of the situations may constitute either absolute or relative contraindications depending on the functional needs, the clinical setting and the level of experience of the surgeon.

To further elaborate on this point, PTK may be indicated in a case of posterior segment diseases to improve the visualization and help in their management. For example a case of silicon oil filled eye with band keratopathy or an eye with a corneal opacity with retinopathy requiring laser photocoagulation would be definitely benefited by PTK (e.g. the case shown in photograph 30 and 31, colour plate 6; had diabetic retnopathy but the corneal opacity hampered retinal visualization).

The corneal thickness is to be considered vis-a-vis the depth of the lesion and the intended ablation depth. The desired depth of the lesion should be less than 100 microns. But now some surgeons prefer PTK to penetrating keratoplasty for deeper pathologies as long as the remaining corneal thickness is more than 250 microns. This is because of better results and less complications with the former. *Glaucoma needs special mention because after PTK long term use of steroids is required to avoid/manage corneal haze. This may aggravate or precipitate glaucoma.*

UNDERSTANDING THE FUNCTIONAL NEEDS AND EXPECTATIONS OF PATIENT

PTK would also be considered successful if the patient is satisfied with regard to his expectations from the surgery. For ensuring achievement of this objective, one has to:

1. Understand the patient's subjective complaints and what is expected by him/her after the treatment.
2. Assess the corneal pathology.
3. Figure out the probable outcome after PTK.
4. Explain and discuss the *probable outcome* with the patient.

The above exercise would avoid patient dissatisfaction and give confidence to the patient as well the surgeon and the general population at large, about the technique of PTK. This point is made clear by the following examples:

1. In a case with *recurrent corneal erosion*, visual acuity is not the prime concern but the painful

episodes of erosions are to be given attention because the former is generally not much affected. The patients with a focal/limited disadherence of the epithelium (see RCE syndrome, vide supra) can be assured of prevention but the ones having EBMD or generalized disadherence should not be given 100% assurance. This is because the current technique of PTK treats only the 6 mm optical zone. The **pancorneal ablation** technique by Kremer and Blumenthal has shown 100% prevention of recurrent erosions.

2. Similarly in eyes with *bullous keratopathy* the primary concern is relief of pain.
3. Many patients of *band keratopathy* are concerned about vision but all are disabled by pain and glare. The later symptoms are taken care of by PTK in all patients but visual acuity may not improve upto the satisfaction because of the primary disease or failure to clear the calcific band due to resistance to ablation.
4. Patients of *corneal dystrophies* may have symptoms of erosions in addition to decreased visual acuity and would expect an improvement in both. A probable assurance regarding visual outcome may be given after assessing the type, depth, etc. of the pathology and other prognostic factors (vide supra) but prevention of erosions may not be always guaranteed. Table 11.1 gives the functional goals which are aimed at in different conditions.

PREOPERATIVE REFRACTIVE ERROR OF THE PATIENT

The main undesired effect most often faced after PTK is that of induced refractive changes which may be significant in certain eyes. A myopic eye is the ideal situation for PTK, as ablation of the optical zone of the cornea causes flattening. Though a *hyperopic shift* is the commonest refractive change, occasionally myopic shift or irregular astigmatism may also occur. These are discussed under *complications* and *refractive changes*. The patient should be told about these and the possible need for corrective glasses or contact lenses. Therefore he/she should be ready to accept them.

EVALUATION OF THE RISKS AND BENEFITS TO THE PATIENT

A large data on PTK research points towards high degree of safety of the technique (vide supra) in comparison to any other available surgical technique. The results are also far superior to those achieved after any other surgical or conservative management. The only problem faced is that of change in the refraction. *Majority of the patients experience a shift in the refraction towards hyperopia.* If the preoperative refraction of the patient is hyperopic and the required ablation is deep, it is better to think again before this case is taken for PTK. It would be of more concern if it is known that the postoperative hyperopia would not be acceptable to the patient.

Therefore, if the corneal thickness permits, there are no major contraindications for healing, no predisposition to keratitis and glaucomatous damage, nothing is lost if PTK is performed after discussing with the patient in detail. But of course 100% guarantee as regards to safety cannot be given, as is true for any other major or minor procedure on the eye.

PREOPERATIVE INTRAOCULAR PRESSURE

The preoperative intraocular pressure measurement is important not only from the glaucoma point of view but also because of the fact that the postoperative management requires use of topical steroids for a long period to prevent the development of corneal haze. Topical steroids are known to produce iatrogenic glaucoma, therefore this parameter needs a constant supervision throughout the follow up period. Table 12.1 summarizes the parameters to be evaluated before PTK.

Table 12.1: Parameters to be evaluated for PTK

Preoperative Evaluation

1. UCVA and BCVA (Snellen's)
2. Comprehensive slit-lamp biomicroscopy
3. Depth of lesion: Haag-Striet
   Optical Pachymetry
4. Keratometry
5. Central corneal thickness:
   * Ultrasound pachymetry
   * Orbscan pachymetry
   * Haag-Striet pachymetry
6. Schirmer test and tear-film Break–up time (BUT)
7. Corneal topography
8. Direct and indirect ophthalmoscopy
9. IOP: applanation (where ever possible)
10. Corneal sensations
11. Distribution of the corneal pathology

Chapter 13

PRK and PTK: Pretreatment of the Surface

For procedures involving surface ablation of the cornea like excimer laser PRK and PTK, the corneal surface needs removal of the epithelium to save laser energy and for smoother ablation. The opinion on this issue differs among different surgeons.

In case of LASIK, wavefront-giuded LASIK and LASEK, the epithelium is not debrided because the ablation is done on stromal bed after raising a partial thickness corneal flap or an epithelial flap in the latter case.

PRETREATMENT FOR PRK PROCEDURE

Epithelial Debridement

Some researchers feel that the epithelium should be removed in case of smooth surface before performing refractive excimer laser ablation. This is suggested for following two reasons.

1. To decrease the energy needed for ablating the required amount of tissue.
2. Because the differential ablation rate of epithelium, nuclei and cytoplasm might lead to uneven stromal ablation.

Methods of Epithelial Debridement

Whenever required, the following methods can be used for removal of the epithelium:

1. Mechanical removal
2. Removal with excimer laser
3. Isopropyl alcohol removal

Mechanical Removal of the Epithelium

Mechanical removal of the epithelium may be done using one of the following instruments.

1. A blunt spatula
2. An iris repositor
3. Number 15 Bard-Parker blade
4. The 'Pallikaris circular nylon brush', which has automated rotatory movements. This removes the epithelium quickly and neatly.

The following points are to be noted when employing the mechanical method of epithelium removal.

1. The area of epithelial debridement is 1 mm more than the desired ablation zone diameter.
2. The time taken for the epithelial removal should not be > 2 minutes to avoid stromal tissue dehydration.
3. Blunt instruments are ideal for epithelial removal but they may take longer time (from 1-2 minutes).
4. The sharp instruments complete the debridement faster but have the risk of producing an uneven and rough surface, leading to irregular ablated surface in the end.
5. The removal is done from the periphery of the demarked zone to avoid unnecessary removal of

the epithelium that occurs during the opposite process.
6. The debris is cleaned with a dry cellulose sponge. No fluid is used to remove it because this will result in tissue overhydration leading to decrease in ablation rate and undercorrection.
7. The central epithelium or pieces of epithelium should not be left in the central part till the end. This would result in this area becoming more hydrated that may predispose to central steep island formation.

Removal with the Excimer Laser

The epithelium removal with the excimer laser is done in the *plano mode*, the depth of ablation set at about 50–60 micron. The end point of epithelial removal is marked by the cessation of the *blue fluorescence* produced by ablation of this tissue, which is visible in the dark room.

Diadvantages of laser epithelial removal

1. The end-point of epithelium removal may be difficult to determine visually.
2. If the epithelium is thinner than the preset ablation, ablation of the stroma would also occur and result in overcorrection.
3. If the epithelium is thicker, undercorrection may result.

Alternatively the ablation depth for the laser removal may be set at 40 micron and supplemented by mechanical removal of the remaining epithelium.

Advantages of laser epithelial removal

1. The centration problem is decreased because any decentration in ablation is detected during the ablation of the epithelium before the refractive ablation begins.
2. Postoperative pain may be less and healing time reduced because the area of de-epithelization is less.
3. The laser removal does not apply any mechanical pressure and is of advantage in cases of post-PK treatment.

Isopropyl Alcohol Removal

The use of *70% isopropyl alcohol* applied for 30 seconds to 2 minutes has been employed for epithelial removal. It causes an increased inflammatory response and has *damaging effect* on keratocytes. A lower concentration of 18% with application time of about 20 seconds has been used to mitigate this problem.

Studies have shown that epithelial removal with low concentrations of alcohal results in a smoother stromal surface in comparison to mechanical removal[7-11]. This would help in achieving a more regular ablated surface and improved visual results after refractive surface ablation like PRK and customized-PRK.

Transepithelial Ablation

Others have suggested that transepithelial ablation through the intact epithelium using it as a template has good results. *In cases of retreatment the epithelium acts as a masking agent to smooth the underlying irregular stromal surface.*

Transepithelial ablation utilizes a modified algorithm for PRK. Slight overcorrection and higher incidence of the central steep islands may occur with the transepithelial approach but no statistically significant difference has been reported in comparison to cases where the epithelium is removed before commencing the refractive ablation.

DURING PTK PROCEDURE

Smooth Surface

In case of smooth anterior surface, the epithelium can be removed either mechanically or with the excimer laser. One of the methods of mechanical epithelial removal given above may be utilized.

During the laser epithelium removal the epithelium is left intact and only the debris and cellular remnants are removed with a wet cellulose sponge. The epithelium is removed with excimer laser with the the 'plano-mode' before ablating the Bowman's layer and corneal stroma.

Irregular Surface

In case of PTK, when anterior stromal surface is irregular, the epithelium in situ acts as a smoothing agent and is not removed. In such case, some surgeons advocate *removal* of the epithelium manually *only over focal corneal excrescences* and leaving it in situ in the depressed areas, to help prevent excessive ablation around the lesion.

Suggested readings

1. Gimbel HV, De Broff BM, Beldavs RA et at: Comparison of laser and manual removal of corneal epithelium: J Ref Surg 1995; 11: 36-41.
2. Johnson DG, Kezirian GM et al: Removal of corneal epithelium with PTK technique during Multizone multipass PRK. J Refract Surg 1998; 14(1): 34-38.
3. Campos M, Nietsen S, Szerenyi K et al: Clinical follow-up of PTK for treatment of corneal opacities, Am J Ophthalmol 1993; 115: 433-440.
4. Chamon W, Azar DT et at:, PTK: Ophthalmol Clin North Am 1993; 6: 399-413.
5. Campos M, Nielsen S, Szerenyi K et al: Clinical follow-up of PTK for treatment of corneal opacities. Am J Ophthalmol 1993; 115: 443-440.
6. Sher NA, Bowers RA, Zabel RW et al: Clinical use of 193-nm excimer laser in the treatment of corneal scars. Arch Ophthalmol 1991; 109: 491-498.
7. Vinay B. Agrawal et al: Alcohol vs. mechanical epithelial debridement before excimer laser surgery. J Cata Ref Surg 1997; 23: 1153-1159.
8. Jenkins L: A comparison between the use of 18% alcohol and simple scraping for epithelial debridement. Propceedings of the Third Annual UK International Ophthalmic Excimer Laser Congress. Eye News 1996; 3(2): Suppl 7-8.
9. Carones F, Fiore T, Brancato R: Mechanical vs. alcohol epithelial removal during photorefractive keratectomy. J Ref Surg 1998; 15: 556-562.
10. Shah S, Doyle SJ, Chatterjee A et al: Comparison of 18% ethanol and mechanical debridement for epithelial removal before PRK. J Ref Surg 1998; 14 (Suppl): S212-S214.
11. Zhao J, Nagasaki T, Maurice DM: Role of tears in keratocyte loss after epithelial removal in mouse cornea. Invest Ophthalmol Vis Sci 2001; 42: 1743-1749.

Chapter 14

PTK: Treatment Strategies

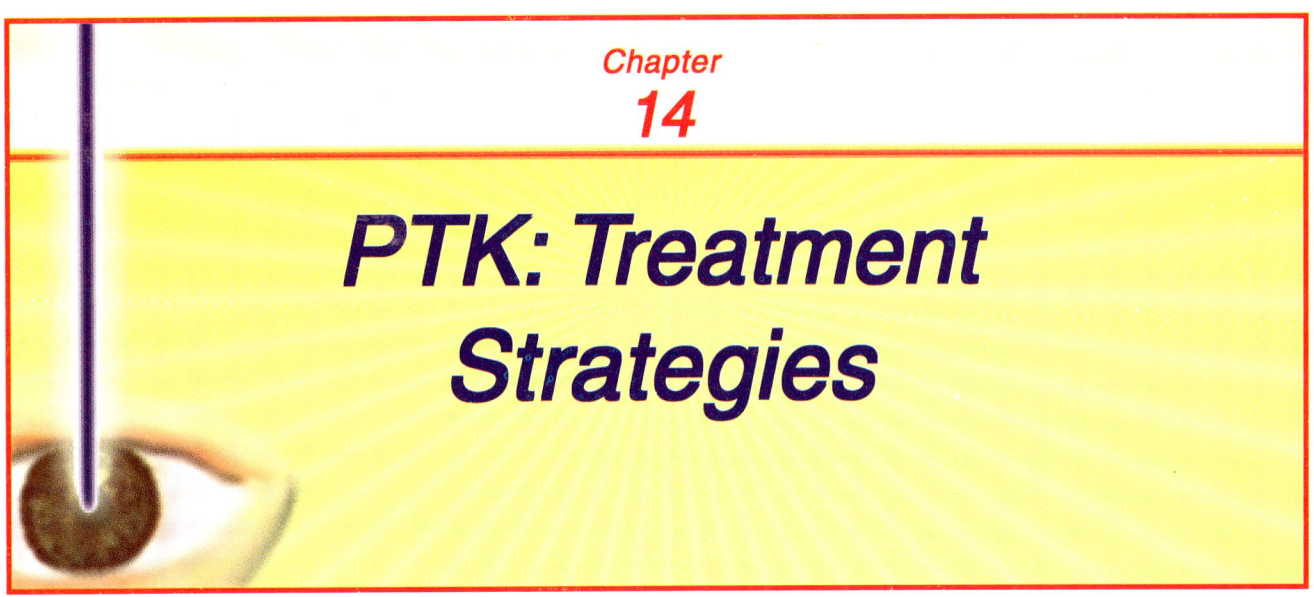

TREATMENT OF IRREGULAR SURFACE

In case of phototherapeutic, keratectomy if the irregular surface is ablated as such, the resultant surface would be a *true replica of the original contour*. This is because:

1. The laser beam ablates an area of at least 1-2 mm for spot scanning and larger in case of a large beam system. It acts equally on the tissue within this area and hence would remove same amount of tissue from the raised as well as the depressed sites.

2. The diseased cornea has different pathological tissues. They have different ablation rates and hence would be removed up to different depths with the same number of laser pulses. The *result would not be a smooth surface, which is an important objective of PTK*.

3. *Raised lesions, scarred tissue* and *calcium* require the surrounding cornea to be protected while removing these lesion using the excimer laser. In the latter cases, scar and calcium deposits have low ablation rates and require more number of laser pulses for their removal.

During the *'extra treatment'* of these lesions, those having a low ablation rate (e.g. *calcium*), an appropriate agent should *shield the surrounding tissue* while the irregularity if still being removed (Fig. 14.1 and 14.2).

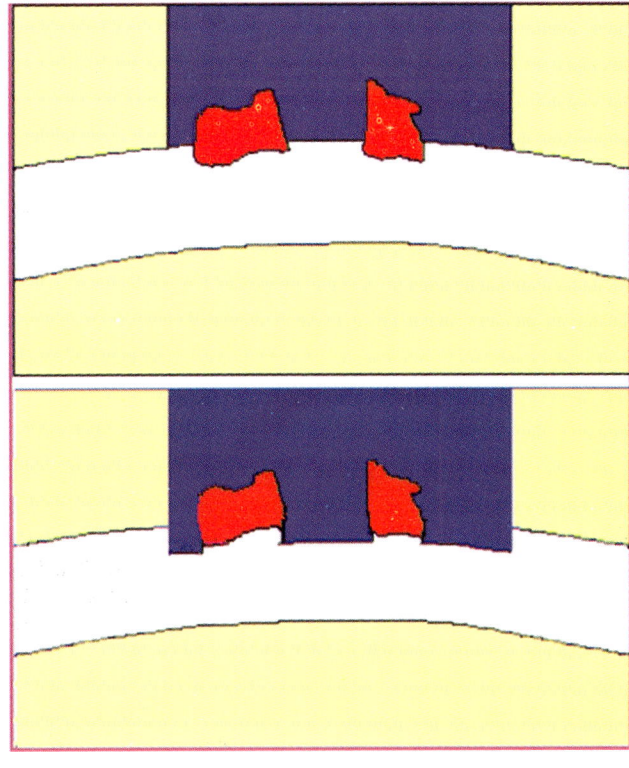

Fig. 14.1: Ablation of 'calcium deposits' with excimer laser without the use of a masking fluid. Corneal tissue has higher ablation rate as compared to calcium and is removed early by laser while the lesion remains unablated.

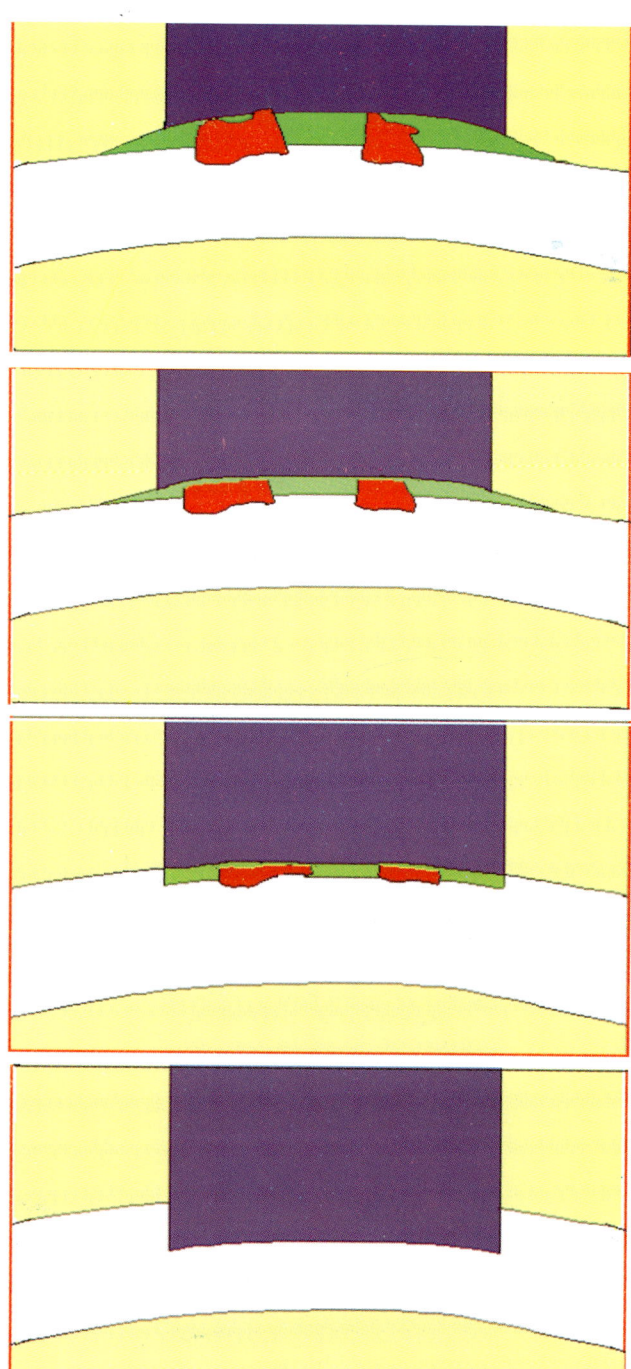

Fig. 14.2: Use of a suitable masking agent ensures that the normal corneal tissue is shielded from the laser action, while the 'calcium deposits' are being removed by the excimer laser. The result is an optically smooth surface after excimer laser ablation.

MASKING AGENTS/WETTING AGENTS/ COUPLING FLUIDS

These are substances that are used in case of surface irregularities to fill up the **valley's** and keep the **peaks** exposed during ablation and thus help in achieving smooth corneal surface after ablation (Fig. 14.3). An ideal masking agent should have the following properties.

1. It should have the same ablation rate as that of the corneal tissue.

    If its ablation rate is more, it would need frequent applications.

2. It should have optimum viscosity and surface tension.

    a. A low viscosity substance runs off and pools up towards the periphery of the curved surface.
    b. Those having high viscosity/surface tension:
       i. Do not have *good contour-following*.
       ii. May not fill deeper part of the irregularity.
       iii. May also coat the elevations, thus negating the purpose of the masking agent.
       iv. May form droplets on the surface.
           The end result in these above situations (a and b) is an irregular surface after ablation.

3. It should be non-toxic to the corneal tissue.

COMPARISON OF DIFFERENT MASKING AGENTS

Kornmehl and colleagues, in a study of various masking fluids, compared the effect of 0.3% hydroxypropyl methyl cellulose (HPMC) with 0.1% *Dextran-70*; 1% *carboxymethyl cellulose*, 0.9% *saline* and *no masking fluid*; and found that:

1. Use of HPMC and Dextran 70 results in smoothest ablation
2. No masking fluid or 0.9% saline produce most severe surface irregularities.
3. The effect of 1% carboxymethyl cellulose is in between.

Hydroxypropyl Methyl Cellulose (HPMC)

1. Lower viscosity HPMC

HPMC of lower viscosity than 1% would run off the surface easily and would not achieve the effect of the masking agent.

Fasano et al reported that 0.3% HPMC used as masking agent produces smoother ablations as compared to no masking agent. They also suggested a slower repetition rate to allow time for the valleys to be filled and to give the operator time for intraoperative adjustments.

2. One percent HPMC

Gartry and colleagues are of the view that 1% HPMC is a better masking agent than 2% HPMC because of :
a. Low viscosity.
b. The ease to fill up the valleys.
c. Similar ablation rate as the corneal tissue.

But it tends to run off towards the periphery, which could cause lesser ablation at the periphery. To prevent the meniscus effect of 1% HPMC, the edge should be blotted with cellulose sponge.

Moreover, 1% HPMC is *not a suitable agent in case of* irregularity formed by inclusions such as *calcium*, which have lower ablation rate than the corneal tissue and 1% HPMC, thus making the use of masking agent futile. *Adjustable shields* are recommended for such cases.

3. Two percent HPMC

Two percent HPMC is too viscous to properly fill the valleys and it might stay on the peaks also. Hence it is not an ideal masking agent.

Polyvinyl Alcohol

Use of polyvinyl alcohol as a masking fluid has been found to give similar effect as that of 2% HPMC.

The 'Biomask'

Scott et al used the 'BioMask'—a mixture of cross-linked and non cross-linked porcine collagen, as a masking agent. They found it to be a good masking agent for PTK.

PTK: ABLATION TECHNIQUES

In a case of phototherapeutic keratectomy, the treatment strategies are decided depending upon the following:

1. Type of pathology
2. Distribution of the pathology
3. Refractive status of the eye
4. Associated change in corneal sensation
5. Functional need of the patient

Depending upon these considerations, one of the following treatment strategies may be used:

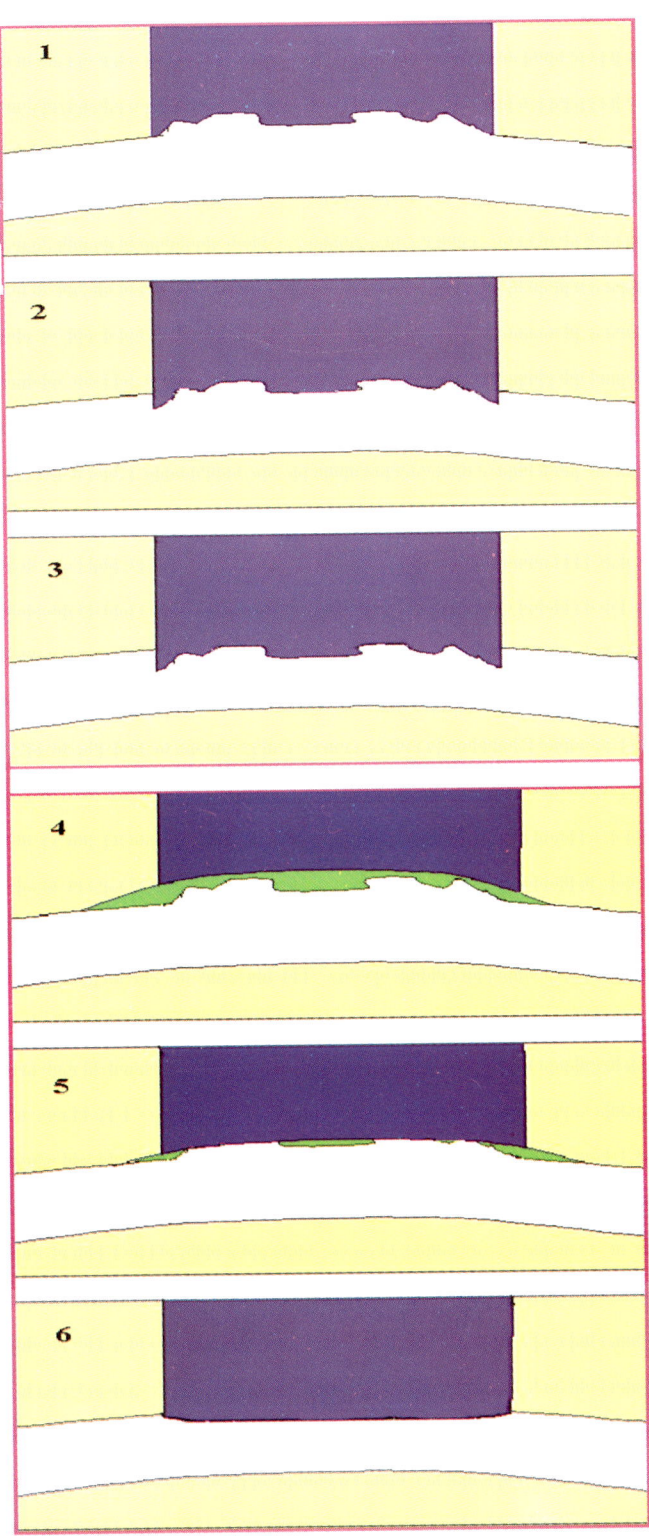

Fig. 14.3: Ablation without (top three figures) and with (lower three figures) the use of a masking agent. Use of a suitable masking agent makes sure that the laser does not reach the depressed areas until the elevations are completely removed. This results in a smooth surface after ablation.

1. Large area photoablation
2. Manual superficial keratectomy combined with large area PTK
3. Focal smoothening
4. Basement membrane ablation
5. Pan-corneal ablation

LARGE AREA PHOTOABLATION

The most common ablation pattern used for removal of superficial corneal pathologies is *large area ablation.* This is because mostly the conditions requiring PTK, such as degenerations, dystrophies, corneal irregularities (pathological or iatrogenic), are *diffuse or complete in distribution.*

It involves treatment of central *6 mm optical zone* of the cornea that would be *sufficient to clear the visual axis.* The edge of a zone smaller than this is likely to fall within the pupillary area *under the scotopic conditions,* which may cause disturbing glare and halos during night driving.

Various *developments* have taken place in the technique of PTK laser delivery to the eye over the past years. All the efforts are *to avoid the hyperopic shift,* which is the most common and the only disturbing undesired outcome bothering the surgeons. Following account deals with six types of large area ablation techniques.

Point and Shoot Technique

Previously used technique for PTK, in which the eye was stationary could be described as point and shoot technique. A large beam laser was used. It resulted in an abrupt edge at which increased epithelial hyperplasia and corneal fibrosis resulted. Decreased energy at the periphery (derby shape) further increased this problem (Fig. 7.4). The results were significant hyperopic change and unacceptable corneal scarring at the periphery.

Standard Taper Technique (Stark and Chamon)

In this technique, a 0.5 mm transition zone is created between the normal and the ablated stromal surface as a **default setting.** This is achieved by delivering few laser pulses after increasing the iris aperture at the end of the ablation.

This technique, again is not successful in producing a smooth transition at the edge and uniform re-epithelization. Therefor it is unable to avoid the problem of hyperopia.

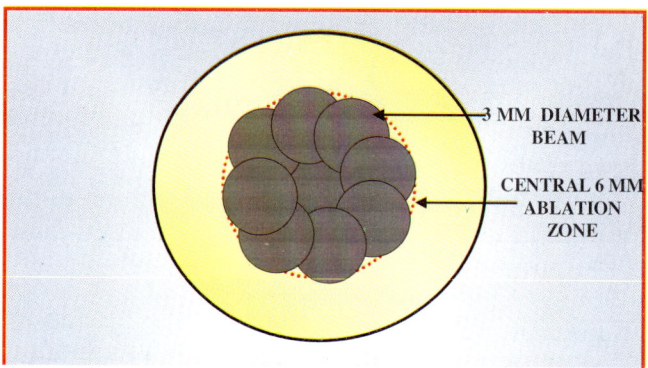

Fig. 14.4: Overlapping zone ablation. Creation of such patterns during full treatment would produce an irregular surface

Modified Taper Technique (Stark and Chamon)

In this technique described by the same authors, a ring shaped ablation pattern at the periphery of the ablated zone is created. This results in a corneal contour simulating a convex surface (lens).

During this procedure, the eye is moved in a circular fashion so that the *circumference of the ablation zone is treated with a 20 µm deep, 2 mm diameter spot size* of beam. They reported that use the of this technique induced less hyperopia as compared to the standard taper technique.

This type of taper can be easily carried by the scanning laser beam systems which are in common use these days.

Smoothening Technique

In an attempt to create a smooth transition zone, *Sher and colleagues* had used a smoothing technique in which the 'eye' was moved in a circular manner *under the large beam ablation* to avoid the sharp transition zone.

This technique was abandoned because the resultant ablation was unpredictable.

Later, the above researchers suggested a technique of *combined ablation* in which they used a *secondary set of pulses* to steepen the peripheral part of the ablated cornea in order to correct the hyperopia, similar to the 'modified taper' technique of Stark and Chamon.

Overlapping Zones vs. Single Zone Ablation

Gartry and colleagues in their report on the results of first series of PTK for superficial corneal pathologies, reported that the use of overlapping ablation zones

(Figs 7.2 and 14.4) resulted in irregular astigmatism. They recommended use of large single axial zone of ablation.

Polishing Technique

This technique was suggested by *Dannial* and colleagues, while reporting the results of FDA trial study for PTK. The patient's 'head' was held by the surgeon and moved in a brisk controlled circular manner in order to polish the corneal surface. This is similar to the smoothing technique of Neil Sher.

MANUAL SUPERFICIAL KERATECTOMY COMBINED WITH LARGE AREA PTK

There are a number of clinical situations where superficial keratectomy should be combined with excimer laser photoablation. This approach facilitates the ablation in a number of ways.

1. It *de-bulks* the pathological tissue and thereby saves the laser energy and hastens the procedure.
2. The pathological tissue may be resistant to excimer laser ablation. Continued attempt to remove such tissue by laser would result in the formation of deep gutters into the surrounding corneal tissue (e.g. raised scars, calcium plaques). After manually removing such tissue, the troughs created in the stroma can be filled by a masking fluid and ablation is then carried on to smoothen the surface.
3. Some disorders are conventionally amenable to the surgical blade. Here the laser ablation is aimed to provide a perfect, optically clear and smooth surface (e.g. pterygium, nodules).

Removal of calcium thoroughly by chelating agents before laser ablation in case of BSK is another example of a *combined manual and laser treatment.*

The following corneal conditions are some of the examples where this combined treatment approach need to be employed:

1. Salzmann's nodules
2. Keratoconic nodules (without significant corneal thinning)
3. Spheroidal degeneration
4. Band keratopathy
5. Pterygium
6. Superficial dense scar

FOCAL LASER SMOOTHENING

If the corneal pathology is focal in distribution, one may not opt to treat the entire 6 mm optical zone by deep ablation. This would otherwise mean removing the surrounding corneal tissue in an attempt to remove the focal lesion, which would lead to avoidable change in refraction after the the ablation.

The strategy employed here is different. The focal lesion is first de-bulked by superficial keratectomy. Then a small laser beam is used to smoothen the surface focally, while the surrounding normal corneal tissue is protected from being ablated with the help of a masking agent. It is to be noted that this type of treatment is not suitable in case the lesion is deep seated because the focal ablated area would cause irregular astigmatism. It is best reserved for focal, superficial, raised lesions, e.g.

1. Salzmann's nodule
2. Keratoconic nodule
3. Some focal corneal opacities
4. Focal irregularities.

The *aim of this treatment is not to remove the entire lesion*, but to smoothen the corneal surface which would then have better optical properties in comparison to the untreated one. Nevertheless, in some cases one may also decide to give some more laser pulses, as in large area PTK; if it so appears that this would lead to complete removal of the lesion.

BASEMENT MEMBRANE ABLATION

For the treatment of cases of '*corneal erosion syndrome*', a different treatment strategy is to be followed because of the follwing reasons.

1. Most of these cases *do not require deeper ablation* as the abnormality is located above the Bowman's layer. Since the superficial ablation does not *ablate the stromal tissue*, it avoids the postoperative stromal haze as well as hyperopia associated with deeper ablation.
2. The epithelium can be removed manually which further considerably reduce the laser ablation.
3. Some cases of corneal erosions secondary to corneal dystrophies may need further ablation for associated opacity.

Different studies have employed different treatment protocols for 'basement membrane ablation' which can be divided into following two broad groups.

1. **Focal ablation:** The ablation is restricted to the affected zone of corneal epithelium
2. **Diffuse ablation:** It involves treating the entire surface of Bowman's layer

Focal Ablation

This is carried in the following manner.

1. Focal ablation with intact epithelium: A focal ablation of 40 micron was done over the intact epithelium in case there was no actual erosion present.

2. Focal ablation of the corneal area with erosions (1–5 micron) with direct 30–40 micron deep ablation of the immediately surrounding loose epithelium (in case of localized erosions secondary to superficial microtrauma).

3. Focal 5–7 micron ablation after removal of the loose epithelium.

The recurrence rate of erosions with the above strategy is in the range of 20–30 percent. A similar number of cases are not relieved of their symptoms after the focal ablation PTK. Therefore this technique does not enjoy much favour.

Diffuse Ablation

Two approaches have been utilized for the 'diffuse ablation technique' for recurrent corneal erosions. These are:

1. Diffuse ablaton by simple PTK-mode
2. Combined PTK and PRK technique

Diffuse Ablation by the PTK-mode (Kaplan-Messas)

First total epithelium removal up to the limbus is done. Then the basement membrane is ablated up to a depth of 5–7 microns, from the entire treatment zone surface using the PTK- mode. No recurrence has been reported by the authors up to a mean follow up of 9 months after the *diffuse PTK* technique.

The Combined PRK and PTK Approach

This combined PTK and PRK approach is also called "pancorneal ablation". The pancorneal ablation technique of Kremer and Blumenthal has been described in the next section.

PANCORNEAL ABLATION (Kremer-Blumenthal)

This method reported by *Kremer* and *Blumenthal* from Israel treats the whole corneal surface rather than only the central 6 mm zone. It was utilized for treating cases of *recalcitrant corneal erosions* who were *myopic*. They used *combined PRK and PTK* in the following manner (Fig.14.5).

1. The epithelium was removed up to the limbal zone
2. The central 6 mm optical zone was treated by **PRK-mode** for correcting the spherical and astigmatic components of the preoperative refractive error. The depth of ablation varied on the degree of correction required.
3. The peripheral 3 mm wide zone was treated by **PTK-mode** using 3 mm circular laser beam. Confluent laser spots were applied around the previously treated central zone to ablate up to a depth of 6 micron (up to the surface of the Bowman's membrane).

The rationale behind this 'diffuse pancorneal ablation' is that *recalcitrant cases* of corneal erosions are due to diffuse abnormality of adhesion complexes, although it may manifest as localized erosions. *Therefore it is crucial to treat the entire corneal surface to avoid future recurrences.* In fact they achieved 100% relief of symptoms and 100% prevention of recurrences after a long follow up of their 16 cases (26–42 months). Good *adhesion complexes* are formed after about one and a half year.

Going by the same ideology, even when treating cases of 'recurrent erosion syndrome' who are not myopic, it is wise to follow the same approach of pancorneal ablation. Of course the treatment strategy would change; the central 6 mm zone would not require 'refractive ablation' in this situation. *The entire corneal surface may well be treated in PTK mode.*

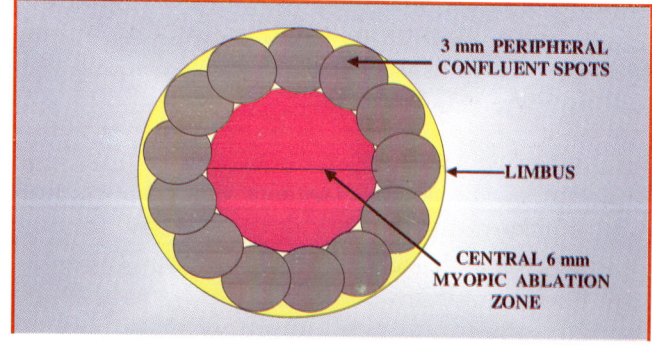

Fig. 14.5: Pancoreal ablation

Suggested readings

1. Kornmehl EW, Steinert RF, Puliafito CA: A comparative study of masking fluids for excimer laser PTK. Arch Ophthalmol 1991; 109: 860-863.
2. Kremer I, Blumenthal M: Combined PRK and PTK in myopic patients with recurrent corneal erosions. BJO 1997; 81 (7): 551-554.
3. Fasano AP, Moreira H, McDonnell PJ et al: Excimer laser smoothing of a reproducible model of anterior corneal surface irregularity, Ophthalmology 1991; 98: 1782-1785.
4. Gartry D, Kerr Muir M, Marshall J: Excimer laser treatment of corneal surface pathology a laboratory and clinical study. Br J Ophthal 1991; 75: 258-69.
5. Stark JW, Chamon W, Kamp MT et al: Clinical follow-up of 193 nm ArF excimer laser photokeratectomy. Ophthalmol 1992; 99: 805-811.
6. Stark JW Chamon W, Azar DT et al: Photo therapeutic keratectomy. Ophthalmol Clin North Am 1993; 399-413.
7. Sher NA, Bowers RA, Zabel RW et al: Clinical use of 193-nm excimer laser in the treatment of corneal scars. Arch Ophthalmol 1991; 109: 491-498.
8. Scott X, Stevens MMD et al: The BioMask for treatment of corneal surface irregularity with excimer laser PTK. Cornea 1999; 18(2) : 155-163.
9. Gallo JP, Raizman MD: PTK for superficial corneal disorders. Int Ophthal Clin 1997; 37: 155-170.

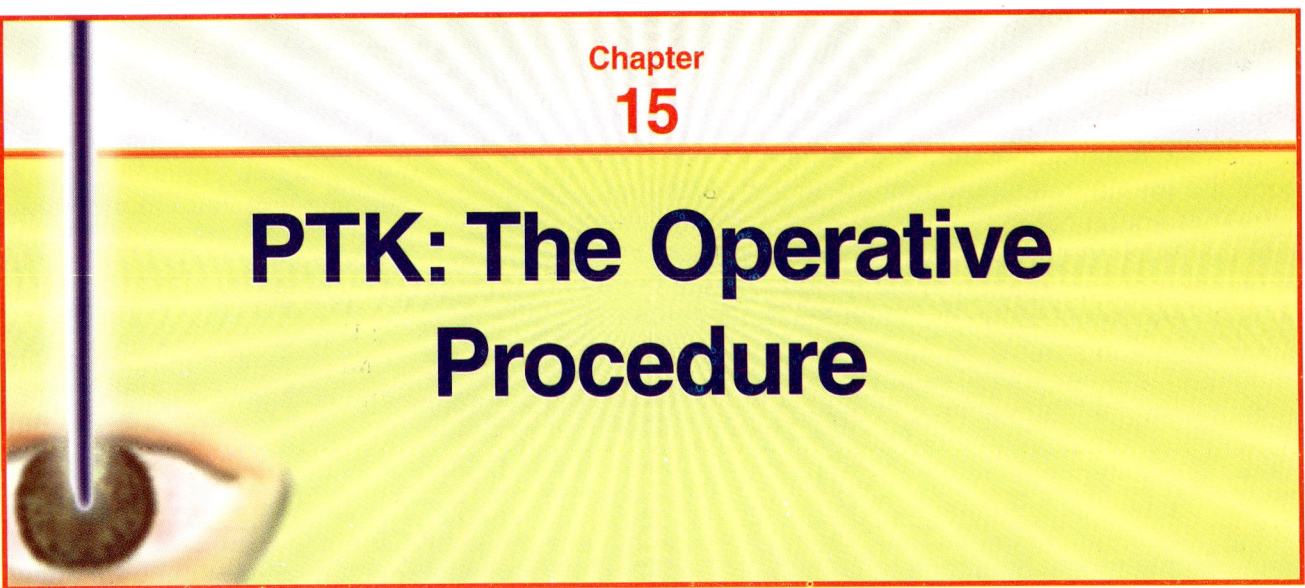

Chapter 15

PTK: The Operative Procedure

PREOPERATIVE CONSIDERATIONS

Like any other corneal surgery, the procedure is carried out in the sterile operating conditions. In addition, the laser system requires the operating room to be air conditioned with proper temperature (15-25° Celsius), humidity (<50%) and suspended particle control.

To avoid the postoperative pain, *premedication* with systemic analgesic and sedative is to be given. *Prophylactic broad-spectrum antibiotic* eye drops are started 1-2days before the procedure. *Oral acyclovir* 400 mg four times daily is also started one day in advance and continued for 10 days, if a herpetic etiology is suspected. This is to avoid recurrence of herpes keratitis.

The patient is explained in detail about the corneal disorders, the available treatment options and the probable outcome of those treatment modalities including the possible complications. Then a written consent to undergo the excimer laser procedure is obtained from the patient. The patient is also made aware of the peculiar sound and some smell like that of burning flesh. This ensures that the patient does not get suddenly alarmed during the procedure.

The patient wears a sterile gown and a cap, while the surgeon undergoes the usual strict rituals followed for other surgeries. The patient washes the face and eyelids with soap and water before entering operating room. An assistant cleans the eye with 5% povidone-iodine solution thoroughly. A broad-spectrum antibiotic drop and local anesthetic drops are instilled and the eye is draped. Other eye is patched to facilitate fixation of the eye undergoing laser ablation. A wire-speculum is put and the patient is instructed to look into the fixating light. The centration of eye is checked. The illumination of the microscope is reduced. This decreases the glare and ensures good fixation by the patient.

The laser system, all electrical connections and other required equipment are checked. The gases in the laser system are checked and the laser output is calibrated to ensure smooth delivery of the laser during the procedure. Data is fed into the computer with regard to the following information.

1. The patient's particulars.
2. Type of ablation—myopic, hyperopic or plano (for PTK)
3. The preoperative central corneal thickness
4. The preoperative refractive error (for refractive correction)
5. The intended depth of ablation /depth of corneal pathology (for PTK)

INTRAOPERATIVE CONSIDERATIONS

Pretreatment of the Surface

Necrosed epithelium, surface plaque and scars, which may significantly alter ablation parameter because of their different ablation rates are removed manually using a blunt instrument.

The normal epithelium is be removed in case of smooth corneal pathologies, but left in-situ in case of irregular pathologies to acts as a masking agent. The removal is carried out manually using an iris-repositor or number 15 Bard Parker blade. The removal is done from the central 7 mm area in case of 6 mm ablation zone.

For LASIK surgery, no surface treatment/epithelial removal is required. In fact, an intact epithelium on the corneal surface is the key for early visual recovery after LASIK.

Centration of the Laser Beam

The eye is draped and an eye speculum is applied. The patient is instructed to look into the fixation light. Centration of the coaxial light is done either by centering upon the center of pupil or by utilizing the **Purkinje-Sanson image** before removal of the epithelium, whose presence helps in its formation. The eye tracker is activated after centration of the light of the microscope. Since the laser beam has the same path as the co-axial light of the microscope, its centration follows automatically.

The centration is crucial for a uniform ablation around the visual axis. The *decentration of the ablation zone or off-axis ablation would result in iatrogenic astigmatism*, which may be troublesome.

In case of 'focal smoothening' of a localized lesion, the surgeon may decide to ablate a particular area more. This may be done by switching the eye tracker off and maneuvering the patient's head.

Method of Centration

The method of utilizing the Purkinje-Sanson image for the purpose of centration of the laser beam should be *discouraged*. This image lies about 4 mm behind the anterior corneal surface and is therefore subject to parallax. This may result in centration error. Moreover many a times the corneal disease or the opacity interfere in proper visualization of this image.

Using the center of the entrance pupil is the best method for centration. This is done by providing a *fixation target* which is *co-axial* with the laser beam and microscope light, assuming that the visual axis and the center of the pupil roughly correspond.

It has been suggested that sighting monocularly, via the eye piece which is coaxial with the fixation target, is best for centration, because by using stereoscopic visualization only 50% of the surgeons were found to site the centration point in one study (*Vozoto and Guyton et al*).

Pilocarpine should not be used to constrict the pupil because it may lead to *pharmacologically induced shift of the pupil.*

Laser Ablation

PTK is carried out using one of the strategies discussed previously *(vide supra)*.

The strategy to be used in a particular case should be carefully worked out beforehand after taking several things into consideration.

The intended *depth of plano* (nonrefractive) *ablation* is fed into the computer, which than decides the number of laser pulses to be delivered. For example, in a case of recurrent corneal erosions, in which the epithelium is removed manually, the intended depth of ablation is about 5–7 microns. For diffuse lesions, the depth of the lesion as assessed by the Haag-Striet pachymeter is the expected depth of ablation.

For lesions with complete distribution, *where the depth is difficult to be assessed*, an arbitrary depth of ablation is taken as 100 microns.

Number of Laser Pulses

For *focal laser*, where *spot mode* is used, the approximate number of laser pulses to be delivered may be worked out by the following formula.

$$\text{Number of laser pulses} = [\text{Height of lesion/Depth}] \times \frac{1}{\text{Ablation Rate}}$$

For a laser system delivering 180 mJ/cm^2 and having an approximate ablation rate of 0.25 μ, this multiplication factor is 4. *But this multiplication factor is not same for other systems having different energy irradiance and hence different ablation rates.* For example, a laser system that has an output about 120 mJ/cm^2 and ablation rate about 0.125 μ, therefore would require more number of laser pulses (approx. double).

For a *scanning/flying* mode of delivery, the number of laser pulses are worked out by the software of the computer based on the ablation rate, diameter of the ablation zone and the desired ablation depth. *Such calculation cannot be done by simple mathematics because the pulses overlap during the scanning.*

Masking Fluid

A suitable masking agent is used during the ablation procedure as discussed in the previous chapter.

Intraoperative Hydration and Removal of Ablation By-products

The ablation rate depends on tissue hydration. Dehydration of the tissue lead to deeper (increased) ablation of the tissue and greater refractive changes for given number of laser pulses. On the other hand excessive use of a fluid (e.g. BSS) leads to shielding effect for the laser energy.

The ablation by-products, which are constantly being ejected out as the ablation proceeds, are also to be removed constantly from the corneal surface. Accumulation of these by-products not only would shield the laser energy but also lead to surface irregularity due to uneven ablation. The incidence of **central steep islands** also increases, if the ablation by-products are not removed at a constant rate, since they tend to accumulate centrally.

Nitrogen Gas-blowing for Removal of Ablation By-products

Historically, earlier scientists had *'used nitrogen gas blowing'* during PRK and PTK to remove the by-products. This caused tissue dehydration resulting in:

1. Increase in ablation rate and hence decreased predictability and variability of refractive outcome.
2. More incidence of corneal haze.
3. Greater roughening of the corneal surface.
4. Detrimental effect on *pseudomembrane* formation, which has a protective effect for the ablated stroma and cells and prevents water entry into the lamellae.

This practice of intraoperative use of nitrogen gas blowing was soon abandoned and is no more in use.

Use of Humidified Air

The use of humidified air during ablation results in dense, finer and continuous pseudomembrane and less corneal haze. It also effectively removes the ablation by products. Therefore it is recommended to use *gas blowing provided it is a humidified one*, to keep the cornea hydrated as well as for removing the ablation by-products.

Use of Cellulose Sponge

Another method commonly employed now is gentle removal of the ablation by–products by a sponge intermittently during the ablation procedure.

Use of Few Drops of BSS (Balanced Salt Solution)

Intermittent use of one drop of BSS during ablation along with the use of the above cellulose sponge procedure works more efficiently to keep proper corneal hydration as well for removing the by–products.

End Point of Treatment

To determine the end point of treatment, the *Shoot and check technique or intraoperative biomicroscopical evaluation* is employed. *This is essential to avoid any overtreatment.* This approach requires to stop the ablation in between and to make an assessment on the slit-lamp as to how much more ablation is needed. Such assessment might have to be done more than once in some cases.

The idea is "not to undertreat the corneal lesion" but to perform minimum tissue ablation just sufficient to remove the lesion or smoothen the surface. This step is essential to:

1. Minimize the refractive change which is more if the depth of ablation is more.
2. Keep the option open for any future treatment by conserving the corneal tissue. Retreatment may be needed, for example, in case of recurrence of a dystrophy or if the corneal clarity is not satisfactory due to any reason.

Points for Successful PTK Treatment

Partial Ablation

Deeper lesions may benefit by excimer laser ablation without removing them completely in the following situations:

1. If the *densest* part of the opacity is located superficially.
2. If the main aim of the ablation is to achieve a smooth surface or to relieve the symptoms of pain, glare, etc. as in a case of band keratopathy.

Paraxial Lesions

Any *'isolated deep paraxial treatment'* is contraindicated to avoid irregular astigmatism.

If the Major Component of Paraxial Lesion is above the Surface

If a lesion located in the paraxial zone is causing irregular astigmatism and needs treatment (e.g. Salzmann's nodule), this can be best achieved by *masking* the normal cornea and treating the focal lesion with a small diameter beam. At the end of treatment, it is also desirable to give minimum ablation to the central 6 mm area after removing the epithelium manually to provide a smooth central surface with good optical function.

If the Paraxial Lesion is Deep but has a Component Extending to the Axial Zone

Such opacities (e.g. following pterygium surgery) can be best treated by **on-axis** ablation to clear the central 6 mm optical zone. Any remaining paraxial component may be ignored.

Avoiding the Hyperopic Shift

The periphery of the ablated zone is to be treated to 'even out' the sharp edge between the ablated and non ablated area. This *'sharp transition' causes flattening* of the optical zone. *Epithelial hyperplasia at the sharp transition edge further aggravates this change.*

Tapering of this sharp edge can be achieved by ablating the 1.5-2 mm peripheral transition zone with about 50-100 additional laser pulses. This may be done in the following ways:

1. By the *modified taper technique* described earlier. The 1.5 mm to 2 mm laser spots may be delivered to the peripheral area by moving the patient's eye in a controlled manner as described by Stark and Chamon. The delivery of the laser spots can be visualized by the secondary fluorescence produced by the ablation. But the manipulation of the eye is seldom accurate to produce a smooth and uniform annulus.
2. The computer may be provided with a software to deliver the additional pulses to the periphery at the end of the ablation.
3. A 4.5 mm contact lens, a sterile filter paper or 2% HPMC or more viscous substance may be used to shield the central cornea and an additional 50-100 laser pulses delivered in the usual 6 mm zone treatment strategy. This would ablate only the peripheral unshielded circular area.
3. Using secondary hyperopic photorefractive excimer laser keratectomy (PRK).

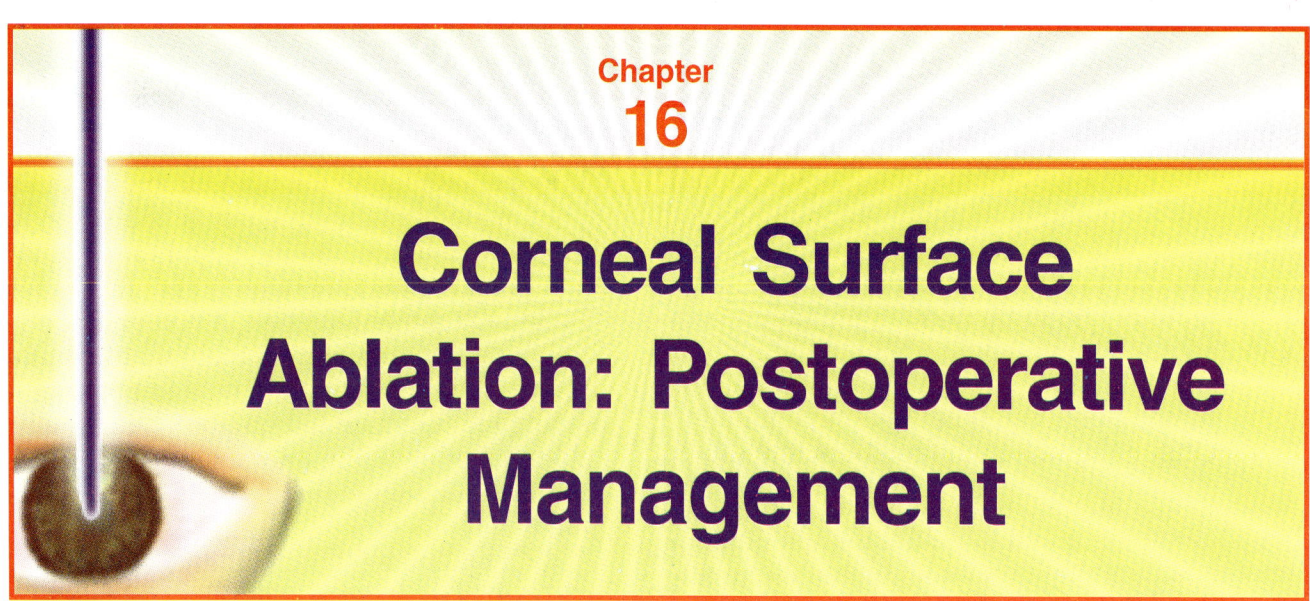

Chapter 16
Corneal Surface Ablation: Postoperative Management

The postoperative care after excimer laser corneal surgery is as crucial for successful results as the preoperative selection of the cases.

The following account pertains, in particular to corneal surface ablation, e.g. PTK and PRK, though the general management and the *pharmacological modulation* of refractive outcome apply to all excimer laser surgeries.

Keratorefractive surgeries where the corneal surface is not violated, e.g. LASIK, wavefront LASIK and LASEK, need to be cared in a different way because of the intact surface, special care of the corneal flap related aspects and virtually absence of postoperative pain and corneal haze.

If the ablated corneal surface is not properly cared, it may turn out to be irregular with epithelial healing abnormalities. The cornea may develop *haze* or even an *opacity* as a result of unwanted *abnormal healing response*. Last but not the least, disaster may strike in the form of *infectious keratitis* in a poorly managed case because the *surface is raw* for many days.

Therefore the postoperative care revolves around the following:

1. Postoperative pain
2. Epithelization of the ablated corneal surface
3. Prophylaxis against infectious keratitis
4. Minimizing the postoperative inflammation and corneal haze
5. Minimizing the hyperopic shift through pharmacological modulation in case of PTK.
6. Minimizing the regression of the effect through pharmacological modulation in case of refractive surgery.

POST OPERATIVE PAIN

Post-ablation pain is common and prominent feature during first 12–36 hours after corneal *surface ablation*. It is quite severe in some cases and might require systemic analgesics and/or sedatives. Following medications are used for the management of postoperative pain.

Topical NSAIDs

Most surgeons, find use of topical nonsteroidal anti-inflammatory agents such as *diclofenac sodium or ketorolac*, to be sufficiently effective in controlling the postoperative pain.

1. *Philips and Szerenyi et al* showed that there is a rapid and sustained increase in PGE_2 following excimer laser photoablation in comparison to mechanical keratectomy. The PGE_2 response is significantly decreased by diclofenac. This paved the way for the use of systemic NSAIDs also for post-ablation pain in the eye.

    Another finding was that *diclofenac sodium*, used topically, *reduces corneal sensitivity*.

2. Local *anesthetic effect* of topical diclofenac sodium has also been reported by Zaidman *et al* after excimer laser corneal ablation.
3. Use of diclofenac has not been found to exacerbate acute Herpetic keratitis or prolong shedding of virus, unlike corticosteroids.
4. Many other also have reported that diclofenac sodium, topically applied, reduced post–excimer laser treatment discomfort and pain.
5. *Ekdhal and Stein* reported analgesic effect with topical ketorolac trimethamine 0.5% after excimer laser photoablation of the cornea.

Topical *indomethacin* has not been found to have any significant analgesic activity in the eye.

Topical Steroids

Independent studies by Eiferman et al and Sher et al showed that steroids have no significant effect in reduction of pain. These researchers treated one eye with fluromethalone 0.1%, cycloplegic and contact lens and other with the same regimen plus diclofenac sodium 0.1% after PRK photoablation of both eyes.

They found markedly less pain in the eye having diclofenac treatment.

Topical NSAID have less adverse effect on corneal epithelial healing after excimer laser ablation as compared to topical steroids.

EPITHELIZATION OF THE ABLATED SURFACE

Rapid and adequate covering by a healthy epithelium is not only highly desirable but also essential because of the following reasons:

1. For a quick visual recovery, the corneal surface must normalize as soon as possible.
2. Excimer laser ablation leaves behind a raw surface open for a number of pathological insults. The cornea needs to be protected during this period of recovery.
3. Even if no infection takes place, *inflammation and abnormal healing* would leave behind various grades of opacities and uneven surface which would nullify the very objective of the surgery.
4. An intact corneal surface is required not only in cases of recurrent erosions but in all cases of PTK to avoid complications arising because of persistent epithelial defects.

Management of the Ablated Surface

Bandage Contact Lenses

The use of the bandage soft contact lenses is contraindicated because of the following reasons:

1. They predispose to infectious keratitis
2. Patients who are given contact lenses *must be examined daily* on the slit-lamp.
3. Use of *NSAIDs and contact lens* following excimer laser ablation of cornea has been shown to cause the formation of *sterile stromal infiltrates*. These cause acute pain, redness, lacrimation, ring-like opacities and even stromal melting (see under *complications* for details).
4. Patients undergoing PTK in this part of the world are found be of poor hygiene and low socio-economic background who cannot be expected to maintain a good lens hygiene.
5. Its presence *gives a feeling of pseudo- security to the surgeon* as well as to the patient.
6. Moreover the patient might ignore its presence and come back only because of the complication.

Eye Patching

The application of a pad and bandage for 24–48 hours is advocated by most surgeons. But the epithelium does not regenerate to cover the whole surface (6 mm wide area) within this period*. Practically it is found to take about one week. It is, therefore imperative to continue the eye patching till the complete re-epithelization. Topical medication needs to be continued throughout this period of eye patching.

This is the procedure which was followed during our PTK study (*vide infra*). The patient was given an eye patch after careful cleaning of the lid and periocular area with betadine very frequently during the early postoperative days. Slit-lamp examination was done to look for remaining epithelial defect, any infiltration, etc. Antibiotic drops, topical NSAID and lubricating drops were instilled at intervals and an eye patch was given.

The patient's relative was instructed as to how to instill the prescribed topical medications by gently lifting the eye patch on the inner canthal side without removing

---

*The healing response of the epithelium in response to wounding begins after 5 hours. Cellular migration from the edges is at the rate of 60-80 micron/hour. (Smolin G: *The cornea*, third edi: page 31)

it. Patients who were unable to follow this and had persistent epithelial defect were given sub-conjunctival injection of gentamycin and dexamethasone and reviewed after 24-48 hours. None of the patients following this regime developed any complication relating to healing or infection.

There are different opinions about the use of antibiotics like ciprofloxacin, NSAIDs and steroids in the immediate postoperative period due to differing reports of their effect on epithelial healing. The first two should be used as a must to prevent an infection and inflammation respectively.

The steroids might have to be added early depending on the severity of inflammation (see below).

Use of diclofenac sodium 0.1% has not been shown to delay corneal re-epithelization following excimer laser photoablation in rabbit model.

Srinivasan reported that topical NSAID have less adverse effect on corneal epithelial healing after excimer laser ablation as compared to topical steroids.

Hanna et al reported that early use of topical steroids in the presence of large epithelial defect might lead to delayed epithelial healing.

POSTOPERATIVE INFLAMMATION AND CORNEAL HAZE

Postoperative inflammation and development of corneal haze is *invariable after corneal surface ablation* such as PTK and PRK. This results due to healing response and the ensuing stromal remodeling *(vide supra)*. It jeopardizes the visual results and needs to be controlled. Following agents are used for the management of postoperative inflammation and haze.

Topical Steroids and Corneal Haze

Research has documented the role of topical steroids in reducing corneal haze after excimer laser photoablation in rabbit model. This is due to the effect of steroids on stromal remodeling. The use of steroids causes reduction in fibroblast proliferation, decrease in new collagen and proteoglycan matrix formation which are responsible for appearance of corneal haze.

Retrospective clinical studies by many surgeons (e.g. *Tuft SJ, Zabel and Marshall, Zabel & Tuft, Seiler, Sher et al, Cubert E,* etc.) have documented the beneficial effect of topical steroids in reducing corneal haze following excimer laser photoablation of the cornea. It is also felt that no use or early discontinuation of topical steroids is associated with significant corneal haze.

Use of topical **fluoromethalone** has been reported to reduce stromal infiltration with polymorphonuclear cells (PMNs) after photoablation of the cornea. The finding is important since the steroids might have to be used for prolonged period because the stromal remodeling may continue for a year or longer (average 6 months). Prolonged use of topical steroids may result in precipitation of glaucoma and cataract formation. Topical fluoromethalone has much lower penetration into the anterior chamber and therefore this is associated with a lower incidence of steroid induced glaucoma and cataract as compared to dexamethasone.

Some recent studies have questioned the beneficial effect of topical steroids and do not advocate routine postoperative use of topical steroids.

Prospective double blind studies by *Gartry, KerrMuir & Marshall and O'Brart & Lohman* have failed to find any conclusive beneficial effect of topical steroids on corneal haze after excimer laser corneal surface ablation. They have suggested the use of **plasmin and plasminogen-activator inhibitors** for prevention of corneal haze due to their effect on stromal remodeling.

Concurrent use of Topical Steroids and NSAIDs

Concurrent use of topical steroids and NSAIDs appears to have more beneficial effect in reducing corneal haze. This effect was more pronounced with flurbiprofen than with diclofenac sodium.

Topical use of NSAID and contact lens without concurrent corticosteroids is found to be associated with development of 'sterile stromal infiltrates'.

Topical NSAIDs Alone

A higher incidence of corneal haze is reported with the use of topical NSAID alone without topical steroids following excimer laser ablation.

Newer Agents

Other newer agents such as **Interferon-alpha-2b** and topical **Mitomycin-C** are also being studied for their role to reduce corneal haze produ photoablation, in addition to **plasn activator inhibitors.**

In a study in rabbit model *Nassrala et al* in 1995 reported that, use of topical diclofenac sodium alone resulted in less corneal haze. Added combination with fluromethalone topically did not result in further decrease in corneal haze.

In spite of the conflicting views, it appears prudent at the present moment, that both, topical fluoromethalone and one of the NSAIDs be used for many months to keep the corneal haze under control. Frequent monitoring of intraocular pressure and the degree of the corneal haze itself should be taken into consideration to modify/decide about discontinuing such treatment.

PROPHYLAXIS AGAINST INFECTIOUS KERATITIS

The ablated corneal surface is prone to develop infectious keratitis because it lacks the protective cover of the epithelium and because of any carrier stage of organisms due to bad ocular hygiene of the patient having the corneal disorder. Therefore it is essential to use a broad-spectrum topical antibiotic till the re-epithelization is complete and may be for few more days after it. The eye lids and the periocular area also should be frequently cleaned with betadine postoperatively.

MINIMIZING THE UNDESIRABLE REFRACTIVE CHANGES

The hyperopic shift after PTK and the regression of effect after PRK are found to be associated with (among other factors discussed elsewhere) *epithelial hyperplasia* and excessive keratocyte response leading to laying down of *extracellular matrix* and synthesis of new collagen (type III) over the ablated stromal surface. These changes are associated with corneal haze and refractive change.

The thickness of this new collagen increases with deeper amount of ablation. PRK involves deeper ablation of the central zone as compared to the periphery, thereby leading to increased healing through exaggerated keratocyte activity centrally. This is thought to be one of the factors responsible for decrease in corneal flattening effect leading to regression/myopic shift, seen more frequently with greater amount of attempted correction.

The *'plano'* ablation in PTK without tapering the edge causes a similar effect in the periphery of the ablated zone leading to the hyperopic shift. The exaggerated epithelial hyperplasia in the periphery of the ablation zone in response to the abrupt edge effect also contributes to the corneal flattening and hyperopic shift after PTK. This hypothesis is proven by the fact that the hyperopic shift decreases significantly with *tapering off* of the edge of the ablation zone.

Pharmacological modulation of the stromal healing response by the postoperative use of topical steroids, NSAIDs and other agents on long term basis has been shown to minimize these refractive changes by many clinical studies.

The use of topical steroids avoid the regression of myopia and maintains a hyperopic shift. Their discontinuation results in loss of this effect that had been previously achieved in many patients of PRK on this therapy. The steroids achieve this effect by:

1. Decreasing the fibroblastic activity and laying down of the extracellular matrix and new collagen.
2. Controlling the stromal remodelling.
3. Inhibiting the *hyaluronan* expression by epithelial and stromal cells. The hyaluronan is a high molecular weight disaccharide polymer that draws water and increases corneal hydration and thickness. This mechanism is thought to cause delayed regression after PRK.

TOPICAL ANESTHETICS

Experimental studies on *healing of corneal epithelial defects* have shown that only topical *piperocaine* 2% and *lidocaine* 2% are found to *allow normal regeneration* of the epithelium. Tetracaine 0.5% delays healing slightly. Oxybuprocaine 0.4%, butacainesulphate 2%, cocaine 4%, dibucaine 0.1%, proxymetacaine 0.5% and phenacaine 1%—all cause impaired healing of the corneal epithelium.

Repeated instillation of benoxinate, lidocaine or tetracaine can result in loss of microvilli and disruption of plasma membrane of the epithelial cells. This is seen as stippling of the cornea on slit-lamp examination. Proxymetacaine can cause severe immediate hypersensitivity type of allergic reaction, with acute intense epithelial keratitis.

Suggested readings

1. Aquavella J, Gasset A, Dohlmann C: Corticosteroids in corneal wound healing. Am J Ophthalmol 1964; 58: 621-626.
2. Arshinoff S, D'Addario D, Sadler C, et at: Use of topical nonsteroidal anti-inflammatory drugs in excimer laser PRK. J Cataract Refrat Surg 1994; 20 (Suppl): 216-22.
3. Corbett MC, O'Brart DPS, Marshall J: Do topical steroids have a role following excimer laser photorefractive keratectomy? J Refrac Surg 1995; 11: 380-7.

4. Caubert E: Cause of sub-epithelial corneal haze over 18 months after photorefractive keratectomy for myopia. Refract Corneal Surg 1993; 9 (Suppl): S65-S70.
5. Epstein RL, Laurence EP et al: Relative effectiveness of topical ketorolac and topical diclofenac on discomfort after radial keratotomy. J Cataract Refract Surg 1995; 21: 156-9.
6. Fitzsimmons T, Fagerholm P, Harfstrand A et al: Steroids after excimer surgery decrease corneal hydraulic acid content. Invest Ophthalmol Vis Sci 1992; 33 (Suppl): 766.
7. Gartry Ds, Kerr Muir MG, Marshall J: The effect of topical corticosteroids on refraction and corneal haze following excimer laser treatment of myopia: an update. A prospective, randomized, double masked study. Eye 1993; 7: 584-90.
8. Gartry DS, Kerr Muir M, Marshall J: Excimer laser photorefractive keratectomy: 18 month follow-up. Ophthalmology 1992; 8: 1209-1219.
9. Gartry D, Kerr-Muir M, Lohmann C et al: The effect of topical corticosteroids on refractive outcome and corneal haze after photorefractive keratectomy. Arch Ophthalmology 1992; 110: 944-952.
10. Gebhardt B, Salmeron B, McDonald M: Effect of excimer laser on energy growth potential of corneal keratocytes. Cornea 1990; 9: 250-210.
11. Harr D, PRK: No pain, major gain. Ocular Surgery News 1992; 12: 73-74.
12. Herschel MK, McDonald MB, Ahmed SD et al: Voltaren for treatment of discomfort after excimer ablation. Invest Ophthalmol Vis 8ci 1993; 34 (Suppl): 893.
13. Lohmann CP, Marshall J: Plasmin and plasminogen-activator inhibitors after excimer laser photorefractive keratectomy: new concept in prevention of postoperative myopic regression and haze. Refract Corneal Surg 1993; 9:300-302.
14. Lohmann CP, Obart D, Patmore A et al: Plasmin-inhibitors and plasminogen-activator inhibitors after excimer laser PRK: new concept in prevention of myopic regression and haze. Invest Ophthalmol Vis Sci 1993; 34 (Suppl): 705.
15. Lobmann C, Gartry D, Kerr-Muir M et al: Haze in photorefractive keratectomy: its origins and consequences. Lasers Light Ophthalmol 1991; 4:15-34.
16. Lipner M et al: NSAIDs shown to dramatically cut post-PRK pain. Ocular surgery news 1994; 21: 58-61.
17. Morlet N, Gillies MC, Grouh R et al: Effect of topical interferon-alpha 2b on corneal haze after excimer laser PRK in rabbits. Refract Corneal Surg 1993; 9: 443-51.
18. McGhee GNJ et al: Pharmacokinetics of Ophthalmic corticosteroids. Br J Ophthalmol 1992; 11: 681-4.
19. Nassaralla SA et al: Effect of diclofenac on corneal haze after PRK in rabbits. Ophthalmology 1995; 102: 469-74.
20. Szerenyi K, Wang XW, Lee M et al: Topical diclofenac treatment prior to excimer laser photorefractive keratectomy in rabbits. Refract Corneal Surg 1993; 9: 437-42.
21. Srinivasan BD et al: Corneal re-epithelization and anti-inflammatory agents (Review), Transactions of the American Ophthalmology Society 1982; 80: 758-822.
22. Szerenyi K, Sorken K, Garbus JJ et at: Decrease in normal human corneal sensitivity with topical diclofenac sodium. Am J Ophthalmol 1994; 118: 312-5.
23. Stein R, Stein HA. Cheskes A et at: Photorefractive keratectomy and post-operative pain. Am J Ophthalmol 1994; 117: 403-5.
24. Talamo J, Gollamudi S et al: Modulation of corneal wound healing after excimer laser keratomileusis using topical mitomycin C and steroids. Arch Ophthalmol 1991; 109: 1141-1146.
25. Campos M, Abed HM, Mc Donnell PJ: Topical fluorometholone reduces stromal inflammation after PRK. Ophthalmic Surg 1993; 24: 654-657.
26. You X, Zheng X, Bergmanson JPG et al: Manipulation of post-PRK stromal remodelling in rabbit corneas with corticosteroids. Invest Ophthalmom Vis Sci 1994; 35(Suppl): 2015 (abstract).
27. Cerruti S, Traverso CE, Murialdo U et al: The efficacy of topical corticosteroids in reversing the regression of refractive effect after myopic PRK. Invest Ophthalmom Vis Sci 1994; 35(Suppl): 2019 (abstract).
28. Marques EF, Leite EB, Cunha-Vaz JG: Corticosteroids for reversal of myopic regression after PRK. J Ref Surg 1995; 11(Suppl): S302-S308.
29. O' Brart DPS, Lohman CP et al: The effect of topical corticosteroids and plasmin inhibitors on refractive outcome, haze and visual performance after PRK: A prospective, randomized, observer-masked study. Ophthalmology 1994; 101: 1565-1574.
30. Fitzsimmons TD, Fagerholm P et al: Steroid treatment of myopic regression: Acute refractive and topographic changes in excimer PRK patients. Cornea 1993; 12: 358-61.

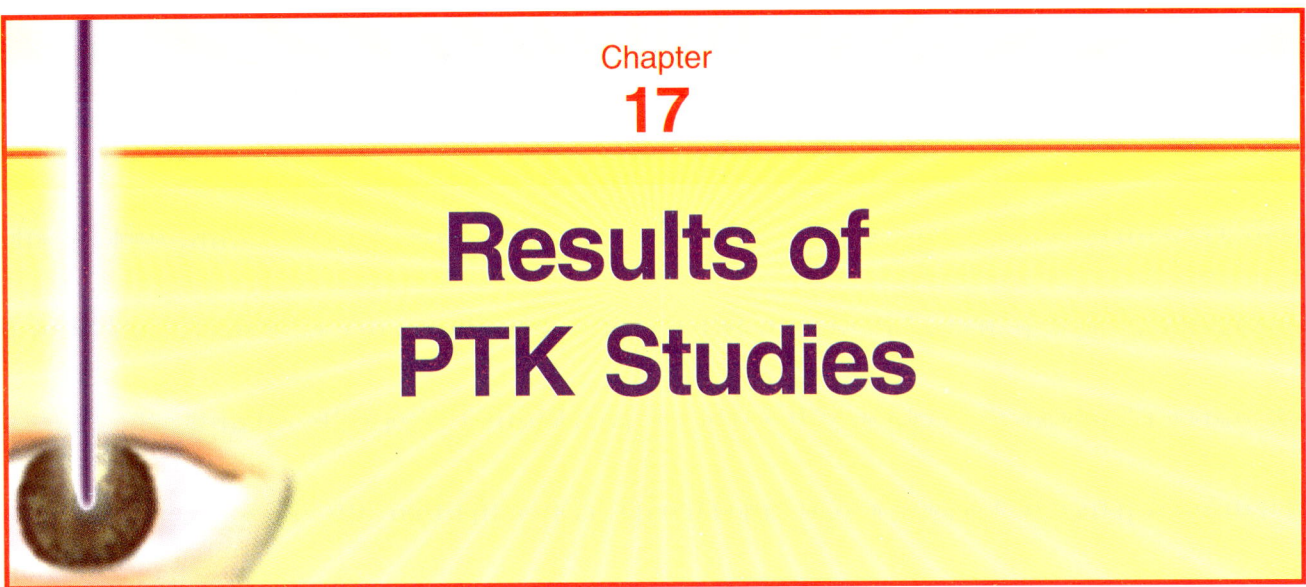

Chapter 17

Results of PTK Studies

INTRODUCTION

A prospective study on efficacy of the PTK for superficial corneal disorders was conducted for the first time in this subcontinent. Review of the literature had reveled only one study from India on PTK at the time of commencement of our study, which was a *retrospective review* of 11 patients of PTK. It was reported by Rao et al from Southern part of India.

No report was available on tear-film changes after PTK in the world literature at the time of commencement of our study. The method of search utilized was through internet using PTK, phototherapeutic keratectomy, excimer laser and tear- film studies as different reference key words. Later, one report on 'ocular surface changes' after PTK was found in the year 2000, published by Dogru et al.

MATERIALS AND METHODS

Goal of the Study

The goals of this prospective study were the following.
1. To improve visual acuity
2. To provide a healthy and intact corneal surface in addition to relief of the ocular symptoms in cases of recurrent corneal erosions.
3. To determine the change in refraction produced by the depth of the corneal ablation with the ArF excimer laser.
4. To study any change in corneal tear-film status subsequent to PTK.

Place of the Study

Our prospective study population included 48 eyes of 26 male and 14 female patients with age ranging from 13 years to 85 years (mean age 49 years, Table 17.1). All the patients underwent 193 nm ArF excimer laser PTK at Dr. Rajendra Prasad Center for Ophthalmic Sciences (RAPCOS), All India Institute of Medical Sciences New Delhi, between March 1999 to July 2000.

Patient: Inclusion and Exclusion Criteria

The inclusion criteria for our prospective study were various corneal pathologies limited to the anterior one third of cornea, interfering with vision and recurrent erosion syndrome. Patients with more than 100 μ deep involvement of the cornea, heavy corneal vascularization dry eye, lagophthalmos, healing disorders, severe blepharitis, uveitis, systemic auto-immune diseases, advanced diabetes, corneal thickness less than 400 μ, any posterior segment pathology, raised intra ocular pressure, immunocompromised status, ocular infections and corneal conditions not causing visual impairment were excluded from the study. Each patient was explained in detail about the risks and benefits of the various treatment options. Unwilling patients were also excluded from the study.

Table 17.1: Patient data

Patient No. Age/Gender	Diagnosis	Pre-PTK UCVA	BCVA	Refraction	Post-PTK UCVA	BCVA	Refraction	Depth of ablation	Change in sphe. equil.	Change in ref. per10 μ
1. 19, M	N.M.CO	6/36	6/18	+2/+4.5 X 35	6/24	6/5	+5.25/+1.50 X 30	33 μ	+2.0 D	+0.6 D
2. 48, M	N.M.CO	6/18	6/12P	+1.0 X 180	6/9	6/5	+1.25/+0.50 X 170	28 μ	+1.0 D	+0.4 D
3. 13, F	R REC COR.EROS.	6/24	6/12	-0.75/-0.5 X 180	6/9	6/5	-0.50 X 180	35 μ	+0.75 D	+0.20 D
4. 13, F	L REC COR.EROS.	6/12	6/6P	-1.0/-0.75 X 140	6/12	6/5	-0.25/-0.50 X 140	50 μ	+0.87 D	+0.17 D
5. 55, F	PTERYGIUM	6/18	6/12	-1.5 X 38	6/6P	6/5P	-0.25/-0.25 X 5	33 μ	+038 D	+0.12 D
6. 50, M	REC. COR. ERO	6/24	6/24	-2 D. SPH	6/12	6/6P	+1.00/-0.50 X 5	26 μ	+2.0 D	+0.76 D
7. 31, F	R BSK (SMOOTH)	6/60	6/24	+0.5/+1.5 X 90	6/24	6/12	+3.75/-4.00 X 180	80 μ	+0.6 D	+0.07 D
8. 31, F	L BSK (SMOOTH)	6/36	6/18P	+1.0/-1.5 X 15	6/18	6/9	+0.75/-1.50 X 50	80 μ	-0.25 D	-0.03 D
9. 18, M	N.M.CO	6/36	6/18	+0.5/+1.25 X 90	6/24	6/9	+150/+1.00 X 80	82 μ	+1.87 D	+0.23 D
10. 50, M	R SPHERO. DEGEN.	3/60	6/60	+3.0/+0.5 X 180	6/36	6/12P	+5.50/+2.00 X 120	92 μ	+3.25 D	+0.35 D
11. 50, M	L SPHERO. DEGEN.	6/36	6/24	+3.0 D SPH	6/24	6/9	+4.5 D SPH	72 μ	+1.50 D	+0.20 D
12. 65, M	BSK+SPH. DEG.	3/60	6/36	+1.5/+2.0 X 9	6/18P	6/12	+2.5/+2.0 X 90	51 μ	+1.00 D	+0.20 D
13. 78, M	REC.CORN. ERO.	6/36	6/18P	+0.25/+1.75 X 180	6/18	6/9	+1.0/+1.5 X 180	25 μ	+0.87 D	+0.35 D
14. 35, M	R BSK (ROUGH)	6/36	6/36	(+4.5/-1.25 X 17)*	6/36	6/18	REF. NOT POSSI.	40 μ		
15. 35, M	L BSK (ROUGH)	6/60	6/60	(+3.75/-0.75 X 117)*	6/36	6/24	+7/-1.5 X 180	35 μ	+2.87 D	+0.82 D
16. 68, F	BSK	6/60	6/24	+7.0/+1.5 X 180	6/36	6/18	+10 D SPH	80 μ	+2.25 D	+0.28 D
17. 30, F	L GRAN.DYSTROPHY	4/60	6/36	-1.5/-1.75 X 180	6/18	6/6	+0.75/-2.5 X 6	87 μ	+1.75 D	+0.20 D
18. 30, F	R GRAN.DYSTROPHY	6/18P	6/12	-1.25/-0.5 X 31	6/18	6/6	+0.5/+1.50X 123	90 μ	+2.75 D	+0.30 D
19. 65, M	L SALZ. NODULES	6/36	6/18	-2.0/-0.75 X 110	6/18	6/12	+1.5/+2.00 X 90	90 μ	+4.87 D	+0.54 D
20. 65, M	R REC. PTERYGIUM	6/60	6/36	-5.75/-1.25 X 63	6/36	6/24				
21. 18, F	L SALZ NODULES	6/60	6/36	-1.75/-3.0 X 37	6/36	6/24	REF. NOT POSSI.	80 μ		
22. 18, F	R SALZ. NODULES	6/18	6/9P	-0.5/-0.75 X 82	6/9	6/6	-0.25/+1.00 X 35	40 μ	+0.87 D	+0.20 D
23. 84, M	R SPHE. DEGENER. BSK (SMOOTH)	6/24	6/18	-0.5/-0.5 X 23	6/24P	6/12	+3.00/-1.00 X 97	50 μ	+3.25 D	+0.65 D
24. 84, M	L BSK (SMOOTH)	6/36	6/36	-1.5/-1.0 X 176	6/24	6/18	+1.75/-2.25 X 3	75 μ	+2.38 D	+0.32 D
25. 22, F	N.M.CO POST HSV FC ½ M	6/36		-17 D SPH	3/60	6/18	-17.5/-0.75 X 100	50 μ	-0.87 D	-0.17 D
26. 63, M	L GRAN. DYSTROPHY	3/60	6/18P	+3.0/+1.0 X 30	6/36	6/18	+5.0/-0.75 X 60	38 μ	+2.38 D	+0.63 D
27. 63, M	R GRAN. DYSTROPHY	6/36	6/24	+2.75/+0.5 X 100	POST	PTK CORN. ULCER				
28. 65, M	N.M.CO POST HSV	4/60	6/24P	+3.0/+0.5 X 15	6/24	6/18	+6.0/-2.00 X 99	40 μ	+1.75 D	+0.40 D
29. 24, M	REC. CORN. EROS.	6/24	6/18	+0.5/+2.5 X 90	6/24	6/12	+2.50 X 90	35 μ	-0.25 D	-0.07 D
30. 72, M	N.M.CO POST HSV	6/24	6/18P	-1.5 X 160	6/18	6/9	-0.25/-1.00 X 170	20 μ	NO CHANGE	
31. 58, F	NM CO	6/36	6/18	+3.75/+0.75 X 40	6/36	6/18	+4.50/+0.75 X 40	86 μ	+1.00 D	+0.13 D
32. 48, M	SALZ. NODULES	3/60	6/24	-1.0 D SPH	6/36	6/18	+2.00/-1.75 X 180	30 μ	+2.00 D	+0.66 D
33. 85, M	SPHE. DEGENER.	4/60	6/24P	-5.5/-2.0 X 94	3/60	6/24	-3.50/-1.25 X 29	60 μ	+2.37 D	+0.39 D
34. 48, M	SALZ. NODULES	6/36	6/18P	+1.5 D SPH	6/36	6/18	+6.00/-2.00 X 90	38 μ	+3.50 D	+0.82 D
35. 28, M	CORN. OPACITY	6/60	6/24	-1.5 X 170	6/18	6/12	+4.50/-1.00 X 90	70 μ	+5.00 D	+0.70 D
36. 24, M	N.M.CO POST HSV FC3M	6/24		+1.0/+2.0 X 110	6/36P	6/18	+5.75/-5.00 X 171	60 μ	+1.25 D	+0.20 D
37. 20, M	CORN. OPACITY	6/60	6/36	-3.0 D SPH	6/18	6/9	-0.75 X 90	65 μ	+2.60 D	+0.40 D
38. 25, M	SALZ. NODULES	6/36	6/24	-1.5/-1.0 X 115	6/24	6/18	-0.5/-5.00 X 171	37 μ	-1.00 D	-0.30 D
39. 68, M	BSK(ROUGH BAND)	6/24	6/18	-1.5/-0.5 X 90	6/18	6/9	+1.0/-0.50 X 110	100 μ	+2.50 D	+0.25 D
40. 53, F	NM CO	4/60	6/60	+0.25/+1.0 X 180	6/60	6/36	+1.0/+1.0 X 90	21 μ	+0.75 D	+0.36 D
41. 60, F	PTERYGIUM	6/60	6/36	+1.00/+1.0 X 180	6/18	6/9	+3.5/-0.75 X 95	55 μ	+1.25 D	+0.23 D
42. 55, F	PTERYGIUM	6/36	6/18	+1.00/-1.50 X 165	6/18	6/6P	+1.25/1.00 X 150	26 μ	+0.50 D	+0.19 D
43. 55, F	N.M.CO POST. HSV FCCF		6/60	-4.59/-1.00 X 50	6/36	6/18	-3.00/-1.00 X 80	40 μ	+1.12 D	+0.28 D
44. 68, M	REC. CORN. EROS.	6/36	6/18	-0.50/-2.75 X	6/18	6/6	-0.25/-1.50 X 90	21 μ	+0.87 D	+0.40 D
45. 60, M	N.M.CO	6/60	6/18	+2.00 D SPH	6/12	6/6	+0.75 D SPH	30 μ	-1.25 D	-0.41 D
46. 70, F	PTERYGIUM SCAR FC1M		6/60	-3.50 D SPH	6/36	6/18	-1.50/-0.50 X 80	50 μ	+1.75 D	+0.35 D
47. 55, F	SPHER. DEGENER. FCCF		FC1M	+1.00 D SPH	FC2M	6/60	+2.00 D SPH	30 μ	+1.00 D	+0.30 D
48. 70, M	GRAN.DYSTROPHY FC2M		6/36	+2.50/-5.50 X 85	6/60	6/24	-0.50/-1.50 X 180	60 μ	-1.20 D	-0.20 D

(* Approximate refraction)

BSK = Band shaped keratopathy
NMCO = Nebulomacular corneal opacity
SALZ. NODULES = Salzman's nodules
REC. CORN. EROS. = Recurrent corneal erosions
SPHER. DEGENER = Spheroidal degeneration
GRAN. DYSTROPHY = Granular dystrophy

HSV = Herpes simplex virus
R = Right eye
L = Left eye
SPHE. EQUIL. = Spherical equivalent
REF. = Refraction
CO = Corneal Opacity

Preoperative Evaluation

A detailed preoperative evaluation was performed in each case which included uncorrected and best corrected Snellen's visual acuity, manifest refraction, central corneal thickness by ultra sonic pachymetry, intra ocular pressure (applanation, wherever possible), keratometry, direct and indirect ophthalmoscopy, corneal topography and evaluation of tear-film status by Schirmer test, tear-film breakup time and Rose -Bengal staining. A detailed slit-lamp examination was done to exclude any associated anterior segment disease. The depth of corneal pathology was measured using a Haag-Striet optical pachymeter. Pre-operative photographs were taken on the slit-lamp.

Preoperative Medication

A broad spectrum antibiotic drop was started one day preoperatively. Patients with suspected history of herpes simplex keratitis, those having decreased corneal sensation or otherwise with known herpetic disease in the past, were started on oral acyclovir 400 mg 4 times a day, started one day in advance and continued for another 9 days post-PTK. This step was taken in view of reports of reactivation of hepetic keratitis in some of such cases if PTK was done without the cover of acyclovir. An oral analgesic tablet such as *diclofenac sodium* or *combiflam* was given an hour before performing the surgery. The procedure was carried out under tropical anesthesia using 0.5% proparacaine.

Equipment and Methods

The ArF excimer laser (Chiron Technolas Keracor 217 C, scanning laser system), was used for ablating the cornea with a scanning mode. The treatment zone was confined to 6 mm central optical area of the cornea. The centration of the laser beam was ensured by asking the patient to fixate on the coaxial light target and by using the eye-tracker.

Manual removal of the epithelium was done in case the corneal surface was irregular and with the laser beam in case of smooth surface. Superficial manual keratectomy was performed to de-bulk nodules raised above the surface. De-bulking the elevated pathology permitted lesser use of the laser energy to smooth the cornea.

A suitable masking agent was used to fill in the valleys on the corneal surface in order to carry out a smoother ablation of the cornea.

In most cases, a *general large area PTK* of the central 6 mm zone was done using the scanning laser beam. In a few cases, *focal laser smoothening* of the elevated lesions was done.

Cases of recurrent corneal erosions were treated by 6 mm zone, 5–7micron *basement membrane ablation* after removing the epithelium manually.

In cases of pterygium, the fibrovascular growth was removed a few days in advance. Excimer laser PTK was done to smooth the optic zone by a general large area ablation. PTK was not combined with manual removal of the pterygium because of the risk of blood interfering in smooth ablation.

In the cases of BSK, the calcium deposits were removed before-hand, as much as possible, with usual EDTA chelation method.

At the end of the central ablation, 50–100 laser pulses (depending upon the ablation depth of the case) were delivered to the periphery to blend the edges of the ablated area.

Intraoperative Assessment

Wherever required, the patient was examined on the slit-lamp after about 75% of the planned ablation had been achieved. Additional ablation was performed, if necessary, to remove the bulk of the pathology from the visual axis. This step is crucial for avoiding over treatment particularly in situations when the depth of the pathology reaches upper limit of the permitted ablation.

POSTOPERATIVE CARE

Follow up Examination

Postoperatively all patients were examined daily for any epithelial defect. After cleaning of the eye with providon idoine, pressure patching was done daily till complete epithelization of the cornea. Subsequently, examinations were done at 1 week, 1month, 2 months, 3 months and 6 months for corneal haze and all other preoperative parameters.

Medication

Patients were given 0.3% ciprofloxacin and tropical NSAID eye drops 4 hourly, and 0.1% fluoromethalone eye drops QID after the epithelization was complete. This treatment was carried on for a period of 2 weeks after which the antibiotic drops were tapered off and stopped after 4 weeks. The steroidal and non-steroidal anti-inflammatory drops were continued 2–3 times for

6 months to minimize corneal haze. Intraocular pressure was carefully monitored at every post-operative visit with applanation tonometry.

RESULTS

Method of Assessing Visual Acuity

The follow-up ranged from 3 months to 12 months (mean 9 months). The preoperative BCVA and cycloplegic refraction were obtained within few days of the surgery. At each follow-up visit, all preoperative parameters were obtained. The Snellen's visual acuity values were converted to log MAR values to obtain the mean pre and post-PTK values. The arithmetic mean of the log MAR values was then re-converted into Snellen's fraction.

Method of Analysis

Wilcoxon's signed rank test was applied for analyzing the significance of change in values. One way analysis of variance (one way AOV) test was used to determine change during follow-up period.

Visual Acuity

The pre and post-PTK Snellen's UCVA and BCVA of the patients are shown in Tables 17.2 and 17.3 respectively.

Table 17.2: Uncorrected Snellen's visual acuity

Visual acuity	Pre-PTK (No. of eyes)	Post-PTK (No. of eyes)			
		1 month	2 month	3 month	6 month
6/6 - 6/9	0	3	3	3	4
6/12-6/18	4	12	13	12	15
6/24-6/60	30	28	28	29	25
<6/60	14	5	4	4	4
Mean	6/60	6/30	6/24p	6/24p	6/24p

Table 17.3: Best corrected visual acuity

Visual acuity	Pre-PTK (No. of eyes)	Post-PTK (No. of eyes)			
		1 month	2 month	3 month	6 month
6/5	0	1	3	4	4
6/6-6/9	1	12	14	16	17
6/12-6/18	14	22	21	19	19
6/24-6/60	32	12	9	8	7
<6/60	1	1	1	1	1
Mean	6/27	6/15	6/15	6/15	6/12

Uncorrected Visual Acuity (UCVA)

None of the patients had pre-operative uncorrected visual acuity in the 6/6 to 6/9 group and only 4 of 48 eyes had 6/12 to 6/18. After PTK 4 eyes had 6/6–6/9 and 15 eyes 6/12–6/18 visual acuity.

The number of eyes having <6/60 uncorrected visual acuity decreased from 14 before PTK to 4 at sixth postoperative month and those with 6/24 to 6/60 UCVA decreased from 30 to 25. The number of eyes having > 6/9 UCVA increased from 1 to 21.

A comparison between pre and six month post- PTK uncorrected visual acuity is shown in Fig. 17.1. The UCVA improved during the first three post operative months. It was apparently unchanged after the third month (Fig. 17.2). The mean uncorrected visual acuity improved from 6/60 before PTK to 6/24p (gain of 2.5 ± 2.2 lines) at sixth postoperative month.

It improved by *2 or more lines* in 62% of the eyes at 1 month, 71 % eyes at second month and 73% of eyes at third and sixth month of follow-up. Loss of >2 lines occurred in one eye (2%) and the UCVA remained unchanged in 6 of the eyes (13%).

A total of 83% eyes experienced gain in UCVA (Table 17.4).

Best Corrected Visual Acuity (BCVA)

The preoperative mean best corrected visual acuity was 6/27. It improved to 6/12 at sixth postoperative month.

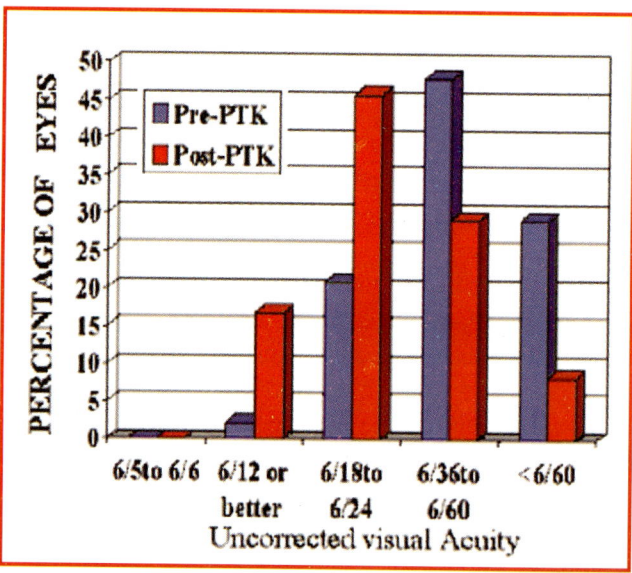

Fig. 17.1: Uncorrected visual acuity pre-PTK (blue bars) and six months after PTK (red bars)

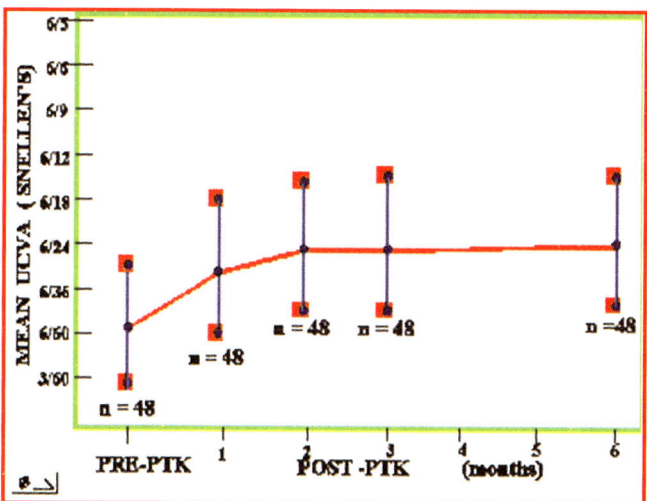

Fig. 17.2: Uncorrected visual acuity pre-PTK and during six months of follow-up; 'n' denotes the number of patients at each time. Points on either side of the mean represents ± one standard deviation.

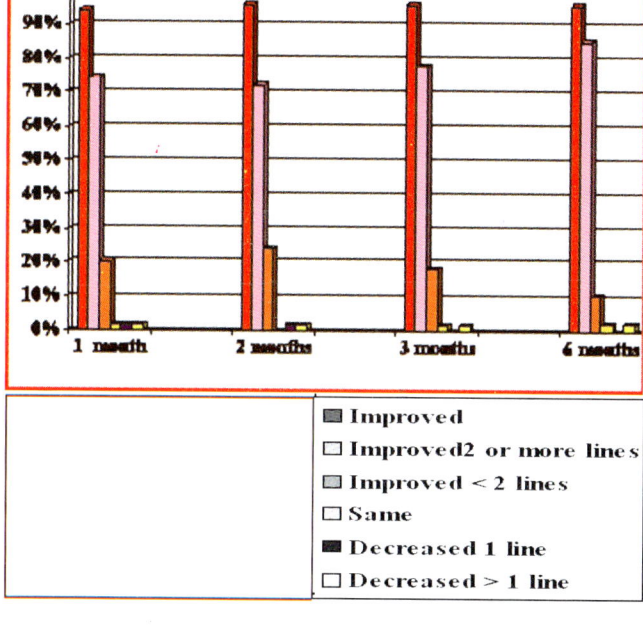

Fig. 17.3: Change in best-corrected visual acuity after PTK from baseline

The *mean change in BCVA* was 2.5 ± 2.4 lines at one month, 2.6 ± 2.4 lines at month two, 2.9 ± 2.4 lines at month three and 3.0 ± 2.5 lines at month six. The change was significant at all post-operative intervals (P= 0.00). A gain of two or more Snellen's lines at sixth post-operative month was achieved in 85% eyes treated by us (Table 17.5 and Fig. 17.3).

Pre-operatively only one eye had 6/9 or better BCVA. Twenty one eyes achieved this level after PTK. Forty eyes (83.5%) were having 6/18 or better BCVA post-operatively as compared to only 14 eyes in this group before PTK. One eye lost vision due to corneal infiltrates and was advised penetrating keratoplasty. Figure 17.4 shows correlation between pre and six month postoperative functional visual acuity. The change in the best corrected visual acuity seemed to stabilize at 3 months as shown in Fig. 17.5.

For *assessing the efficacy of phototherapeutic keratomy in improving visual acuity*, improvement in the UCVA is as important as improvement in the best

Table 17.4: Change in uncorrected visual acuity from baseline

Follow-up Month	No. of eyes	Mean change in Snellen's Lines	SD	Max. Loss of Lines	Maxi. Gain of Lines	Improved			Same	Worsened	
						< 2 Lines	2 or More	Total		< 2 Line	2 or > Line
1 Month	48	1.8	2.4	-6	6.5	10%	62%	72%	15%	0	13%
2 Month	48	2.1	2.1	-6	7	10%	71%	81%	15%	2%	2%
3 Month	48	2.3	2.1	-6	7	10%	73%	83%	13%	2%	2%
6 Month	48	2.5	2.2	-6	7	10%	73%	83%	13%	2%	2%

Table 17.5: Change in best corrected visual acuity from baseline

Follow-up Month	No. of eyes	Mean change in Snellen's Lines	SD	Max. Loss of Lines	Maxi. Gain of Lines	Improved			Same	Worsened	
						< 2 Lines	2 or More	Total		< 2 Line	2 or > Line
1 Month	48	2.5	2.4	-9	7	17%	77%	94%	2%	2%	2%
2 Month	48	2.6	2.4	-9	6.5	19%	75%	94%	2%	2%	2%
3 Month	48	2.9	2.4	-9	6.5	15%	81%	96%	2%	0%	2%
6 Month	48	3.0	2.5	-9	7	11%	85%	96%	2%	0%	2%

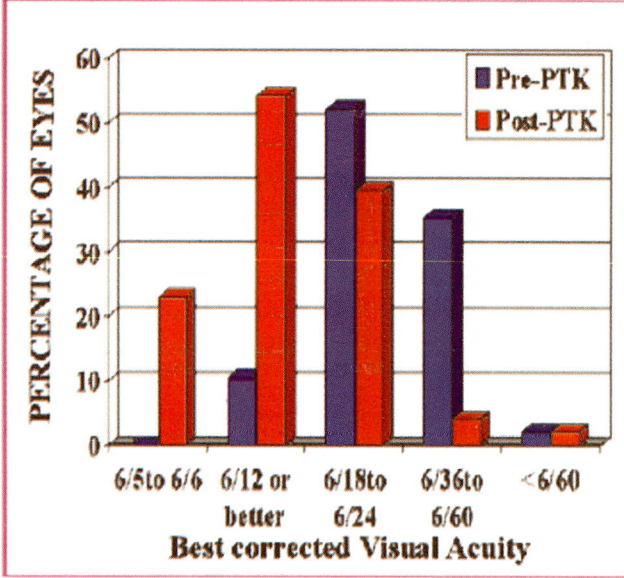

Fig. 17.4: Pre- and postoperative BCVA

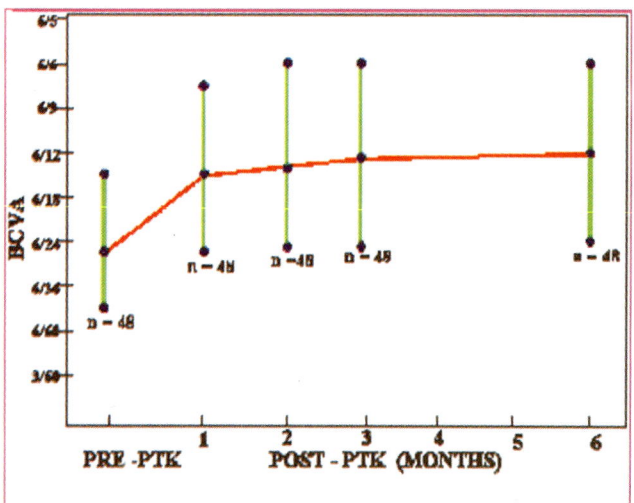

Fig. 17.5: Best-corrected visual acuity pre-PTK and during six months of follow-up; 'n' denotes the number of patients at each time. Points on either side of the mean represents ± one standard deviation

corrected visual acuity, because wide refractive changes do occur after this procedure, thereby causing a decrease in the uncorrected visual acuity.

The procedure is a clear success only when there is a significant improvement in both uncorrected as well as best corrected visual acuity whereas decrease in both means a total treatment failure. An eye with improved best corrected visual acuity but worsened uncorrected visual acuity is to be considered an equivocal result.

In this study we found that the mean uncorrected visual acuity improved at all postoperative intervals till six months (P= 0.00 at all intervals, Wilcoxon signed rank test). Thirty nine of the forty-eight eyes (81%) had improvement in both uncorrected and best corrected visual acuity. One eye worsened in both (patient no. 27). In six eyes (no. 4, 14, 23, 29, 33 and 34) best corrected vision improved but uncorrected vision remained same and one eye (no. 31) did not improve in both. One eye (no. 24) had improvement in BCVA but decrease in UCVA.

Figure 17.6 shows the comparison between pre-operative and six month postoperative uncorrected and best corrected visual acuities respectively.

Change In Refraction

Spherical Equivalent

Pre or post-operative refraction was not possible in 4 eyes. Two eyes (no.14, 15) with BSK had irregular corneal surface pre-operatively. Refraction could be obtained in one of them (no. 15) after surgery. One eye (no. 21) developed irregular corneal surface and other (no. 27) developed corneal opacity after PTK.

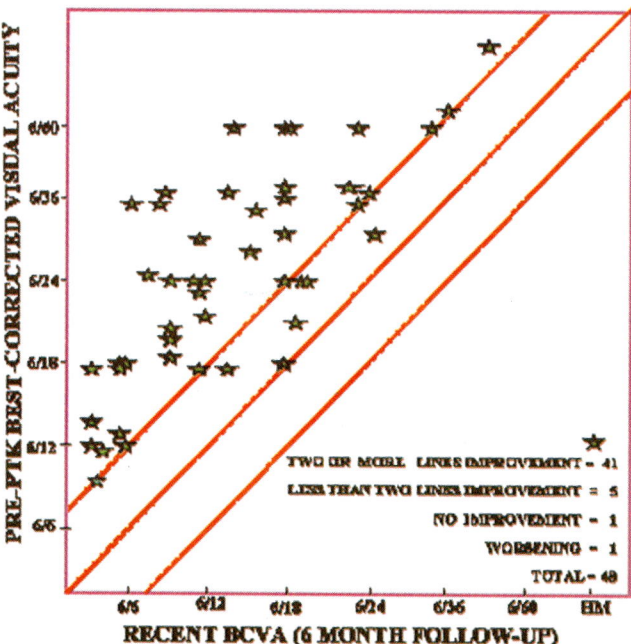

Fig. 17.6: Scatter-gram showing correlation between pre and postoperative uncorrected visual acuity. Values above or below the central line represent improvement or worsening respectively, from the baseline. Diagonal lines above and below the central line represent improvement or worsening by more than 2 lines.

Most patients showed changes in spherical and cylindrical power and shifts in axis of cylinder. Mean pre–and post-operative spherical equivalent was determined for all patients, wherever possible. The mean change in manifest spherical equivalent showed a hyperopic shift of 1.56 ± 1.57 D at 1st post-operative month; 1.48 ± 1.47 D at 2nd month; 1.35 ±1.47 D at the 3rd month and 1.30 ±1.44 D after 6 months (Fig. 17.7).

Thirty six out of 44 eyes, in which refraction could be obtained, experienced *hyperopic shift* (Fig. 17.8). The pre-operative mean spherical equivalent of manifest refraction was 0.33 ± 2.82 diopters. It changed to 2.33 ±3.12D at 1 month; 2.2 ±3.1 D at 2 month; 2.0 ±2.96 at three month; 2.0 ±2.93D at 6 month (range 0.38D to 5.0D).

Seven eyes (no. 8,19,25, 29, 38, 45, 48) showed a mild *myopic shift* in the spherical equivalent. At six month after PTK, it ranged from 0.25D to –1.63D (mean –0.97 D). One eye did not show any change in the spherical equivalent after PTK (no.30).

Fluctuations in refractions occurred during the initial follow up. Although there seemed to be a slight improvement in hyperopia during the first three post-operative months, the overall change was not significant (P=0.43, One way AOY). The refraction became stable after 3 months in most patients (Fig. 17.7).

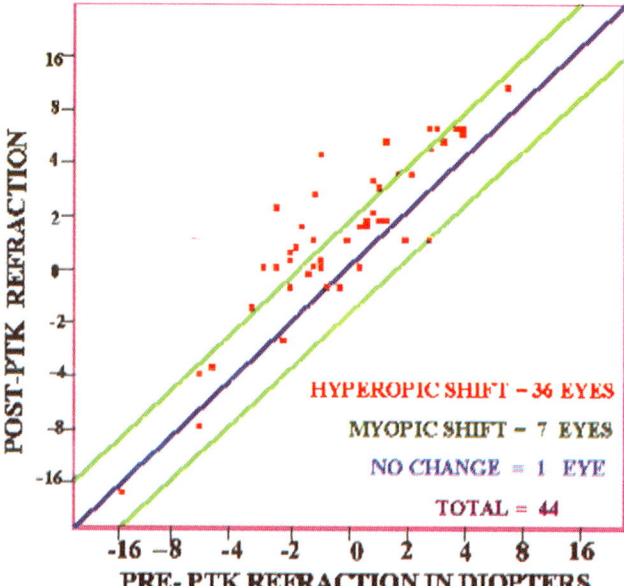

Fig. 17.8: Scatter-gram of manifest refraction (spherical equivalent) before and six month after PTK. Points on the central line represent no change. Points above and below the central diagonal line represent hyperopic and myopic shift respectively. Diagonal line (green) on either side represent change of two diopters

Change in Astigmatism

Change in the astigmatism of manifest refraction was considered without taking the vector change into consideration. Fourteen eyes (32%) had no change in the amount of astigmatism. Thirteen eyes had a mean increase of 1.5 D in astigmatism (range 0.25D to 4 D). Fourteen eyes (32%) had decrease in manifest astigmatism. Three eyes had no cylinder pre–as well as post-operatively. Twenty-two of the 41 eyes having cylindrical power (53.65%) showed change in the axis of cylinder after PTK, from 2° to 80° as compared to pre–PTK cylinder axis.

None of the patients with recurrent corneal erosions had any change in the magnitude or axis of cylinder power.

Change In Keratometry

We could obtain pre as well as post-operative keratometry in 37 of 48 eyes (pre-operative keratometry in 39 and postoperative in 40). In six eyes pre–as well as postoperative keratometry measurements were not possible. In three eyes (no. 10, 11, 21) post-operative keratometry readings became possible but could not be

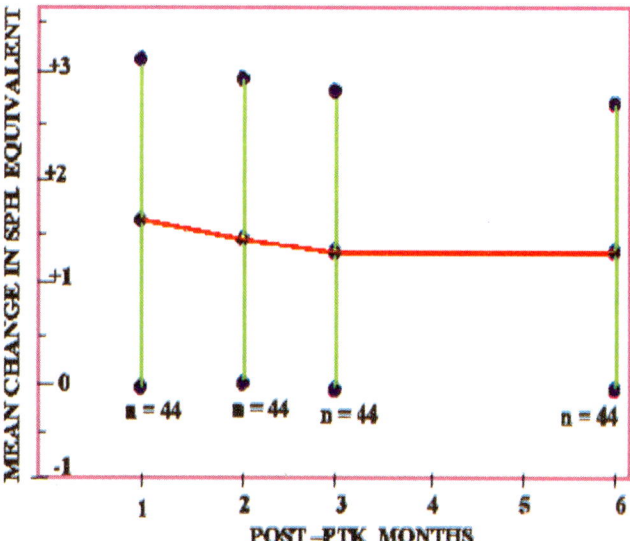

Fig. 17.7: Correlation between change in spherical equivalent and time after surgery. For each time, the change is calculated as the difference between pre- and postoperative spherical equivalent; 'n' denotes the number of patients at each time

obtained in two eyes (no. 27, 33) because of irregular corneal surface after excimer laser photo-ablation (Table 17.6a).

The post-operative change in keratometry correlated well with the observed change in refraction (Fig. 17.7 and 17.9). The keratometry showed flattening of the

Table 17.6a: Keratometry changes from baseline at different months after PTK

Patient No. Age/gender	Pre-PTK mean keratometry	Post-PTK mean keratometry				Change in keratometry			
		1 month	2 month	3 month	6 month	1 month	2 month	3 month	6 month
1. 18 M	38.47 D	35.90 D	36.50 D	36.60 D	36.70 D	-2.37 D	-1.97 D	-1.87 D	-1.77 D
2. 48 M	43.75 D	42.50 D	42.50 D	42.30 D	42.30 D	-1.25 D	-1.25 D	-1.40 D	-1.40 D
3. 13 F	44.00 D	43.50 D	43.50 D	43.20 D	43.20 D	-0.50 D	-0.50 D	-0.80 D	-0.80 D
4. 13 F	44.87 D	44.20 D	44.20 D	44.00 D	44.00 D	-0.67 D	-0.67 D	-0.87 D	-0.87 D
5. 55 F	46.02 D	45.87 D	45.70 D	45.67 D	45.67 D	-0.15 D	-0.32 D	-0.35 D	-0.35 D
6. 50 M	48.00 D	45.00 D	45.60 D	45.70 D	45.70 D	-3.00 D	-2.40 D	-2.30 D	-2.30 D
7. 31 F	43.12 D	41.30 D	42.60 D	42.50 D	42.50 D	-1.82 D	-1.52 D	-1.72 D	-1.72 D
8. 31 F	44.35 D	43.70 D	44.20 D	44.62 D	44.62 D	-0.65 D	-0.15 D	+0.27 D	+0.27 D
9. 18 M	42.72 D	40.60 D	40.50 D	40.80 D	40.80 D	-2.12 D	-2.22 D	-1.92 D	-1.92 D
10. 50 M	N.A.	40.30 D	40.40 D	40.62 D	40.62 D				
11. 50 M	N.A.	41.00 D	41.25 D	41.50 D	41.50 D				
12. 65 M	45.43 D	44.30 D	44.40 D	44.62 D	44.62 D	-1.13 D	-1.23 D	-1.18 D	1.18 D
13. 78 M	42.25 D	40.50 D	40.10 D	40.37 D	40.37 D	-1.75 D	-1.15 D	-1.88 D	-1.88 D
14. 35 M	N.A.		Not Possible						
15. 35 M	N.A.		Not Possible						
16. 68 F	43.25 D	40.50 D	41.00 D	41.20 D	41.20 D	-2.75 D	-2.50 D	-2.05 D	-2.05 D
17. 30 F	L 49.00 D	47.10 D	47.50 D	47.37 D	47.37 D	-1.90 D	-1.50 D	-1.63 D	-1.63 D
18. 30 F	R 46.45 D	44.25 D	44.30 D	44.50 D	44.50 D	-2.25 D	-2.15 D	-1.95 D	-1.95 D
19. 65 M	L 45.80 D	40.50 D	41.00 D	41.50 D	41.50 D	-5.30 D	-4.80 D	-4.30 D	-4.30 D
20. 65 M	R Not Possible								
21. 18 F	L Not Possible	44.40 D	44.80 D	45.00 D	45.00 D				
22. 18 F	R 42.00 D	40.32 D	41.00 D	41.20 D	41.20 D	-1.68 D	-1.00 D	-0.80 D	-0.80 D
23. 84 M	R 44.40 D	40.50 D	40.75 D	41.25 D	41.25 D	-3.90 D	-3.65 D	-3.15 D	-3.15 D
24. 84 M	L 45.27 D	42.50 D	42.80 D	43.10 D	43.10 D	-2.77 D	-2.47 D	-2.17 D	-2.17 D
25. 22 F	44.62 D	46.00 D	45.80 D	45.30 D	45.35 D	+1.38 D	+1.18 D	+0.68 D	+0.72 D
26. 63 M	L 44.50 D	41.50 D	42.00 D	42.20 D	42.20 D	-3.00 D	-2.50 D	-2.30 D	-2.30 D
27. 63 M	L 45.24 D		Not Possible						
28. 65 M	42.85 D	41.50 D	41.00 D	41.12 D	41.12 D	-1.35 D	-1.85 D	-1.73 D	-1.73 D
29. 24 M	42.00 D	40.90 D	42.70 D	42.25 D	42.25 D	-1.10 D	+0.70 D	+0.25 D	+0.25 D
30. 72 M	41.49 D	40.87 D	41.25 D	41.37 D	41.37 D	-0.62 D	-0.24 D	-0.12 D	-0.12 D
31. 58 F	47.35 D	44.30 D	45.80 D	46.10 D	46.30 D	-3.05 D	-1.55 D	-1.25 D	-1.05 D
32. 48 M	R Not Possible		Not Possible						
33. 85 M	41.75 D		Not Possible						
34. 48 M	L Not Possible		Not Possible						
35. 28 M	44.37 D	40.10 D	41.75 D	41.95 D	42.37 D	-4.27 D	-2.62 D	-2.42 D	-2.00 D
36. 24 M	45.00 D	41.00 D	41.50 D	42.60 D	42.65 D	-4.00 D	-3.50 D	-2.40 D	-2.35 D
37. 20 M	43.74 D	41.12 D	41.87 D	41.25 D	41.37 D	-2.62 D	-1.87 D	-2.49 D	-2.37 D
38. 25 M	41.40 D	42.25 D	42.37 D	42.70 D	42.50 D	+0.80 D	+0.93 D	+1.30 D	+1.10 D
39. 68 M	43.00 D	40.27 D	40.50 D	40.87 D	40.87 D	-2.73 D	-2.50 D	-2.13 D	-2.13 D
40. 53 M	42.50 D	42.00 D	42.12 D	42.25 D	42.25 D	-0.50 D	-0.38 D	-0.25 D	-0.25 D
41. 60 F	46.00 D	44.37 D	44.50 D	44.75 D	44.75 D	-1.63 D	-1.50 D	-1.25 D	-1.25 D
42. 48 F	46.75 D	45.87 D	46.00 D	46.25 D	46.25 D	-0.88 D	-0.75 D	-0.50 D	-0.50 D
43. 43 F	44.87 D	43.25 D	43.50 D	43.75 D	43.75 D	-1.62 D	-1.37 D	-1.12 D	-1.12 D
44. 68 M	45.68 D	44.50 D	44.62 D	44.87 D	44.87 D	-1.12 D	-1.06 D	-0.81 D	-0.81 D
45. 60 M	43.56 D	44.37 D	44.50 D	44.75 D	44.75 D	+0.81 D	+0.94 D	+1.20 D	+1.20 D
46. 70 F	45.31 D	43.00 D	43.37 D	43.50 D	43.50 D	-2.31 D	-1.93 D	-1.81 D	-1.81 D
47. 55 F	Not Possible		Not Possible						
48. 70 M	43.62 D	45.50 D	45.00 D	44.75 D	44.75 D	+1.88 D	+1.38 D	+1.13 D	+1.13 D

corneal curvature in the eyes which experienced postoperative hyperopic shift, steepening in those with myopic shift. The mean pre-operative keratometry was 44.22 D (± 2.02 D).

The mean keratometry changed to 42.52 ±2.26 D at first month; 42.84 ± 2.14 D at second month; 42.97 ± 2.10 D at third month and 43.00 ±2.12 D at sixth postoperative month (Fig. 17.10). There appeared to be slight decrease in the *corneal curvature flattening* during the first three post-operative months, the change was not significant (P=0.5081). The keratometry reading became stable at six months in most of the eyes.

Corneal Haze

Corneal haze was graded according to the method of slit lamp examination given by Gartry et al (see chapter 5). Mild (1+) to moderate (2+) corneal haze was noticed in most patients during the first month after PTK. It increased during the second and third month and decreased subsequently. No corneal haze was noticed at sixth month (Table 17.6b).

Corneal Clarity

Although, improvement in best corrected visual acuity is one good way of evaluating the efficacy of phototherapeutic keratectomy, it may be masked by other co-existing confounding conditions such as cataract. To judge the efficacy of PTK, another way is to find the change in the corneal clarity after this procedure.

We examined the pre–and six month post-operative corneal clarity in all patients according to the guideline given in Table 17.7.

The first three postoperative months were not included for this assessment because of the corneal haze appearing during this period which could have altered the corneal clarity scores making it difficult to decide whether the clarity score is low due to the presence of any residual corneal pathology itself.

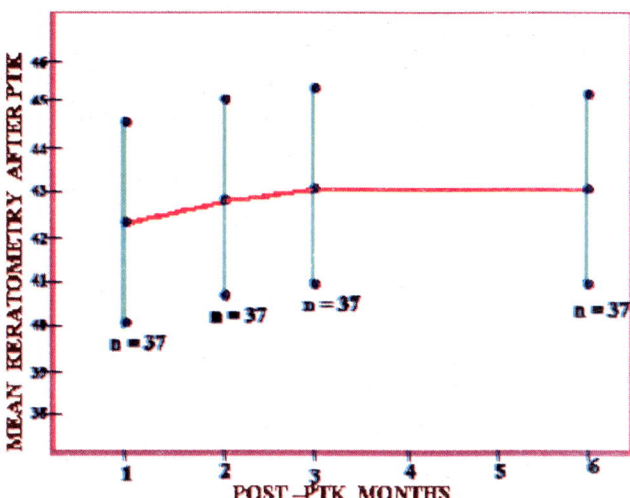

Fig. 17.10: Correlation between *mean keratometry* and time after surgery. For each time, mean keratometry is calculated as the difference between pre- and post operative average keratometry. *n* denotes the number of patients at each time. Results represents mean ± standard deviation

Table 17.6b: Post-operative corneal haze

Postoperative Month	Number of eyes	Grade of haze (mean ± SD)
1	48	1.7 ± 0.4
2	48	2 ± 0.7
3	48	1.2 ± 0.5
6	48	0

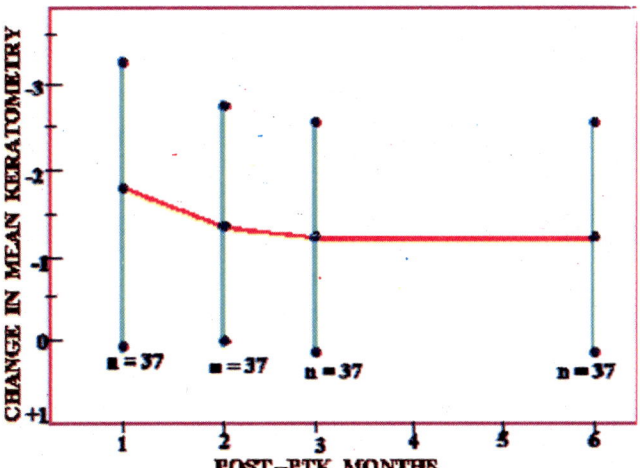

Fig. 17.9: Correlation between *change in mean keratometry* and time after surgery. For each time, change in mean keratometry is calculated as the difference between pre and post operative average keratometry; 'n' denotes the number of patients at each time. Results represents mean ± one standard deviation

Table 17.7: Slit lamp examination of corneal clarity

Grade	Description
4	Totally clear cornea
3	Iris details not obscured by opacity
2	Iris details hazily seen
1	No iris details seen
0	Total obscuration of view

Since the corneal pathology was not distributed uniformly, the area with maximum opacity and least clarity was considered while deciding the scores, both pre–and post-operatively. The pre-PTK mean corneal clarity was 1.1 ± 0.8, which improved to 3.1 ± 0.9 at sixth post-operative month (Table 17.8). This improvement was significant (P = 0.00).

Table 17.8: Pre and six month post-PTK corneal clarity

	Pre-operative	6 month post-PTK
Mean	1.1	3.1
SD	0.85	0.86
Median	1.0	3.0
Minimum	0	1.0
Maximum	3.0	4.0

Epithelial Healing and the Tear-Film Changes

Epithelial healing occurred within 5 to 7 days in 91.7% of the eyes. Re-epithelization was delayed to 8th to 10th day in 4 eyes. These 4 eyes belonged to patients in the older age group and had a relatively bad ocular surface. The patients of recurrent corneal erosions had normal epithelial healing within 5–7 days after PTK. They were by and large symptom free and none of them developed recurrence of corneal erosions upto a follow-up period of 8 to 12 months.

The tear-film status was determined by Schirmer, test tear-film breakup time and Rose Bengal staining of the corneal surface before and after phototherapeutic keratectomy.

The measurement of tear secretion was done by the *Schirmer basic secretion test* to rule out any reflex tearing because of pathological cornea.

The pre-operative mean BUT was 10.9 ± 4 seconds. It improved significantly after PTK (P = 0.00). At 6 month, the mean post-operative basic tear secretion was 14.7 ± 3.0 mm and the mean BUT was 17.7 ± 3.7 seconds.

In any individual case the improvement of break up time from sub-normal to normal signifies a healthy and intact corneal surface and a stable tear-film. Some of our patients had sub-normal BUT and staining of the corneal surface with Rose Bengal stain pre-operatively. After PTK, none of them had either sub-normal BUT or any corneal staining at any follow-up period.

These results indicate improvement not only of the parameters where these were within normal limits, but also change of a poor corneal surface with unstable tear-film in diseased cornea to one which is healthy and stable.

Depth of Ablation and The Refractive Changes

We tried to find a correlation between the depth of corneal ablation and the change in spherical equivalent. The ablation depth was 25 μ to 100 μ in different patients. The mean change in spherical equivalent per 10 μ of corneal ablation was 0.28 ± 0.27 D (range -0.3 D-0.82 D). Figure 17.11 shows correlation between the change in spherical equivalent of manifest refraction and the depth of corneal ablation. It is seen that majority of the points are not clustered around the diagonal line, meaning thereby that *no definite linear* relationship existed between the two.

The above finding of '*no definite correlation between the ablation depth and the refractive change*' should be understood through the following knowledge.

The central optical zone of the cornea is mainly responsible for its refractive power. The refractive change by excimer laser ablation depends on the *pattern of change in the corneal curvature of this central optical zone.*

This change in the corneal curvature depends upon
1. The ablation zone diameter
2. The depth of ablation
3. The centration of the ablation zone with relation to the visual axis
4. The vertical shape of the curvature with relation to the visual axis. This depends upon:

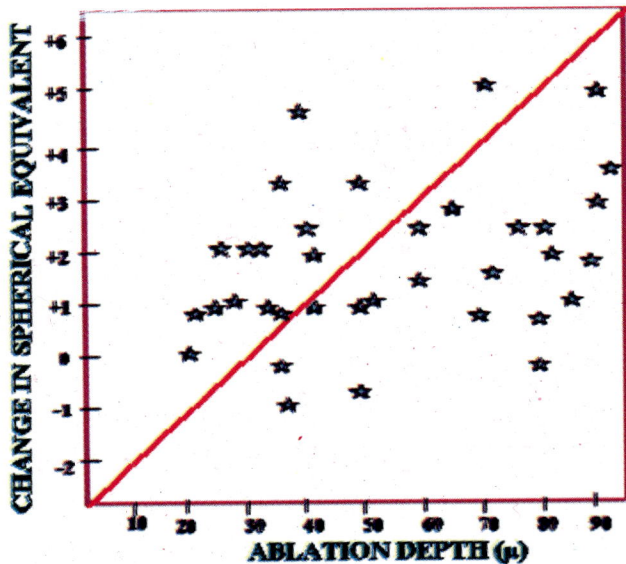

Fig. 17.11: Correlation between depth of ablation in microns and change in the spherical equivalent. Change in spherical equivalent is calculated as the difference between pre- and post operative manifest spherical equivalent

a. Whether ablation is more in the centre or in the periphery.
b. Whether ablation is more in one particular meridian

Smaller zone with sharp edges would flatten the cornea more than a relatively larger zone with tapered edges. Ablation of the paracentral area would cause steepening of the cornea or may also result in irregular astigmatism. Greater depth of uniform (plano) ablation and steep edge of the ablated periphery were found to be associated with higher degree of hyperopic change (Chamon et al).

Marita et al also reported greater risk of hyperopic shift with deeper ablation and scan mode of ablation.

Munnerlyn had calculated that removal of *5 micron of tissue from a 4 mm central optical zone* by the excimer laser would lead to *one diopter* decrease in the corneal power. Hence, without controlling all other possible parameters which would lead to refractive changes, it would not be plausible to expect a *definitive linear* correlation of refractive changes with ablation depth alone.

PTK Results According to Subgroups

Different corneal conditions have been reported to respond differently to excimer laser phototherapeutic keratectomy. We analyzed the best-corrected visual acuity and the corneal clarity scores of each diagnostic subgroup. The results are summarized in Table 17.9. All groups experienced an improvement in BCVA as well as in corneal clarity scores throughout the follow-up. The improvement in both the parameters was significant in all subgroups except the eyes with granular dystrophy where the mean improvement in BCVA at six month was 1.5 lines (P = 0.312) and improvement in the mean corneal clarity was from score 1.0 to score 3.0.

The **pterygium subgroup** experienced the maximum gain in BCVA (mean gain of 4 lines). Band keratopathy subgroup improved more than the eyes with Salzmann's nodule. The difference in mean BCVA between these subgroups was analyzed by Kruskal-Wallis test. There was significant difference at every follow-up in the mean pre and post-PTK BCVA (P=0.003).

The change in corneal clarity score from the baseline is not representative criteria when deciding the difference in outcome among different subgroup as compared to the corneal clarity itself. In recurrent corneal erosions the initial corneal clarity may not be affected so much, therefore any significant change is not expected. In eyes with spheroidal degeneration the final corneal clarity is 2.3, although the change in clarity is almost same as in the eyes with recurrent erosions (Table 17.9).

Post-PTK Complications

Refractive Changes

The most common undesired outcome after PTK was seen in the form of refractive changes. This has already been discussed.

Infiltrative Keratitis

One eye developed significant loss of vision due to infiltrative keratitis. This was the only eye which had

Table 17.9: Functional and anatomical results in different diagnostic sub-groups

Sub Group	No. of eyes	Pre-PTK BCVA	Post PTK BCVA (mean)				Corneal clarity (mean) (at 6 month)		Mean improvement (at 6 month)	
			1month	2months	3months	6months	Pre-PTK	Post-PTK	BCVA	clarity score
Pterygium	5	6/30	6/12	6/9p	6/9p	6/9p	1.6	3.6	4.5 lines	2.0
Corneal Opacity and scars	8	6/24	6/12	6/12	6/9p	6/9p	1.4	3.3	3.5 lines	2.9
Post herpes keratitis scars	5	6/30	6/15p	6/15p	6/15p	6/15	1.1	3.0	3.0 lines	2.9
Recurrent Corneal Erosions	6	6/15p	6/6p	6/6p	6/6p	6/6p	2.3	3.8	3.0 lines	1.5
Granular Dystrophy	5	6/18p	6/18p	6/18p	6/18	6/15	1.0	3.0	1.5 lines	2.0
Salzmann's Nodules	6	6/24	6/15	6/15	6/12p	6/12p	0.7	2.5	2.5 lines	1.8
Spheroidal Degen.	6	6/36p	6/18p	6/18	6/18	6/18	0.7	2.3	3.5 lines	1.6
Band Keratopathy	7	6/30	6/15p	6/15p	6/15	6/12p	0.6	3.0	3.5 lines	2.4
Pterygium	5	6/30	6/12	6/9p	6/9p	6/9p	1.6	3.6	4.5 lines	2.0

decrease in visual acuity (Colour plate 10, photograph 52). This complication occurred during the second postoperative week. This patient was not maintaining follow-up after the PTK. He hailed from Rajasthan and had been prescribed a *bandage contact lens*, NSAID drops and ciprofloxacin drops but no local steroids. He presented with symptoms of pain, redness, watering and photophobia already present for five days when seen by us. This lapse was inspite of the risk being explained to him about use of contact lens and the importance of immediate check-up/consultation in case of any such symptoms. Examination showed stromal infiltrates present in the form of an incomplete ring in the periphery of the ablated zone.

The patient was treated on the lines of bacterial keratitis in an urgent manner. The Gram staining, and culture sensitivity for an infective organism from the corneal scrapring/biopsy were negative.

The eye showed no response to the standard regime of corneal ulcer management. Corneal biopsy taken later showed non-specific inflammatory cells and fibroblasts.

This case appears to be similar to the case of *sterile stromal infiltrates,* described by *Teichmann et al*, which was seen on the fourth postoperative day as a ring of infiltrates, in a patient using bandage contact lens and topical NSAID without concomitant use of topical steroid (vide infra).

DISCUSSION

The success of excimer laser corneal surgery depends on its capability of precisely removing corneal tissue without causing significant collateral damage and leaving behind smooth, clear and healthy corneal surface with quick and adequate epithelium regeneration having normal adhesion complexes. Till recently there had been a large number of clinical studies from the western world which have reported the success of 193nm ArF excimer laser phototherapeutic keratectomy in treating various superficial corneal disorders.

Although surgical success in removing the pathological condition from corneal surface is an important goal of PTK, *functional success* in terms of improved vision is equally desired from the patient's point of view. Overall functional success in improving the best corrected visual acuity in 50-80% of the eyes has been reported by various authors.

Gartry et al were the first to perform series of PTK in 25 sighted human eyes, for rough and smooth band keratopathy. They reported visual improvement in 64% of the eyes. All patients also had improvement in pain and glare disability.

Neel Sher et al treated 33 sighted eyes with corneal scars due to various causes. They achieved improvement in BCVA in 50% of the treated eyes. Two or more Snellen's lines were gained in 44% and improvement in corneal clarity was achieved in 50% of the eyes.

Campos and colleagues treated 18 eyes with corneal opacities due to different anterior corneal pathologies. Improvement in corneal clarity was reported in 77.7% eyes; improvement in uncorrected visual acuity in 60% and improvement in best-corrected visual acuity in 50 % eyes. Sixteen percent eyes were considered treatment failure.

Stark and Chamon performed PTK on 27 eyes with anterior corneal disorders and 4 eyes with surgically induced myopia. Overall improvement in BCVA was obtained in 76% eyes. Seventy percent of the 27 eyes which underwent PTK, had improvement in 2 or more Snellen's lines. Since 18.5% (5 eyes) improved with rigid gas contact lenses, a two-line improvement can be presumed to have occurred in 51.5% eyes only.

Rapuano treated 28 eyes having diverse corneal pathologies with excimer laser PTK. Fourteen eyes achieved more than 2 line improvement in BCVA. Overall improvement in BCVA was reported in 80% of the eyes treated by Marita Amm et al and in 84.6% of the eyes with corneal dystrophy by Orndhal et al.

The largest series published so far is that of Maloney et al. They treated 232 eyes of corneal vision loss with PTK at different centers and followed for one month to two years. They reported improvement in best corrected visual acuity of 2 or more lines in 45% eyes and worsening in 10% eyes. Significant improvement in UCVA in about 50% eyes and worsening in 17% to 28% of the eyes was found. Improvement in corneal clarity was reported in 50% to 70% eyes and worsening in 5% to 10% of the eyes.

Our visual results are a clear therapeutic success. Overall 96% of the eyes achieved improvement in BCVA; 85% eyes gained two or more lines at sixth postoperative month. Improvement in UCVA was achieved in 83% eyes; 73% gained 2 or more lines at sixth postoperative month. Loss of best-corrected vision occurred in one eye and loss of UCVA in two eyes. The patient (eye no. 27) who lost both BCVA and UCVA significantly had already developed corneal infiltrates in the ablated zone forming an incomplete ring in the midperiphery. Investigations were unhelpful in proving an infective etiology. The eye was treated with standard intensive antibiotic regimen as for corneal ulcers without any improvement, ultimately resulting in an opacified cornea. The biopsy showed non-specific inflammatory cells and fibroblasts.

There had been few reports in the literature on sterile corneal infiltrates after photo-ablation of the cornea. Sher et al reported high incidence of sterile infiltrates (9%) in 240 of there patients treated over a period of three years. They noted an association of use of contact lens and topical NSAID without the concurrent use of topical steroids. It was suggested that this combination without topical steroids causes cyclo-oxygenase inhibition leading to increased amount of arachidonic acid and increased formation of *leukotrienes,* which are potent chemotac-tants for polymorphoneuclear leucocytes.

In a survey report of 17 surgeons in Canada, Teal et al reported 30 such cases after PRK, presenting with pain, redness and lacrimation on the second post-operative day. The infiltrates most frequently were in the shape of a paracentral immune ring placed inferiorly. They also found an association with combination of contact lens and NSAIDs. Teichmann et al described a case similar to ours after PTK. He noted a Wessely-type, incomplete dense white ring at the margin of the ablated zone on the fourth day. The patient was using bandage contact lens. The authors suggested that it could be an antigen antibody reaction involving the heat shock proteins (HSP) produced locally at the margin of the ablated zone and the pre-existing circulating antibody against bacterial HSPs. We have been routinely using topical steroid drops post-operatively and discontinued the use of bandage contact lenses for speedy re-epithelization after this case. The use of bandage soft contact lens for expediting regeneration of the epithelium after PTK has been condemned by others also because of increased risk of sterile as well as non-sterile corneal infiltrates.

Our results are different with regard to the outcome of excimer laser PTK in different corneal conditions. Corneal disorders leading to superficial opacity such as granular and lattice dystrophies have been found to be the best candidates for PTK. We did not achieve statistically significant improvement in mean BCVA in eyes with granular dystrophy (Table 15 .9). This is because of loss of 9 Snellen's lines in one eye (no. 27). Other four eyes in this group had gain of 3, 3, 3.5 and 7 lines respectively. Most difficult cases to treat are said to be those with corneal scars and band shaped keratopathy. Irregular astigmatism and low functional and anatomical success rates have been reported in these conditions. The scarred corneal tissue and calcium deposits have decreased ablation rate and sometimes are even resistant to ablation with excimer laser. We obtained good results in both the conditions. The best results achieved by us were in the pterygium subgroup followed by post-herpetic and superficial scar sub-groups. In these diagnostic sub-groups the majority of the patients were young adults.

The nebulomacular corneal opacities that caused significant loss of vision were mostly superficial, hence easy to tackle with PTK. The photographs given in Colour plates 4-9 depict the results in some of these eyes. The other condition where good results have been reported is Salzmann's nodule. In this subgroup our results were third best. Our cases had bad ocular surface, in addition to this degenerative disorder which was possibly responsible for the comparatively lesser improvement in most of these eyes.

The *success of PTK depends on careful patient selection and detailed pre-operative evaluation* as well as on the skills of the surgeon and technique of PTK. Diverse corneal conditions are to be tackled differently. In the band keratopathy sub-group many eyes had a smooth band. In the other eyes with thick calcium deposits, removal of as much of calcium as possible was done by chelating with EDTA application while protecting the normal cornea before performing excimer laser PTK. Frequent applications of an appropriate masking agent are needed in such cases to avoid irregular corneal surface after laser ablation. Similarly frequent intra-operative use of a masking agent which has ablation rate near to that of scar collagen (such 1% HPMC), is necessary during treatment of corneal scars, though at the cost of laser energy. In recurrent corneal erosion syndrome the aim is to prevent the recurrence of the condition. A success rate of 75% to 100% has been reported in treating this condition with excimer laser PTK. In our study, none of the 5 patient had recurrence of corneal erosions after a follow up of 8 to12 months. Recurrent corneal erosions following trauma related focal disorders may be taken of by the usual 6mm area central corneal ablation but those cases which are secondary to epithelial basement membrane dystrophy (EBMD) are due to diffuse pathology and need to be tackled by *pan-corneal ablation* as described by Kermer et al. The central 6mm zone is treated first in the usual manner followed by 3mm confluent zone in the periphery ablated to a depth of 6μ.. By this technique a hundred percent success was reported in preventing recurrence of corneal erosions after a follow up of 26 to 42 months.

We could not establish a *definite correlation between the ablation depth and the refractive change.*

Munnerlyn calculated that removal of 5μ of corneal tissue from a 4mm central optical zone by the excimer laser would lead to 1 diopter flattening of the cornea. It has not been possible as yet to establish a mathematical correlation between the depth of corneal tissue removed and change in diopteric power of the cornea without controlling the defferent factors involved for the refractive change.

This finding should be understood through the following knowledge. The central optical zone of the cornea is mainly responsible for its refractive power. The refractive changes by excimer laser ablation depends on the *pattern of change in the corneal curvature* of this central optical zone. This change in the corneal curvature depends upon the ablation zone diameter, the depth of ablation, the centration of the ablation zone with relation to the visual axis, the vertical shape of the curvature with relation to the visual axis (i.e. whether the central area or the periphery is more ablated and whether ablation is more in one particular meridian). Smaller zone with sharp edges would flatten the cornea more than a relatively larger zone with tapered edges. Ablation of the paracentral area would cause steepening or may result in irregular astigmatism. Greater depth of uniform (plano) ablation and steep edge of the ablated periphery are found to be associated with higher degree of hyperopic change (Chamon et al). Marita et al also reported greater risk of hyperopic shift with deeper ablation and scan mode of ablation.

Hence, without controlling all other possible parameters which would lead to refractive changes, it would not be plausible to expect a *definitive linear* correlation of refractive changes with ablation depth alone.

There has been only one report on the *ocular surface changes after excimer laser* phototherapeutic keratectomy. Dogru et al found favorable effect of PTK on the ocular surface by improving the stability of tear-film and ocular surface health through attainment of regular corneal surface. We report similar results in improvement of tear-film stability and integrity of the corneal surface by excimer laser PTK in various superficial corneal disorders. This is because of regeneration of a healthy, regular and complete epithelial layer after PTK.

Mean *hyperopic shift* of +2.85 D to 8.0 D has been by different studies (+2.5 D by Gartry et al; +5.4 D by Hersh et al; +6.3 D by Chamon et al using the '*standard taper*' and +2.0 D using the '*modified taper*' techniqu*e*).

In our study, we found *hyperopic shift* in 36 of the 44 eyes in which refraction could be obtained; ranging from +0.38 D to +5.0 D of spherical equivalent *(mean +1.67D)*. This induced hyperopia is much less as compared to that reported by the previous studies and *did not become an unacceptable sequelae* of excimer laser PTK for most of our patients. *Myopic shift* found in seven of the eyes (patient no. 8, 20, 25, 29, 38, 45, 48) was mild ranging from –0.25D to –1.63D of spherical equivalent (mean –0.66 D). Patient number 8 (smooth band), patient no.25 (HSV scar) and patient no.29 (corneal opacity with erosions) had the pathology located more in the para-central area, therefore received more off-axis treatment in an attempt to clear it.

The surgical success of PTK relates to obviating the need for penetrating of keratoplasty in patients with superficial corneal dystrophies and scars. Because most patients with corneal dystrophies would require more then one keratoplasty in their life time and PTK is the least aggressive procedure with fast recovery and good results; it has been recommended as the initial surgery in patients with anterior stromal involvement. In the case of recurrence of dystrophy a repeat procedure can be performed till the corneal thickness is not less than 250 microns. PTK is very effective in restoring vision in a way that is easier than lamellar or penetrating keratoplasty. It also would not produce high or irregular astigmatism.

Thus we conclude that

1. *Excimer laser PTK is a safe and effective modality for treating superficial corneal disorders of a wide range in selected group of patients.*
2. *The patient should be ready to accept the refractive changes, particularly hyperopia,* until an algorithm is developed in future to give simultaneous refractive ablation along with PTK.

Chapter 18

Nonsurgical Methods of Refractive Correction

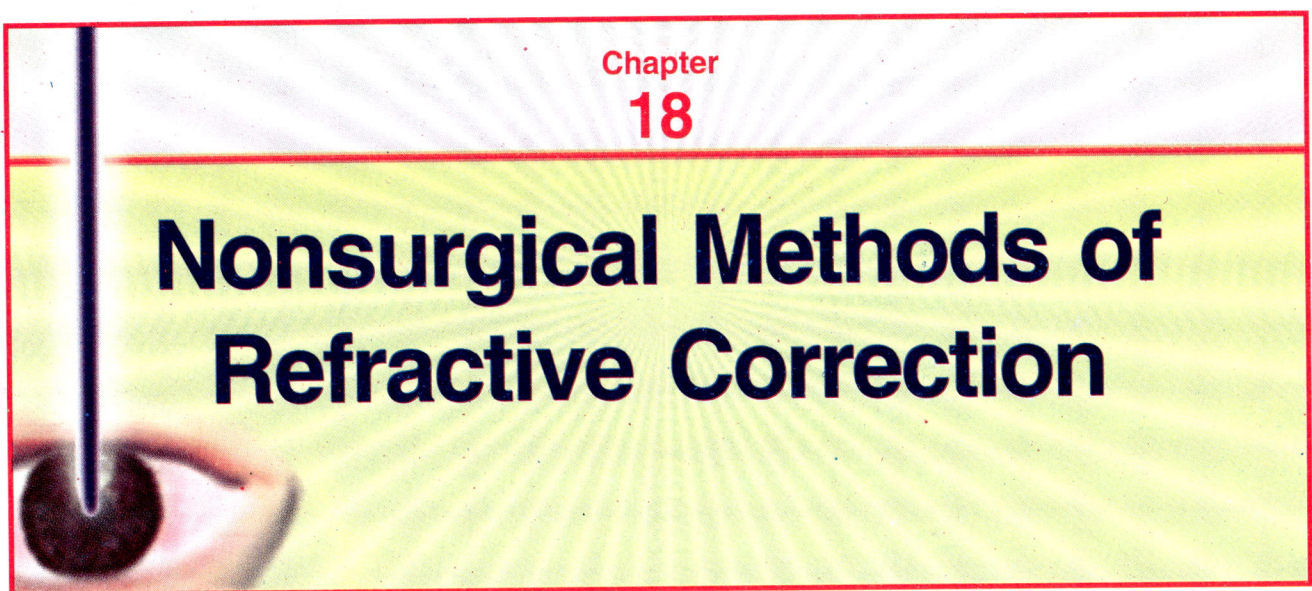

The conventional non-surgical, optical methods of visual rehabilitation are spectacles and contact lenses. The use of spectacle glasses has been known for the last few centuries, while the contact lenses are relatively newer tools in the armament of the ophthalmologist.

In general, these modalities of refractive correction are quite satisfactory because the majority of cases suffer from refractive errors that fall within mild to moderate range, which is easily correctable without any optical or other problems. However, there are definite limitations, particularly in case of severe forms of refractive errors, of these non-surgical methods of refractive correction. In addition, the use of contact lens is associated with a high incidence of well defined complications, some of which are potentially vision threatening.

USE OF THE SPECTACLE LENSES

The use of the spectacles is associated with the following problems:

GENERAL PROBLEMS WITH SPECTACLES

1. Degradation of the retinal image due to spherical and chromatic aberrations and decentration of the lenses results in suboptimal visual acuity particularly with higher power lenses.
2. Alteration in the size of the image.
3. Decrease in the visual field.
4. Continuous use of spectacles even in low degree of ammetropia may be associated with the feeling of discomfort, tightness on the temples and vague dull aching or even eye aches even when the correction is proper.
5. The disparity created by the altered relationship between the accommodation and convergence leads to asthenopic symptoms.
6. The reflections and glare produced at the lens surface may not be avoidable many a times even with the use of best antireflective coatings. This problem can be sometimes very troublesome particularly during night driving.
7. Recent use of glasses or a sudden increase in the power of the lenses is not well tolerated. The adjustment may sometimes take months.
8. Some types of refractive errors are not amenable to the spectacle lens correction, e.g. irregular astigmatism and post surgical refractive errors such as after penetrating keratoplasty, etc.
9. *Visual rehabilitation with spectacles may be poor in extreme degrees of refractive abnormalities.*

Although the patient gets adjusted to many of the above problems, yet he has to undergoing avoidable discomfort of various degree during this adjustment period.

In contrast to the supposedly common and routine problems listed above, there are a large number of special difficulties encountered with the use of spectacle lenses in cases of the high refractive errors, astigmatism and anisometropia.

PROBLEMS WITH THE USE OF HIGH-POWER GLASSES

The user faces a number of significant optical problems with high power spectacle lenses. These are:

Distortion of the Image

Distortion of the retinal image takes place due to refraction by the periphery of the lens (spherical aberrations). The distortions can be of the following types:

1. Pincushion effect by convex lenses.
2. Barrel effect by the concave lenses.
3. Oblique image due to cylindrical lenses.

Altered Image Size

The alteration in the size of the retinal image formed by the high powered lenses leads to *false spatial orientation*. This happens despite the objects being familiar to the user. An object is perceived to be closer due to the larger image size produced by a plus lens and visa versa. This may lead to clumsiness in the daily working routine even to the extent of knocking down the objects due to *defective hand-eye coordination*.

For the same reason, negotiating the stairs swiftly may be difficult. Driving may become troublesome.

Prismatic Effect

The prismatic effect produced by refraction at the peripheral part of a high plus power lens gives rise to the **ring scotoma** and the **jack-in-the box** phenomenon. These effects associated with a **decreased visual field** make the day to day activity troublesome. Driving becomes impossible and hazardous.

PROBLEMS IN CASES OF ASTIGMATISM

1. Use of cylindrical lenses for high astigmatic errors makes the objects appear distorted. This effect may give rise to intolerable distress.
2. When the axis of the cylinders in the two eyes are not parallel (the difference being >20°), the following additional distortions in the retinal image are produced by high power cylinders:

- Rectangles appear as rhomboids in shape.
- *Rotatory deviation* causes the linear objects to appear as slanting and the flat surface as a slope. These effects cause significant inconvenience in daily life.

3. Irregular and iatrogenic astigmatism (e.g. after PK, cataract and other ocular surgeries) are difficult to manage with spectacle lenses.

PROBLEMS IN CASES OF ANISOMETROPIA

Spectacle correction of anisometropia produces troublesome symptoms due to aniseikonia. **Aniseikonia** is the difference in the size of the retinal images of two eyes of the patient suffering from anisometropia.

1. Each diopter difference between the two eyes produces about 2% difference in the image size with the corrective lenses worn at an equal back-vertex distance.
2. The maximum tolerable difference in the size of the retinal images is about 5%.
3. A 10.0 D difference in the lens power (e.g. unilateral aphakia or high myopia) would make the image 25% larger/smaller.
4. The *image difference may be symmetrical in all dimensions and meridional or asymmetrical in astigmatic aniseikonia.*

Hering-Hillebrandt horopter deviation is produced when the image is progressively larger in one direction and smaller in the opposite direction of the horizontal visual field (usually larger in the temporal than in the nasal field). This situation results in an array of symptoms due to the following.

1. Distortion of the *space* or spatial disorientation.
2. Impairment of binocular vision.

Spatial Disorientation

The disorientation of the space lead to confusion, difficulty in driving and aviation. The problem is *aggravated by fatigue* and in surroundings *where monocular clues for depth perception are absent* to guide the patient.

Impairment of Binocularity

The unequal images perceived by the two eyes result in the impairment of binocular vision with variable symptoms depending upon the degree of impairment, such as:

1. Blurred vision.
2. Difficulty in fixation.
3. Eye strains and headache.
4. Nervous manifestations.
5. A tendency to diplopia or actual diplopia.
6. Heterophoria or even manifest squint.

These symptoms arising from the impaired binocularity are aggravated by activities such as reading, looking at the moving objects, watching TV or a movie and by traveling and driving.

The above situations, therefore, become unsuitable for spectacle correction because either the patient develops intolerance to them or the refractive error is primarily not amenable to this modality of refractive correction.

USE OF CONTACT LENSES

Though, contact lenses are able to take care of the decreased visual field, alteration of image size and the aberrations arising from the peripheral part of the spectacle lenses due to their close proximity to the eye, they also have certain limitations and complications.

LIMITATIONS OF CONTACT LENSES

1. Contact lenses cannot be used in cases of:
   a. Inflammatory conditions of the eye, e.g. blepharitis, conjunctivitis, uveitis, keratitis, stye, chalazion, and other inflammatory diseases of the meibomian and lacrimal system.
   b. Conditions like pinguecula, pterygium and limbal dermoid.
   c. Corneal anesthesia due to any reason.
   d. Dry eye.
   e. Vascularization of the cornea.
   f. Patients with poor blinking and lagophthalmos.
   g. Pregnant women and those on oral contraceptives (due to corneal edema).
   h. Patients with impaired manual dexterity.
   i. Patients with poor personal hygiene.
   j. Patients engaged in occupations where chemical fumes, dirt and other toxic agent are present, which can be absorbed by the contact lens.
   k. Hot and dry atmospheric conditions.

2. Contact lenses have their limitations in correcting some types of refractive errors:
   a. Rigid gas permeable (RGP) contact lenses can correct < 1.0 D of astigmatism. Their results in cases of 1.0-2.0 D of astigmatism are variable.
   b. Soft toric–contact lenses are used for higher degrees of astigmatism and for astigmatism due to cause other than the corneal curvature. In spite of the best designs of these *toric contact lenses,* stabilization of the axis of contact lens in the desired meridian is a problem.
   c. The visual results of contact lenses in case of irregular astigmatism are about 60%.
3. The range of refractive errors that can be tackled is less in comparison to excimer laser refractive surgery.
4. They need meticulous care everyday for insertion, removal and maintenance (cleaning and sterilization).
5. The CL 'wearing-time' is limited (depending on the O_2 transmissibility and wettability of the CL).
6. Use of contact lenses has recurring expenditure. They may be lost during handling or a change might be required because of intolerance/allergy to a particular material or due to surface irregularities caused by wearing-out and deposits.
7. The problem of alteration of the image size is not alleviated totally for high refractive errors. For example in an aphakic patient of 12.0 D, the image size disparity is reduced from 30% to 6%, which is still in the trouble zone of aniseikonia.
8. The *disparity between accommodation and convergence is further aggravated* in myopes after contact lens wear in comparison to spectacle wear.

COMPLICATIONS OF CONTACT LENS WEAR

As stated earlier contact lens wear may be associated with definite complications, some of which are potentially vision threatening. The complications are listed in Table 18.1.

Poor Vision

Other than improper correction, following are the reasons for poor vision after CL wear.

1. Faulty lens designs pertaining to the peripheral curve, edge design and improper fit and decentration.

Table 18.1: Complications of contact lens wear

1. Poor vision
2. Spectacle blur
3. Induced astigmatism
4. Over wearing syndrome
5. Acute painful red eye
6. Chronic red eye
7. Allergic reaction to preservatives
8. Acute lens intolerance
9. Corneal abrasions
10. Corneal edema
11. Corneal warpage
12. Corneal hypoxia
13. Tight lens syndrome
14. Corneal neovascularization
15. Microcystic epitheliopathy
16. Dendritic keratitis
17. Punctate keratitis
18. Sterile stromal infiltrates
19. Three and nine O' clock staining
20. Dellen
21. Superior limbic keratitis
22. Microbial keratitis including Acanthamoeba keratitis
23. Giant papillary conjunctivitis

2. The tear meniscus formed at the lower edge of an upward decentred CL, if it obtrudes over a relatively larger size pupil in mesopic condition, can give rise to *ghost images, multiple images* or *double vision.*
3. The additional accommodative requirement with the use of minus lenses can lead to decreased near vision.
4. *Corneal edema* and *warpage* of the cornea after longer period of CL wear may result in progressive decrease in the visual acuity.

   Spectacle blur, i.e. impairment of vision on spectacle wear after discontinuing the CL, is due to these factors. These effects are common occurrence after prolonged use of RGP lenses and less with the soft CL. The corneal edema may clear after some time of the discontinuation of the contact lens.

   The *corneal warpage may persist for month*s or become permanent in its severe form *resulting in astigmatism.* Corneal warpage is uncommon with soft lenses.
5. Deposits of proteinaceous material, bio-film or cosmetic and atmospheric pollutants.
6. Insertion of the contact lens into the wrong eye.

Acute Painful Red Eye

The causes of an acute red eye include.

1. Allergy to chemical preservatives, particularly thiomersal.
2. **Acute soft lens intolerance** in the form of significant epithelial edema, necrosis and ulceration of the surface developing *within a few hours* of a soft lens wear.
3. Abrasion of the cornea by finger nail or the lens itself on insertion.
4. Epithelial edema suddenly resulting in surface abrasion, when it becomes severe enough after certain period lapse. This is called **'over wearing syndrome'**.
5. Breakdown of the cysts, if the epithelium has developed *microcysts* as a consequence of CL wear.
6. Infective keratitis.

Chronic Red Eye

An eye which is chronically inflamed can be the result of a number of conditions. These conditions can be one of the following.

1. Corneal hypoxia, sometimes causing even frank neovascularization.
2. Damaged lens.
3. Deposits on the lens.
4. Poorly fit lenses: *Tight Lens Syndrome.*
5. Rreaction to the solution, which can be either toxic or hypersensitivity reaction to the preservatives.
6. Giant papillary conjunctivitis (GPC).
7. Superior limbic keratoconjunctivitis (SLK).

Superior Limbic Keratoconjunctivitis (SLK)

Causes of SLK

1. Chemical sensitivity reaction: thiomersal.
2. Poorly fit lens.
3. Soft contact lens use.
4. Toxic reaction to solutions.

Clinical Features of SLK

1. The condition is usually bilateral but often asymmetric.
2. Causes foreign body sensation, blurring of vision, photophobia and mucoid discharge.
3. There are micropapillae on the superior tarsal conjunctiva, giving it a diffuse velvety appearance.

4. Papillary hypertrophy of the superior limbus and hyperemia of the superior bulbar conjunctiva.
5. The superior cornea shows punctate erosions, subepithelial opacities and micropannus.

Dendritic Keratitis

1. This condition is characterized by dendritic corneal lesions.
2. It is essential to exclude herpes simplex keratitis.
3. The lesions in CL-related dendritic keratitis are thinner and usually bilateral. Herpes keratitis is unilateral.
4. A correct diagnosis is crucial because topical steroids, which are the treatment of this condition, are contraindicated in viral keratitis.

Punctate Keratitis

Cause of Punctate Keratitis

1. CL related mechanical injury.
2. Chemical toxic reaction.
3. A dry eye condition.
4. Tight fit lens.
5. Tight lids.

Treatment

1. Discontinue the contact lens.
2. Prophylactic antibiotic drops.

Three and Nine-O' Clock Staining and Dellen Formation

1. It is commonly seen in lens wear specially with rigid lenses.
2. If severe, it can lead to dellen formation.
3. It can result in secondary degeneration leading to localized scarring and vascularization.

Treatment

1. Artificial tears and blinking exercises.
2. Lens with a thinner edge or larger diameter.
3. Change the fit to ensure adequate lateral movement.

Microcystic Epitheliopathy

1. This condition results due to corneal hypoxia and is a common feature of hard contact lens wear.
2. It can occur with soft lens wear also.
3. The microcysts rupture on wearing the lens, resulting in acute red painful eye.

Management

1. Discontinue the use of the contact lens.
2. Revert to a lens with better oxygen permeability.
3. Decrease the contact lens wear-time.

Sterile Stromal Infiltrates

1. These are usually asymptomatic.
2. Usually small, peripheral opacities.
3. Located within the epithelium, subepithelially or in the anterior stroma.
4. Result of chemical sensitivity or sometimes sensitivity to staphylococcal antigen.
5. No epithelial defect is seen.
6. Disappear after lens wear is discontinued.

Management of Sterile Stromal Infiltrates

1. Refit with a flatter lens and use non-preserved saline.
2. These cases should be treated as an infective one as it difficult to differentiate them from early infective keratitis.

Corneal Hypoxia

Prolonged CL wear, use of lenses with low O_2 transmissibility and extended lens wear result in corneal hypoxia (see under 'corneal physiology').

Acute hypoxia presents with epithelial erosions (as with PMMA).

Chronic hypoxia presents with punctate staining, epithelial microcysts, stromal edema and corneal neovascularization. It occur with soft or RGP lens wear.

Management

1. Use of contact lens with greater oxygen transmissibility.
2. Reduction in the daily wear time.

Corneal Neovascularization

It is s a potentially serious complication of contact lens wear arising because of corneal hypoxia. It is seen with extended wear and therapeutic contact lens. Occasionally corneal neovascularization can occur with thicker and tight fit daily wear contact lenses.

Findings

Typically, the neovascularization is subepithelial, although stromal vascularization can also occur. The superior limbus is most susceptible. The possible complications include lipid exudation, corneal scarring and intracorneal hemorrhage.

Management

1. Management is as for corneal hypoxia in the milder cases with special reference to the oxygen permeability of the contact lens.
2. The fit of the CL has to be checked, a tight fit lens with improper edge may be contributing to the problem.
3. In severe cases the CL wear may have to be discontinued.

Giant Papillary Conjunctivitis (GPC)

Giant papillary conjunctivitis is a well known complication of contact lens wear. Though it may occur in many other conditions, e.g. AKC, VKC, due to irritation from sutures, foreign body or ocular prosthesis; etc. contact lens wear is an important cause of this condition of significant ocular morbidity and needs a special mention. It is fairly common with lens wear particularly with soft contact lenses. Patients with asthma, hay fever and atopy are at increased risk.

Clinical Features

The symptoms may appear months or even years after beginning lens wear. The early symptoms are increased lens awareness/decreased tolerance, itching after lens removal and blurring of vision. There is increased mucous production characteristically in the morning, after over night use of the CL.

Examination shows the presence of **papillae** on upper tarsus > 0.3 mm in size. In severe form they give rise to the **'cobble stone'** appearance. Fluorescein outlines the papillae and also stains the scarred conjunctiva and apices of the papillae in severe cases. **Trantas' dots**, **limbitis** and **punctate keratopathy** may be seen. Ptosis and bloody tears may sometimes occur.

These associations along with the finding of a **coated lens** are diagnostic of GPC.

Pathophysiology

Immunological reaction to altered, coated lens surface with proteins or to the lens material itself and *mechanical factor* such as trauma from the lens edge causing release of neutrophlic chemotactic factor from traumatized conjunctival epithelial cells are thought to be responsible in the development of this condition. Tear from patients show IgE, IgG, IgM and complement, reduced lactoferrin and normal lysozyme levels.

Management

1. *Early Stage*
   a. Discontinue the present contact lens.
   b. Lens replacement with special attention to the design and material.
   c. Meticulous lens care and hygiene using non-preserved solutions, heat sterilization or 3% H_2O_2 is needed. Bi-weekly enzymatic treatment of lens may be required.
   d. Adjunctive use of 4% chromolyn sodium eye drops four times daily.

2. *Moderate Stage*
   a. Discontinue use of the contact lens and reassess after 3-4 weeks.
   b. Usually improvement occurs. In this case the patient can be refit with a lens of different polymer and design.
   c. *Frequent lens change may be needed subsequently every 1–2 months.*
   d. The lens care and use of chromolyn sodium is continued as above.

3. *Severe Stage*

At this stage the management is difficult. Same regime is followed as for moderate stage.
But the CL change is to be done weekly.

Bacterial Keratitis

Microbial keratitis is a serious, potentially blinding complication of contact lens wear. The following obeservations have been made for cases of bacterial keratitis in contact lens users.

1. Almost 40% of all cases of microbial keratitis occur in contact lens wearers.
2. Extended wear soft contact lens and overnight use puts the user at an increased risk, almost 10–15 times more than that for daily-wear.
3. The annual incidence of infective keratitis is about 3 cases per 10,000 even for daily-wearers. This means about 3–5 cases per 1000 of the extended-wearers, which is quite a significant figure.
4. Aphakic contact lens wearers have 6–9 times higher risk.

The pathogen responsible for bacterial keratitis is most commonly *Pseudomonas aeruginosa*. Other agents are *Staphylococcus* and *Streptococcus pneumoniae*.

The suspected corneal infection in contact lens wearers is to be treated as an emergency situation. It should ideally be prevented at all costs.

Prevention of Corneal Infections

1. Avoid over-wear of contact lens.
2. Follow lens care instructions carefully.
3. Never insert lens without disinfection.
4. Always wash hands prior to insertion.
5. Discontinue wear if red eye develops.
6. Avoid swimming with lenses on.
7. Never use saliva for cleaning the lens.

Treatment of Bacterial Keratitis

Treatment of a case of bacterial keratitis is with intensive, fortified, broad spectrum topical antibiotics, at least two in number e.g. an aminoglycoside (tobramycin 1.5%) and *cephazolin (5% to 10%)* every ½ an hour for initial few days and then 1–2 hourly on improvement. Treatment should be guided by Gram staining and culture and sensitivity. Subconjunctival injections may be needed sometimes.

Acanthamoeba Keratitis

- *Acanthamoeba keratitis* is a dreaded, but fortunately rare complication of contact lens wear.
- It is a ubiquitous free-living protozoa that survives in hostile environmental conditions.
- Almost 85% of infections are seen in contact lens wearers.
- Use of tap water or separate distilled water and salt tablets rather than the commercial preparation of saline solution leads to increased risk.
- The sources of infection are home made solutions, tap water, saliva and '*cases*' for keeping the contact lens.
- The management is extremely difficult and the prognosis poor.

Suggested readings

1. Smolin Gilbert: In "The Cornea": Scientific foundation and clinical practice; Third edition, 1994, Little Brown and Company USA.
2. Bennet AJ, Rabbetts RB: Clinical Visual Optics, Butterworths, London, 1984.
3. Abrams D: Duke Elder's Practice of Refraction (Churchill Livingstone: Edinburgh 1993 tenth edition).
4. Tsubota K, Laing RA: Metabolic changes in corneal epithelium resulting from hard contact lens wear. Cornea 1992; 121: 11.
5. Bonanno JA et al: Effect of rigid contact lens on O_2 transmissibility on stromal pH in the living human eye. Ophthalmology 1987; 94: 1305.
6. Weed KH, Fond D, Potvin R: Discontinuation of contact lens wear. Optom Vis Sci 1993; 70 :140.
7. Silbert JA: Anterior segment complications of contact lens wear Churchill Livingstone: Edinburgh 1994.

Chapter 19

Photorefractive Surgeries: Indications and Patient Evaluation

WHY PHOTOREFRACTIVE SURGERY?

For a long time the refractive surgeries had been considered by the medical fraternity as cosmetic surgeries due to lack of awareness of certain hard facts. Surveys have shown that the 'cosmetic' appearance forms a less important reason in the list of the patient. The reasons given by the patients seeking excimer laser surgery are listed below.

1. Desire to improve unaided vision (about 86 %).
2. Freedom from spectacles (about 84 %).
3. Problems with contact lenses (about 73 %).
4. Gain unaided vision to be able to participate in sports (about 70 %).
5. Cosmetic reason (about 60 %).
6. Expense of spectacles or contact lenses (27 %).

The need to get rid of the glasses or contact lenses may arise due to multiple reasons.

To Avoid Dependence on the Corrective Appliances

The desire of the patient with refractive disorder to do away with the lenses is to be understood in terms of the psychological aspects arising from the handicap that the user experiences due to the constant dependency. This applies more to the sufferers of higher degree of ammetropia. Thus, often than not, this desire is more than a cosmetic reason: a longing to experience the world freely, even in the absence of these *prosthesis*, without which one is unable to have this privilege.

Intolerance to the Spectacles

The intolerance to spectacles can develop due to different reasons (discussed in the previous chapter) such as the following.

1. Optical aberrations, aniseikonia and loss of binocularity in anisometropes of higher degree.
2. Improper fit, decentration and relatively uncomfortable frames are responsible for intolerance in cases of even low refractive errors.
3. Constant wearers of spectacles, who devote much time for near work, can best describe the discomfort of different magnitude arising due to inharmonious relation between the accommodation and convergence that has developed after months or years.

Intolerance and/or Complications Due to Contact Lenses

1. The user may develop intolerance due to problems relating to the design, fit, hypoxia related corneal problems or allergic phenomenon such as allergic conjunctivitis and giant papillary conjunctivitis.
2. The intolerance may be due to poor visual rehabilitation (see previous chapters for details).

3. The user may find a contact lens to be much more cumbersome to use and maintain.
4. There may be inability to use the spectacles in contact lens users (**spectacle blur**).
5. The complications may be serious enough to warrant their withdrawal.

Inability to Provide Visual Rehabilitation

There may be certain situations where the spectacles and contact lenses are unable to provide visual relief to the patient, e.g. post surgical refractive errors, very high refractive errors, high and irregular astigmatism.

ADVANTAGES OF PHOTOREFRACTIVE PROCEDURES

The excimer laser has evolved as a magical tool in the hands of the keratorefractive surgeon due to its high precision, efficacy, predictability, reproducibility of cuts and excellent optical results after the corneal surgery. It can be used for keratomileusis of the corneal surface (PRK), keratomileusis of the stromal bed after raising a partial thickness flap (LASIK) or subepithelial keratomileusis (LASEK, after raising an epithelial flap).

Photorefractive surgeries, in particular the latest technique of wavefront-guided LASIK, are able to avoid the dependency on corrective lenses by providing excellent visual rehabilitation, with high degree of predictability, efficacy, reproducibility and safety (more than wearing a contact lens) over a wide range of refractive errors. The *wavefront–guided* or ***customized LASIK*** is able to enter the **supervision zone** of visual acuity, a theoretical, unrealized dream of any refractive surgery.

Now a well informed excimer laser surgeon has enough experience of many years to understand the definite indications and contraindications; has the know-how of the developments and refinements of treatment algorithms and has deep insight into the factors that would lead to stabilization of the refractive outcome. The failure to achieve the results that the excimer laser surgery is capable of providing is because of the learning curve of the surgeon and improper assessment of the cases. It may also be because of over-enthusiasm on part of the surgeon and a less sincere approach than what is desired for such a crucial surgery, due to the growing commercialism.

AIM OF THE PHOTOREFRACTIVE SURGERY

A photorefractive surgeon aims for the following objectives.

To Achieve an Emmetropic State of Eye

The surgeon should know and the patient must be made aware of the fact that it is always not possible to achieve an emmetropic state. This is because of the reasons given below.

1. The degree of refractive error vis-a-vis the corneal thickness might not allow the full treatment due to safety reason.
2. Although the predictability, precision and reproducibility of the excimer laser is very high, the *possibility of achieving emmetropia is never 100%* in view of the reasons given below.

    a. Occasional variation in the energy and intra-operative hydration changes (hence some change in the ablation rate).

    b. There might be errors in the assessment of the preoperative refraction.

    c. Postoperative changes relating to healing, particularly after surface ablation (PRK, hyperopic correction), such as epithelial hyperplasia, stromal remodeling and corneal haze may result in instability of refraction for sometime. These changes may also lead to regression of the achieved correction of myopia.

    d. The **change in the *biomechanics* of the cornea** after LASIK may occur. In LASIK the accuracy of the flap thickness is crucial for leaving a *safe residual bed thickness*. Some of the microkeratomes are known to cut flaps with variable thickness resulting in inadvertently less thick residual stromal bed that may lead to **corneal curvature changes** later on. The residual bed thickness may also be less due to attempted correction of a very high refractive error deliberately planned by the surgeon.

    e. Although the **algorithms**, developed by various companies marketing the different laser systems, have undergone extensive refinements and improvements; to develop the **most perfect** one is still an **unfinished business**. This is more so for treatment of *high astigmatism and hyperopia.*

    f. The results vary considerably depending upon the *system* used (with different claims).

    g. The last but not the least factor is the surgeon's experience, as with any other surgery.

To Provide an Alternative/Decrease Dependence on Lenses

The aim is to provide an alternative to those who are intolerant to the spectacle and contact lenses and to decrease their dependence on these appliances.

If the above facts are realized, then one can easily understand that even in those cases where emmetropia cannot be achieved, the surgeon can still gain the confidence and satisfaction of the patient undergoing the refractive surgery.

This is because *the quality of life* improves. For example if a patient with refractive error leading to uncorrected visual acuity less than the *'work vision'* is left with ±1.0 D of refractive error or 6/12 UCVA (which are the outcome in almost > 90% of photorefractive surgeries), he should be highly satisfied. Moreover, think of a patient who has a refractive error of such a severity that it is difficult to even locate the glasses after he/she wakes up in the morning. For such a patient the morning has never begun.

In these cases, depending upon the central thickness, associated ocular changes and other parameters, the surgeon can aim to correct the maximum possible refractive error without jeopardizing the ocular integrity. The resultant UCVA may turn out to be highly useful to the patient.

Even the cases with not so severe degree of ammetropia, are benefited by the gain of an acceptable UCVA that rids them of their glasses. ***In cases with low myopia, the refractive outcome and visual results are still better and stable with reports of 100% eyes within ± 0.5 D.***

Provide the Benefit of the Latest Technology to the Patient to Fulfill his *Desire*.

The patient may wish to get the benefit of the advancements in the photorefractive surgeries. With the latest technique such as wavefront LASIK, there are reports of better than 6/6 visual acuity and decreased optical aberrations after this surgery.

THE RANGE OF REFRACTIVE CORRECTIONS

Initially the excimer laser keratorefractive surgery was started as corneal surface ablation for correcting low degree of myopia. It was called photorefractive keratectomy (PRK). With improvements in the technology, the range of refractive corrections has increased to include not only the higher degrees of myopia but also other types of refractive errors.

Now the photorefractive surgeries, with newer techniques and algorithms have ventured into the following zones of refractive errors.

Myopia

With the advent of excimer laser refractive surgeries, one important change that is noticeable is the change in the definition of the degrees of myopia. Conventionally < – 3.0 D was called mild, – 3.0 to – 6.0 D moderate and > – 6.0 D as high myopia. With large number of cases of very high degree of myopia being confronted by the refractive surgeons, these limits have changed. Most photorefractive surgeons now define myopia as given below:

Mild myopia	< – 3.0 D
Moderate Myopia	– 3.0 to < – 10.0 D
High Myopia	– 10.0 to < – 15.0 D
Extreme Myopia	– 15.0 D or more

- The definition of *high* myopia given by the laser companies was – 6.0 D at the time of seeking the FDA approval for photorefractive keratectomy (PRK).
- The documented range of myopic corrections is up to – 30.0 D of spherical corrections.
- Commonly – 2.0 D to – 20.0 D of spherical corrections are attempted, but most surgeons agree that – 12 D is the upper safe limit for LASIK. Pallikaris et al in 2002 have reported that –8.0 D is the safe limit, below which no case of corneal ectasia has been seen after review of 2873 cases that underwent LASIK.
- The maximum limit of correction is a function of the *residual bed thickness* (RBT, the unablated stromal thickness). PRK would permit much higher amount of corneal tissue to be removed in comparison to the LASIK surgery in which the corneal flap thickness (average of 160 microns) limits the ablation by the same amount.
- Inspite of the residual corneal thickness remaining in the safe zone, PRK ablation is limited by the more aggressive healing changes and the consequent undesirable refractive effects as the amount of corneal tissue removed increases.
- LASEK increases the attempted range of ablation as for PRK, with the advantages of improved visual results of LASIK by virtue of a thin epithelial flap (about 50–60 micron).

- The final decision on the amount of maximum correction is to be taken on the table by assessing the expected RBT by intraoperative measurement of the flap thickness, the available tissue for ablation and the calculated ablation depth.

The approximate ablation depth is calculated by the Munnerlyn formula given below.

$$\text{Ablation depth} = \frac{(\text{optical zone})^2 \times \text{Diopters}}{3}$$

This formula presumes the excimer laser irradiance to be 180 mJ/cm^2 with an ablation rate of 0.25 μm. The suppliers of different laser systems have developed their own algorithms and the software supplied with the system calculates the expected depth of ablation.

Hypermetropia

- Treatment of hypermetropia involves extending the excimer laser ablation to a large zone of 9.4 mm to 10 mm.
- The initial ablation of the central 5.5–6.5 mm zone is supplemented by a blending treatment of the periphery to produce the steepening of the corneal curvature.
- Such type of ablation pattern is easy to be sculpt by the PRK technique.
- The later modifications in LASIK technique with creation of larger than the usual 9.0 mm diameter flap has allowed treatment of hypermetropia by this method.
- Conventionally +2.0 to +8.0 D of hypermetropic errors have been treated by the excimer laser procedures.
- Rad et al, in 2002, have combined diode laser thermokeratoplasty (DTK) with LASIK to treat hypermetropia up to 10.0 D. This combined approach also reduces the regression of effect which is a frequent problem with the hyperopic correction with photorefractive surgey alone.
- The number of reports on hyperopic treatment, however, are limited in comparison to the vast number of myopic photorefractive surgeries

Astigmatism

- All types of astigmatic errors: simple, compound and mixed; have been treated with excimer laser surgeries.
- Correction of up to 10.0 D of astigmatism has been attempted through different treatment protocols.
- Treatment of the irregular astigmatism involves treatment with *phototherapeutic* (PTK) method. The irregular, steep area / areas are identified by preoperative topography. These areas are treated after protecting the surrounding cornea with a suitable masking agent. This is followed by the required spherical ablation with final smoothening of the corneal curvature.
- The outcome of "photoastigmatic keratectomy" (PARK) is very good in cases of astigmatism up to about 4.25 D (91% within ± 1.0 D) and good in case of higher degrees of astigmatism (up to 72% within ± 1.0 D).
- In the post-surgical astigmatism, the best results are achieved in the post—RK patients (equal to those of primary PARK group) followed by the post-cataract group having 5.0 D of astigmatism. The results of *refractive correction in post—PK patients are also promising* but the visual outcome is compromised by complications like corneal haze, graft failure and irregular astigmatism.

PREOPERATIVE EVALUATION FOR PHOTOREFRACTIVE SURGERIES

Although a careful patient evaluation is a mandatory part of any surgical procedure, it is of immense importance for keratorefractive surgeries. This is because the surgery in this case is an elective one, on an eye which is apparently normal from the patient's point of view. If one has to deliver the goods expected out of such a demanding surgical procedure, an elaborate, thorough, careful and exhaustive assessment is to be carried out involving several aspects. The patient evaluation for photorefractive surgeries has to be done on the following lines.

1. Assessment of parameters concerning and affecting the refractive ablation.
2. Assessment of the patient's suitability for the photorefractive surgery.
3. Assessment of the ocular status and any local or systemic disorder affecting the outcome.
4. Assessment of the benefits *vis-a-vis* risks on an individual basis.

EDUCATION OF THE PATIENT AND INFORMED CONSENT

In this era of high expectations and medical litigations, the first interaction of the excimer laser surgeon with his patient desiring to undergo any photorefractive procedure should begin with a detailed information about the refractive procedures available, the expected benefits and potentials undesirable effects/risks that the prospective candidate might face.

The surgeon must carefully understand the expectations of the candidate out of the proposed excimer laser procedure and make him/her aware of the possible outcomes after a particular procedure (PRK, LASIK, wavefront-guided LASIK or LASEK) based on the previous available reports as well as the experience of the surgeon himself. He should also discuss the nature of the refractive problem of the patient, its natural course (specially the myopia), other available options and risks and benefits of each of them.

The fact may be emphasized that the latest techniques of *excimer laser refractive surgeries* offer the *maximum possible benefits* with *least risk* in comparison with any other available refractive surgery in proper hands with careful selection of the cases. But the surgeon must desist from making any overenthusiastic and overoptimistic claims even in the best prognostic situations because the surgery is being performed on an *apparently* normal eye and *no surgery can be claimed to be absolutely free of any undesirable effects/complication,* however minimal. Moreover, there are *always some postoperative surprises*, inspite of the most sincere efforts of the surgeon. These surprises can occur due to unexpected happenings and machine dependent factors at various levels. This approach would help in avoiding the patient's dissatisfaction as well as any avoidable litigations.

The verbal discussion should be supplemented by other educative materials in the form of booklets and audio-visual means, whatever is available with the surgeon.

The patients in the presbyopic age must be informed of the need for the reading glasses after a successful emmetropic correction.

A written consent is obtained from the patient in the presence of two educated adult witnesses after giving him/her sufficient time to understand all the above aspects of the surgery, in case he / she desires to undergo the offered excimer laser procedure.

PATIENT'S HISTORY

A detailed history is obtained from the patient as follows.

Previous Eye Conditions

History of any previous ocular disorder, ocular surgery or orthoptic treatment should be obtained.

Stability of Refraction

1. *Stability of refraction* is judged by the frequency of spectacle changes over last few years. At least 3 prescriptions for previous 3–5 years must be obtained.
2. The refraction must be stable for at least one year.
3. A stable refraction is crucial before the surgery is undertaken. This would ensure that the post operative regression of effect is not due to myopic progression.
4. The cut off age for photorefractive surgery is generally taken as 18-21 years. By this age most myopes (87% of females and 68 % of males) are stabilized with regard to the progression of their myopia.
5. Progression in the remainder of patients is much slower. Only about 6% of the males show a fast progression of their myopia after the above age limit.
6. Females stabilize earlier than males by about 2 years.
7. These facts about the natural course of the myopia must be told to the patients to avoid any future dissatisfaction and misunderstandings/litigations.
8. *Instability of refraction* is known to occur in pregnancy, breast-feeding (harmonal influence), diabetes mellitus and with exogenous harmonal replacement and steroid therapy.

Systemic Diseases

Any systemic diseases, for example immunocompromized status, diabetes mellitus and collagen disorders, etc. should be ruled out. The collagen vascular diseases are associated with a risk of flap melting. Uncontrolled diabetes and therapy with systemic steroids might affect the healing and therefore the visual results.

Patient's Occupation

The occupation of the patient should be known. Some occupations demand high visual acuity, for example drivers, pilots, employees of armed services, etc. This is essential because some visual problems like loss of

BCVA, halos, glare and diplopia, etc. may occur following the photorefractive surgeries, particularly PRK. Possibility of such eventualities must be discussed with the patients before obtaining consent from them.

Type of Contact Lens

Facts related to the type of contact lens and the duration of its use should be inquired. Any specific problems faced with its use should be known. This is because of the following reasons.

1. Contact lens use changes the refraction of the eye due to corneal edema and /or corneal warpage and therefore hampers the preoperative assessment.
2. A soft contact lens is discontinued for 7 days and a RGP lens for 14 days prior to refractive assessment. *The discontinuation period may extend to 6 months or more in case of corneal warpage.* This is to allow sufficient time for recovery of corneal curvature.
3. If the repeat refraction at the end of this discontinuation period shows a change of >0.5 D, reassessment is postponed for another month till a stable refraction if obtained.
4. Prolonged use of hard contact lens may cause permanent corneal warpage.
5. Any specific problems associated with any type of contact lens should be known because later use of a CL may be needed in case of uniocular correction/ammetropia after surgery or if the full correction of the refractive error was not intended.

ASSESSMENT OF PARAMETERS CONCERNING OR AFFECTING THE REFRACTIVE ABLATION

The list of parameters to be assessed for the photorefractive surgeries is given in Table 19.1.

The Visual Functions

An accurate documentation of all the visual functions namely visual acuity, contrast, colour vision and glare disability, is important for the following reasons.

1. To ascertain the visual potential, particularly in high myopes and to rule out any other associated disorder responsible for the decrease in any of the visual functions.
2. Postoperative comparisons.

Table 19.1: Preoperative evaluations for refractive surgery

1. Refraction
2. Visual acuity: uncorrected (UCVA), best-corrected (BCVA), low-contrast (LCVA) and glare visual acuity (GVA)
3. Near vision in presbyopic subjects
4. Colour vision
5. The pupil diameter
6. Wavefront analysis of higher-order aberrations
7. Ocular muscle imbalance/binocular muscle co-ordination
8. Corneal topography
9. Keratometry
10. Autorefraction
11. Slit-lamp examination
12. Tear-film status
13. Specular microscopy
14. Intraocular pressure
15. Fundus evaluation
16. Indirect ophthalmoscopy
17. Central corneal thickness
18. Corneal sensations

3. To rule out any preoperative decrease in any of the these function. This would avoid future dissatisfactions.
4. The visual acuity is taken under both scotopic and mesopic standardized illumination conditions.
5. A photopic standard illumination about 120-150 candelas/meter^2 must be used to make comparison of the pre and postoperative visual acuity.
6. Patient with decreased contrast may have visual symptoms despite a normal visual acuity after the photorefractive surgery.

Near Vision

The full correction of refractive error or a postoperative hyperopic shift may result in difficulty of near work for patients in the presbyopic age group. The patient must be told of this possibility. The options to avoid this consequence are:

1. The myopic eye may be undercorrected, in consultation with the patient, to an extent to provide a fair degree of near as well as distant vision.
2. The patient may be offered *monovision*, i.e. one eye fully corrected for distance and the other left slightly undercorrected to allow near vision or else only the non-dominant eye be treated for myopia. However the loss of binocularity in this situation

must be explained to the patient, because it results in judgment errors of speed and depth causing problems with driving.
3. The patient can well be comfortable with the reading glasses.

Glare Disability

1. PRK procedure in particular is associated with problems of glare, halos and ghost images due to haze, disparity of pupil size and ablation zone diameter or decentred ablation. Therefore presence of these symptoms preoperatively becomes a contraindication for surgery, specially for PRK. These symptoms might get aggravated to an intolerable level after surgery.
2. The assessment of glare is done by a standard instrument which projects measured amount of light on to the patient's eye in a graded manner. A hand-held device is available for testing glare disability.
3. The patient, specially in the presbyopic age may have glare disability due to a posterior sub-capsular cataract or a peudophake due to posterior capsular opacification.
4. In addition, some subjects might have had symptoms of halos, glare or ghost images due to other reasons.

Keratometry

The assessment of corneal power by modern technique of computerized videokeratography has become a routine for the keratorefractive surgeons these days. But the conventional keratometry has its own place and value in patient evaluation for photorefractive surgeries because of the following reasons:

1. Properly taken readings of the keratometry can corroborate the findings of the true axis in case of corneal astigmatism.
2. It can also helps in diagnosing keratoconus as the cause of an irregular astigmatism.
3. Extremes of keratometry readings should make the LASIK surgeon careful because of the associated flap complications such as a free flap with < 40.0 D and buttonholing with > 46.0 D of keratometry readings.
4. A large difference in the keratometry readings in the opposite meridians should arouse the suspicion of peripheral thinning disorders or keratoconus.
5. However the keratometry can miss early cases of these condition because it evaluates only the 3 mm part of the central cornea.

Refractive Error

The accurate determination of the patient's refractive error is the single most parameter that is so vital for a successful outcome of the photorefractive surgery, among all other factors.

Attention must be paid to many minute details during the process of assessing the refractive error. Some of the points that need to be given importance are given below.

1. The trial frame is to be set in accordance with the interpupillary distance of the individual.
2. The patient must not have a head-tilt and the frame must be placed in a perfect horizontal position with respect to the eyes to avoid wrong determination of the cylindrical axis.
3. If the spherical equivalent is more than -4.0 D, the *back-vertex distance* must be measured and adjustments made accordingly.
4. However, the newer laser systems have the option of making corrections for the back-vertex distance. The correction is incorporated in the software.

Hypermetropia

The use of a cycloplegic is must in cases of hypermetropia. It helps to find out any *latent hypermetropia*, which would remain otherwise unrevealed for full correction.

Myopia

The use of a cycloplegic is not generally recommended in cases of myopia because of increase in the spherical aberration of the optical system in a dilated pupil, increase in the oblique astigmatism and decrease in the *neutralizing power of the lens* which takes care of these aberrations when it is in accommodated shape.

Nonetheless, to take care of the 'pseudomyopia' (increase in the minus power due to excessive accommodation) and overestimation of the myopia, the following regime is followed.

1. The refraction is done asking the patient to look at the distant object such as the 6/12 letters of the Snellen's chart.

2. Fogging of the contralatreral eye is done with a +1.0 D lens if it is not myopic, to make the visual acuity about 6/12.
3. The spherical component is neutralized first, both for spherical as well as cylindrical errors.
4. Any accommodation is eliminated by using plus lenses in small increments till decrease in visual acuity is reported.
5. The possibility of *eating up* of minus lenses is taken care of by adding only the minimum minus lens that improves the visual acuity.
6. A "duchrome test" is performed, using ± 0.25 D spherical lens to make the green *just* clear instead of the red. Addition of a +0.25 D lens should make the red clear. This step also ensures that the myopia is not underestimated.
7. The refraction on the other eye is carried out in a similar manner.
8. Finally a +1.0 D *blur back* test is done in each eye separately to ensure binocular balancing. With addition of plus 1.0 D sphere, the VA should reduce to 6/12 if there is no overcorrection of the minus sphere. If the VA is not reduced to this extent by the **blur back test,** the refractive correction needs to be revised.

Astigmatism

The cylinder axis has to be well defined for treatment of the cases of astigmatism because a 15° of error in determination of the pretreatment axis has been reported to result in as much as 50% less correction.

The following points must be considered when assessing the astigmatism.

1. The accurate determination of the cylinder axis is achieved with the help of the **Jackson cross-cylinder.** The **astigmatic fan** (of Landolt) or the **Maddox V test** are also useful for this purpose.
2. During the final adjustment of the cylindrical power, the spherical component also may require some alteration to make the retinal image sharp.
3. The computerized videokeratography (CVK) axis may differ from the *subjective axis* because the astigmatism may be *lenticular* and not corneal.
4. In cases where the *subjective axis* shows a variation of > ± 5°, the mean of the *subjective axis,* the *CVK axis* and the *axis obtained by autorefractor* may be taken as the final cylinder axis provided the visual acuity remains unchanged or improves with this axis.

The Autorefractor for Determining the Refractive Errors

Although the autorefractor is thought to give reproducible and excellent results in an un-operated eye without any other abnormality, its use as a primary tool for evaluation of the refractive errors prior to refractive surgeries has been underscored due to the reasons given below.

1. The results of the carefully done retinoscopy with fogging/cycloplegia are better than those of an autorefractor.
2. It cannot detect the cases of keratoconus and corneal warpage where the retinoscopy reflex gets distorted, thereby making one to suspect these disorders.
3. It induces *proximal myopia* without cycloplegia.
4. Its usefulness is limited because of inaccuracy in cases of any corneal or lenticular opacities.
5. The postoperative corneas might have surface irregularity due to epithelial disturbances. In this situation the autorefractor may give inaccurate readings.

Ocular Muscle Imbalance

Preoperative detection and management of any binocular muscle imbalance is an essential part of the preoperative evaluation because of the following reasons.

1. The patients may develop manifest squint or even diplopia after a refractive surgery because the prismatic effect of strong glasses is lost after the surgery, thereby converting phoria into tropia if such a condition was present before surgery.
2. An undercorrected anisometrope is also likely to develop this problem if prior detection and proper orthoptic treatment is not given preoperatively.
3. The *accommodative demand* of a myope increases on substitution of the spectacles with the contact lenses and after corneal refractive surgical correction. This would further aggravate any previously untreated accommodative weakness/insufficiency.

Corneal Topography

The computerized videokeratography (CVK) has come as a very important tool in the hands of the excimer laser surgeon for assessing the corneal topography.

1. Modern softwares are able to efficiently document the anterior as well as posterior corneal contour changes with an accuracy of ±0.20 D.
2. Preoperatively the CVK helps in detection of early cases of keratoconus, peripheral thinning of the cornea (e.g. pellucid marginal degeneration and collagen disorders), which are contraindications for excimer laser surgery. Thes are missed by routine keratometry.
3. An average of the astigmatic axis, as determined by subjective refraction, CVK and autorefraction, is taken for treatment of astigmatism (PARK).
4. The topographic information provided by the CVK is vital in postoperative assessments and for planning retreatments. It helps in:
   a. Early detection of many abnormalities.
   b. Establishing the actual cause (diagnosis) responsible for the patients visual symptoms e.g. whether these are due to asymmetric healing, differential regression or true decentration and steep islands or primary undertreatment.

Principle Of Computerized Videokeratography (CVK)

The CVK utilizes the digital video camera in combination with the computer technology to generate images of the corneal topography. The method of computerizes videokeratography essentially involves the following steps.

1. An illuminated placido-type target is projected on to cornea to form an image.
2. This virtual image formed on the cornea is captured by the video camera.
3. The digitalization of this captured image is done by the computer software.
4. The computer software uses complex *algorithms* to *convert the information* from the digitalized images *into measurements of power and radius of curvature.*
5. A *conversion factor* called the "Standard Keratometric Index" (SKI) is utilized by all algorithms for calculating the power and curvature of the cornea from the information provided by the digitalized images.

Presentation of CVK

The data, thus generated by the computer software can be displayed in the form of numerical charts, colour-coded contour maps or as keratoscopic images.

The **colour-coded contour maps** are the commonly used modality to represent the corneal power in which standard colours represent the corneal power in the form of a colour map. Conventionally the warm colours (red and orange) depict higher powers, the cool colours (green and blue) the lower values and the yellow colour represents the medium corneal power. A scale is given on one side of the display/print out for reference, showing the colour representing a particular corneal power (Fig. 19.1).

The colour map makes a better visual impact of the keratometry. *The colour maps can be constructed in three ways.*

1. Fixed colour-to-power scale map
2. The normalized map or automatically adjusted scale map
3. Personalized default adjusted scale map

The Fixed Colour-to-power Scale Maps or Absolute Scale Colour Maps Here the same corneal power is represented by identical colours in all maps thus making the comparisons easy. The incremental steps may range from 0.5 D to 1.5 D. Since the same colour represents a particular corneal power in each map regardless of the incremental value, the comparisons of chronological changes are made easy. These maps also give an idea of the corneal power faster and more readily without a constant referral to the colour code scale provided with the map.

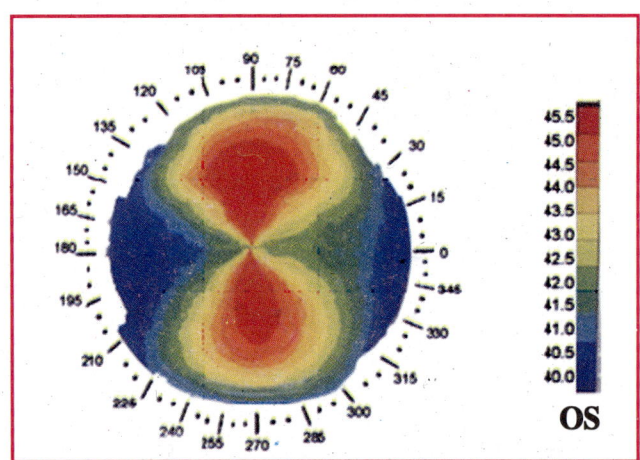

Fig. 19.1: Computerized videokeratography: Colour-coded map showing with the rule astigmatism (WTR). The range of dioptric scale is 40.0 D to 45.5 D with incremental steps of 0.5 D

The 'Normalized maps' or the 'Automatically Adjusted Scale' Maps In these maps the colour representation of the corneal power changes depending upon the incremental value and the range of dioptric power. These maps use the colours and the incremental steps to suit the 'dioptric power range' of an individual's keratometry. For example in a cornea with a power range of 40.0 D to 45.0 D, the incremental value is smaller to cover the small power range within the colour spectrum, the blue would represent 40.0 D and the red 45.0 D. But in corneas with a larger power range (e.g. 35.0 D-48.0 D), the same colours would depict the lowest and highest of these values (Fig. 19.2). Moreover the incremental steps in the later case have to be larger in comparison to the former situation, to cover this range. Thus the same colour represens a different coeneal power in the two cases (Figs 19.3).

Advantages of a Normalized Map

1. It provides *more details* of the overall contour.
2. *Maximizes the visual impact* of the corneal power in a particular case.

Disadvantages of a Normalized Map

1. Areas with the same power are depicted with different colours due to *the use of dissimilar power range and different incremental steps*. This *makes chronological comparisons difficult.*

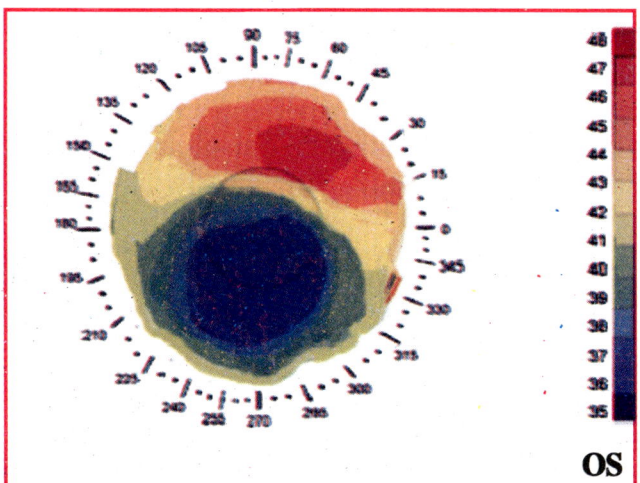

Fig. 19.2: An automatically adjusted or normalized map with power range of 35.0 D–48.0 D and incremental step of 1.0 D. This is showing decentered ablation after phorefractive surgery. The details of the corneal power at different locations are well highlighted

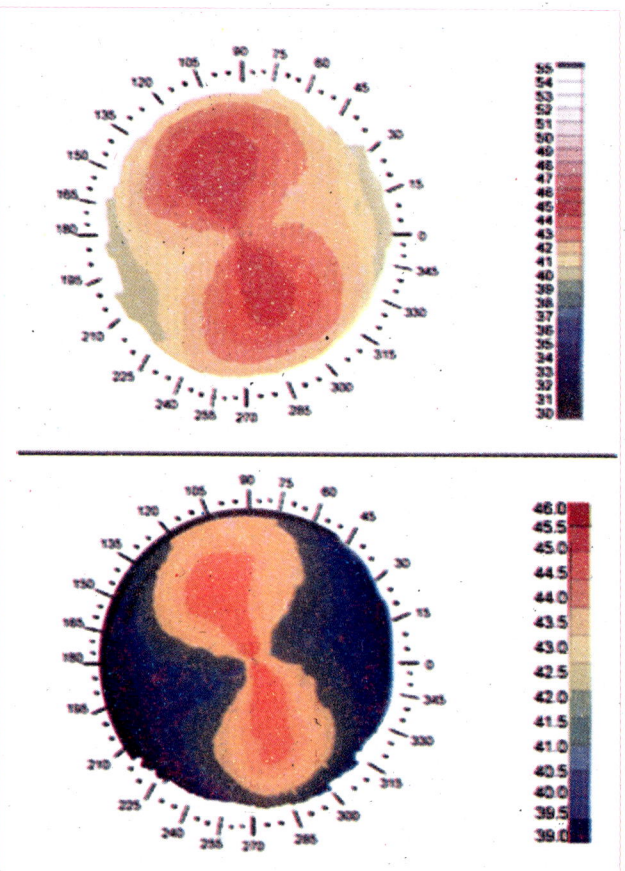

Fig. 19.3: Topography maps of the same cornea with two different dioptric scales. Use of different dioptric scales has greatly changed the appearance of the topographic maps obtained from the same eye

2. The value of the corneal power cannot be readily comprehended from a normalized map. A constant reference to the colour scale has to be made to get the desired information from the map.

The Personal Default Adjusted Scale Map These maps combine the benefit of fixed colour-to-power or absolute scale colour map with the greater details provided by the normalized map. The range of diopteric scale is kept wide and constant for example (30.0 D–55.0 D) in all maps to include extremes of values. The incremental steps are also kept fixed (e.g.1.0 D) to maintain the same colour to corneal power relationship. But these values are chosen as a personalized default setting by the surgeon (Fig. 19.4).

Difference Maps/Subtraction Maps

These maps compare and analyze the chronological changes produced in the corneal topography of the same

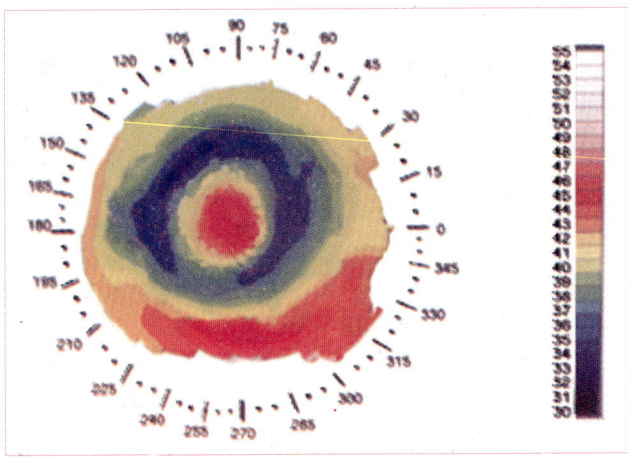

Fig. 19.4: A personal, *default adjusted dioptric scale* topography map

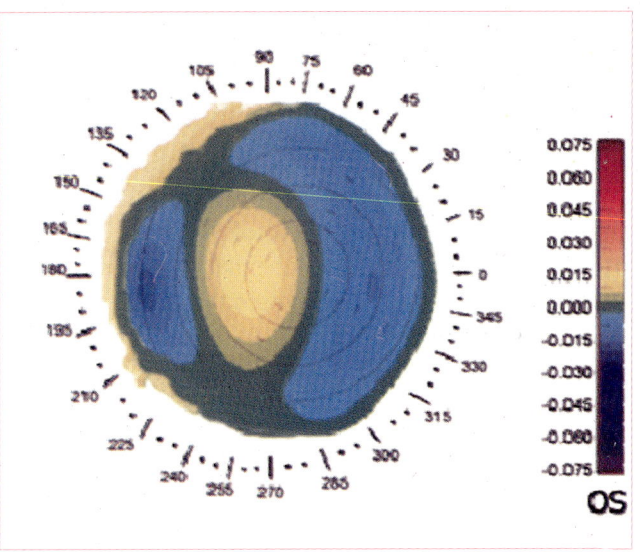

Fig. 19.5: Surface elevation map or tangential map. The map is generated by converting the radii of curvature into true height values to produce the corneal surface profile

eye after the excimer laser ablation. The visual information given by these maps is easy to comprehend and helps in he following ways.

1. Corneal warpage and surface irregularity induced by the contact lenses can be picked up and sequentially followed till improvement before surgery.
2. The postoperative curvature changes can be easily compared and analyzed with the difference maps.
3. Cases of *myopic regression, decentred ablation zone, central steep islands* and *corneal ectasia* can be *picked up early* and timely managed.
4. These maps also help in differentiating cases of focal undertreatment from focal regression.

Elevation Maps or Tangential Maps

The newer CVK systems can produce corneal topography as *true corneal profile* rather than as maps of the corneal power. This is achieved by converting the keratometric values (the radii of curvature) into true height values. Since the digital images are used by CVK, it is possible to provide the details of the total surface profile (Fig. 19.5).

The system uses two extra cameras in the temporal/tangential position to the cornea for '*temporal image grabbing*', thereby providing three dimensional information. The elevation maps are helpful in the following manner.

1. They can detect localized surface irregularities, for example in cases of post-surgical irregular astigmatism, central steep islands and post PRK surface irregularities due to abnormal healing.
2. These maps are then utilized to treat cases associated with visual symptoms.

Two different methods can be used for such treatment.

Using the PTK Mode: Surgeon Controlled Ablation The CVK map is divided into 8 sectors. The map is put behind the oculars in an inverted position at the surgeon's eye level to guide the ablation. The region of low contour/ more initial treatment, shown by the CVK, is masked with a suitable agent while the elevation is being ablated.

Topography-Assisted or Topography-linked Ablation (TOPOLINK) Systems and software have been developed in which the ablation pattern is decided by the machine according to the corneal contour through the utilization of the elevation maps in an individual case. The software of the system calculates the required ablation profile after analyzing the elevation map of a particular case in addition to the required refractive correction fed by the surgeon.

Posterior Corneal Curvature

Newer softwares can provide the information about the posterior surface of the cornea, in addition to the corneal power map and the surface contour (profile). The changes in the posterior corneal curvature can be picked up by serial recordings by CVK after excimer laser surgery to assess the cases of regression and detect early cases of corneal ectasia (Chapter 6).

Normal Corneal Topography

Normally the corneal topography demonstrates the **prolate shape**, i.e. the central cornea is steeper than the peripheral cornea. This is called *positive asphericity*. Only the central part of the cornea is *approximately* spherical, which is evaluated by the keratometery.

Enantiomorphism Enantiomorphism is a phenomenon demonstrated by the normal corneas, in which an individual's corneas are non-superimposable mirror images of each other.

Normal Variations in Topography The variation in the normal prolate topography of the general population is divided into five subtypes. These five subtypes are as follows.

1. **The oval topography appearance**
2. **The round topographic appearance**

The above two patterns are not associated with any significant astigmatism and are included in the same category.

3. **The symmetric bow-tie appearance**
   - The bow-tie appearance is characteristic of an astigmatic cornea.
   - The bow-tie is vertical in case of with the rule (WTR) astigmatism.
   - It is horizontal in a cornea with against the rule astigmatism.
   - It is oriented obliquely in case of oblique astigmatism, with the long axis of the bow-tie in the direction of the steep meridian of the cornea.

4. **The asymmetric bow-tie appearance**

   The asymmetric bow-tie characterizes an astigmatic cornea that has differential power in one particular quadrant, e.g. in keratoconus, corneal warpage induced by a contact lens and peripheral corneal ectatic conditions.

5. **Irregular topographic appearance**

   The cornea shows an irregular topographic appearance after certain disorders like trauma, keratitis, scarring and surgeries like keratoplasty and RK.

CVK: Role In Postoperative Assessment

Computerized videokeratography has a critical role in the assessment and diagnosis of the postoperative topographical corneal abnormalities as already discussed above.

The earliest time when the corneal topography can be obtained after corneal surface ablation (PRK, PTK and PARK), is by the seventh day. However, most patients have surface irregularities related to epithelial healing for a variable period. Nonetheless all patients yield an excellent topographical information by 1 month. Subsequent examinations should be made at third, sixth and twelfth month because the topographical patterns may change up to one year.

The corneal *topography must be obtained as soon as possible* after photorefractive surgery to detect the early abnormalities. Crntral steep islands may present early as undercorrection. Cases of true decentration can be differentiated from asymmetric healing in the early period. Later focal regression may also simulate a decentred ablation zone. These cases, in addition to other cases of focal undertreatment due to *cold spots* in the broad laser beam, can be picked up and differentiated by the CVK only.

Postoperative Topography Maps

The topographical map of the cornea after myopic ablation shows the central blue zone representing marked corneal flattening with surrounding areas of relatively higher power (Fig.15.6). This means that the *prolate corneal contour* with **positive asphericity** converts into an *oblate contour* with **negative asphericity.**

Different authors have described a variety of topographical patterns after PRK. These are summarized in Table 19.2.

The study on post PRK topographical variations by Hersh et al gave the following conclusions.

1. The UCVA was best in the *homogenous pattern* subgroup, The other subgroups showed less UCVA in comparison to the homogenous pattern of topography. It was worst in the *toric against axis* subgroup.
2. There was no statistical difference in the BCVA among the different subgroups based on corneal topography.
3. There was no case of central steep islands in this series.

Slit-Lamp Examination

The slit-lamp examination provides many a useful informations for an eye which is to undergo excimer laser ablation. These additional informations are:

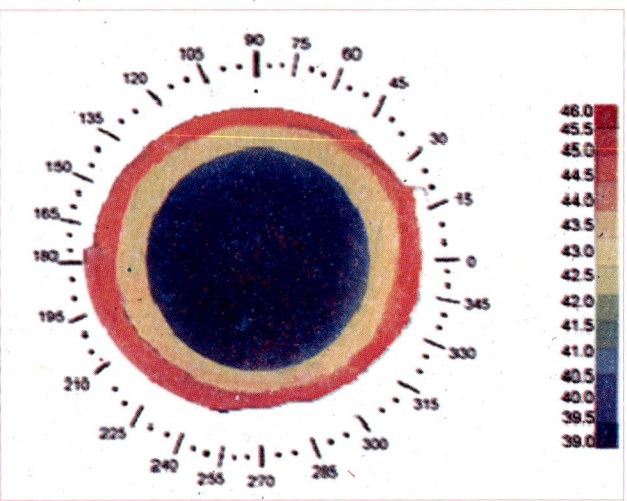

Fig. 19.6: Topography of cornea after myopic PRK. Central part of cornea shows flattening. The corneal power is reduced to 39.0 D in the optical zone. This area of central flattening is surrounded by areas of relatively higher power, i.e. the corneal contour has changed to *negative asphericity*. The ablation zone is well centered and has a smooth appearance. Note a thin rim surrounding the ablation zone coresponds to about 39.5 D–40.0 D, showing a smooth transition of the ablation zone

1. The quality of the tear-film can be directly assessed.
2. Tear-film break up time can be assessed.
3. Dry eye/filamentary keratitis can be diagnosed.
4. Abnormalities/disorders of the lids such as blepharitis and meibomitis can be picked up.
5. Any corneal abnormality, dystrophy or degeneration can be diagnosed.
6. Area of any localized thinning of the cornea and focal stromal haze or decreased translucency can be seen in the optical section of the cornea.
7. Corneal changes induced by contact lens wear are detected.
8. Any early changes suggestive of keratoconus such as Fleischer's ring, Vogt's striae or irregular corneal thickness can be seen.
9. The endothelium can be examined to detect any abnormality.
10. Any lenticular changes like early cataractous changes or *nuclear sclerosis* causing a myopic shift can be picked up and appropriate steps can be taken.

Examination of the Fundus

The posterior pole of the fundus must be evaluated to detect any abnormality of the macula, particularly in high myopes for associated macular changes that might preclude a normal VA. This examination should be done preferably with a +78.0 D or a +90.0 D lens.

Indirect Ophthalmoscopy

Myopes are predisposed to peripheral retinal degenerations and retinal detachments several times more than the general population (see Chapter 6). The retina must, therefore, be thoroughly screened for any suspicious lesions such as holes and lattice, etc. by a retinal surgeon after full dilation. All suspicious lesions must be treated appropriately and surgery postponed for at least few months till the adhesions become strong enough.

Intraocular Pressure

The incidence of primary open angle glaucoma (POAG) is said to be higher in the myopes. In addition PRK is associated with corneal haze during the initial few months. This and the regression of myopia frequently demand long term use of the topical steroids. Any predisposed eyes might develop a rise in the IOP even with the low potency steroids. Therefore the known glaucomatous eye should not undergo the PRK procedure. Glaucoma in itself is a contraindication for the laser refractive surgery because of the decreased future prospective of good vision.

Table 19.2: Topographical patterns after PRK

Moreira et al	Lin		Hersh et al	
1. Multifocal cornea	1. Uniform	(44%)	1. Homogenous	(58%)
	2. Keyhole	(12%)	2. Keyhole semicircular	(2.8%)
	3. Semicircular	(18%)	3. Toric with axis	(17.7%)
	4. Central islands	(26%)	4. Central island	(0%)
			5. Toric against axis	(2.8%)
			6. Irregularly irregular	(13.8%)
			7. Focal topographical Variants	(4.4%)

LASIK surgery, on the contrary is not associated with corneal haze presumably because the epithelial growth factors do not come into the contact of the stroma and induce a healing response in the form of corneal haze. It therefore does not require prolonged treatment with the steroids.

Corneal Thickness

Assessment of the corneal thickness is equally vital as the accurate determination of the refractive error. The amount of safe ablation depends solely on the preoperative corneal thickness. The various aspects relating to the methods of measuring corneal thickness, its variations, the bearing of the *residual thickness* on the postsurgical ectasia and the importance of intraoperative assessment have been discussed in chapter 6 in detail.

Corneal Sensation

Decrease in the corneal sensation might be due to past infection with herpes simplex. Such cases need a concomitant therapy with Acyclovir tablets, 400 mg QID for 10 days. The treatment is starting one day prior to surgery. This has been reported to prevent reactivation of the latent herpes virus after excimer laser surgery.

Corneal Endothelial Count

Though no significant loss of the endothelial cells has been reported after excimer laser surgery, using the spot scanning beam, any preoperative abnormality in count and morphology including any guttate changes should be documented by the specular count, specially in older individuals. The preoperative endothelial count also serves as a baseline for any future references.

Pupil Diameter

The size of the pupil, specially under the mesopic conditions, has a crucial role in the genesis of many disturbing symptoms like glare, colour halos, diplopia and ghost images after excimer laser ablation. The pupil diameter under mesopic conditions must be smaller than the ablation zone diameter. It can be measured by the following methods.

1. The slit-lamp can be used with low illumination and dim room lighting to measure the pupil size by adjusting the slit height.

2. A 'pupil template' also can be used. The patient is asked to look through the different sizes at a distant object and the proper size corresponding to the pupildiameter is noticed. But this may not be an accurate method.
3. Alternatively an *infrared pupillometer* can be used, if available.

Tear-Film Status

Dry eye conditions can cause problems with the healing of the corneal surface after PRK. This surgery itself may sometimes produce dry eye like symptoms because of the surface problems. Therefore this condition is to be excluded by carefully evaluating the tear-film status with the slit-lamp examination, the Schirmer test and the tear-film break-up time (BUT).

The Ultrasound A-Scan and B-Scan

These tests are performed because of the following reasons.

1. The globe of a high myope might have a posterior staphyloma, which can be detected by the ultrasound B-scan.
2. Asymptomatic posterior vitreous detachment (PVD) may be detected by the B-scan. Complete PVD gives an assurance that if no damage has occurred to the retina at present, it is unlikely to do so in the future as the vitreous would exert no retinal traction.

CONTRAINDICATIONS vs. PATIENT'S SUITABLITY: THE FINAL DECISION

After a careful evaluations of the different parameters and any relative or absolute contraindications of the surgery, the surgeons critically evaluates and analyzes the risks and benefits of the surgery.

It is to be understood that **the contraindications of any particular surgery keeps on decreasing with time as the procedure itself undergoes refinement overtime and the surgeon becomes more experienced.** Same is true for the excimer laser refractive surgery. The list of the contraindications has become smaller and the line between the absolute and relative contraindications has become blurred. For example *a thin cornea is not an absolute contraindication for the surgery as long as the postoperative RBT remains > 325 microns.* A cornea with a CCT of about 450 μ can safely have about 8.0-

10.0 D of correction with the PRK procedure (requiring about 100 μ ablation, depending upon the ablation zone diameter). But for LASIK the available tissue for safe ablation would be less after subtracting the 120-160 μ thickness of the flap. Therefore LASIK would be contraindicated in the same case.

Table 19.3 enumerates the relative and absolute contraindications of photorefractive surgery.

A final discussion is held with the patient to have his clear views and expectation in light of the final assessment of the surgeon. A cooling-off time is given to the patient before he/she is asked to sign the consent form.

Some points that must be made very clear to the prospective candidate of a photorefractive surgery are.

1. The outcome of the surgery cannot be guaranteed for 100% results.
2. An approximate idea of the anticipated outcome can be provided based on previous reports and the achieved results of the surgeon.
3. The types of problems/complications and their probability, though may be temporary, should be made known to the patient to avoid patient dissatisfaction, anxiety and litigations.
4. The possibility of a retreatment may arise due to over or undercorrection, abnormal healing response in case of PRK or regression, etc. The approximate rate of such retreatments should be told to the patient.

Suggested readings

1. McGhee CNJ, Orr D, Kidd B et al: Psychological aspects of excimer laser surgery for myopia: Reasons for seeking treatment and patient satisfaction. Br J Ophthalmol 1996; 80: 874-879.
2. Kahle G, Seiler T, Wollensak J: Report on psychological findings and satisfaction among patients one year after excimer laser PRK. Ref Corn Surg 1992; 8 : 286-289.
3. Weed KH, Fond D, Potvin R : Discontinuation of contact lens wear. Optom Vis Sci 1993; 70:140.
4. Bennet AJ, Rabbetts RB: Clinical Visual Optics (Butterworths: London, 1984).
5. Abrams D: Duke Elder's Practice of Refraction (Churchill Livingstone: Edinburgh 1993 tenth edition).
6. Yeow EK, Taylor SP: Clinical evaluation of the Humphrey automatic refractor. Ophthal Physiol Opt 1989; 9: 171-175.
7. Hosaka N: The effect of various eye diseases on the measurment of refractive error using the Nikon autorefractometer. In Brenin GM, Seigel IM, eds, Advances in Diagnostic Visual Optics (Springer-Verlag : Berlin 1983). 75-83.
8. Stevens JD: Astigmatic excimer laser treatment : Theoretical effects of axis misalignment. Eur J Implant Ref Surg 1994; 6: 310-318.
9. Sunderaj P, Villada JR, Joyce PW et al: Glare testing in pseudophakes with posterior capsule opacification. Eye 1992; 6: 411-413.
10. John ME, Howard C: Esotropia following radial keratotomy. J Cataract Ref Surg 1991; 17: 246-247.
11. Rengstorff RH: Variations in corneal curvature measurments: an after effect observed with habitual wearers of contact lenses. Am J Optom 1969; 46: 45-57.
12. Morgan JF: Induced corneal astigmatism with hydrophilic lenses. Can J Ophthalmol 1975; 10: 207-213.
13. Silbert JA: Anterior segment complications of contact lens wear (Churchill Livingstone: Edinburgh 1994).
14. Pimendies D, Steele CF, McGhee CNJ et al: Deep corneal stromal opacities associated with long term contact lens wear. Br J Ophthalmol 1996; 80: 21-24.
15. Epstein D, Frueh BE: Indications, results and complications of refractive corneal surgery with lasers. Curr Opin Ophthal 1995; 6: 73-78.
16. Bogan SJ, Waring GO, Ibrahim O et al: Classification of normal corneal topography based on computer-assisted videokeratography. Arch Ophthalmol 1990; 108: 945-949.

Table 19.3: Contraindications for photorefractive surgery

Ocular Contraindications

1. Unstable refraction over the last one year
2. Progressive myopia
3. Keratoconus
4. Herpetic keratitis / history of herpes infection
5. Corneal diseases
6. Cataract
7. Lagophthalmos
8. Dry eye
9. Uncontrolled blepharitis
10. Uncontrolled uveitis
11. Uncontrolled glaucoma
12. Marked corneal vascularization (bleeding would shield the tissue and decrease laser ablation)

Medical Contraindications: Conditions that Would Affect Healing

1. Collagen vascular diseases
2. Autoimmune disease
3. Immunosuppressed/immunocompromized
4. Pregnant or nursing women
5. History of keloids
6. Diabetes mellitus

17. Corbett MC, O'Brart DPS, Saunders DC et al: The topography of the normal cornea. Eur J Implant Ref Surg 1994; 6: 286-297.
18. Salmom TO, Horner DG: Comparison of surface elevation, dioptric curvature and refractive power maps of an elliptical cornea. Invest Ophthalmol Vis Sci 1995; 36(Suppl): S1032.
19. Chan WK, Carones F, Maloney RK: Corneal topographic maps: A comparison of axial curvature with true instantneouscurvature. Invest Ophthalmol Vis Sci 1995; 36(Suppl): S1032.
20. Corbett MC, O'Brart DPS, Sanders DC et al: The assessment of corneal topography. Eur J Implant Ref Surg 1994; 6: 98-105.
21. Ruiz MJ, Mafra CH, Wilson SE et al: Corneal topographic alterations in normal contact lens wearers. Ophthalmol 1993; 100: 128-134.
22. Gangadhar DV, Talamo JH: The use of computerized videokeratography in keratorefractive surgery. Semin Ophthalmol 1994; 9 (2): 81-90.
23. Doane JF, Cavanagh TB, Durrie DS et al: Relation of visual symptoms to topographic ablation zone decentrations after excimer laser PRK. Ophthalmology 1995; 102: 42-47.
24. Lin DTC: Corneal topographic analysis after excimer laser PRK. Ophthalmology 1994; 101: 1432-1439.
25. Maloney RK: Corneal topography and optical zone location in PRK. Ref Corn Surg 1990; 6: 363-371.
26. O'Brart DPS, Corbett MC, Sanders DC et al: The topography of corneal astigmatism. Eur J Implant Ref Surg 1994; 6: 361-369.
27. Wilson SE, Klyce SD, McDonald MB et al: Changes in corneal topography after excimer laser PRK for myopia. Ophthalmology 1991; 98: 1338-1347.
28. Moreira H, Garbus JJ, Fasano A et al: Multifocal corneal topographic changes with excimer laser PRK. Arch Ophthalmol 1992; 110: 994-999.
29. Hersh PS, Schwartz-Goldstein BH: Corneal topography of phase III excimer laser PRK. Ophthalmology 1995; 102: 963-978.

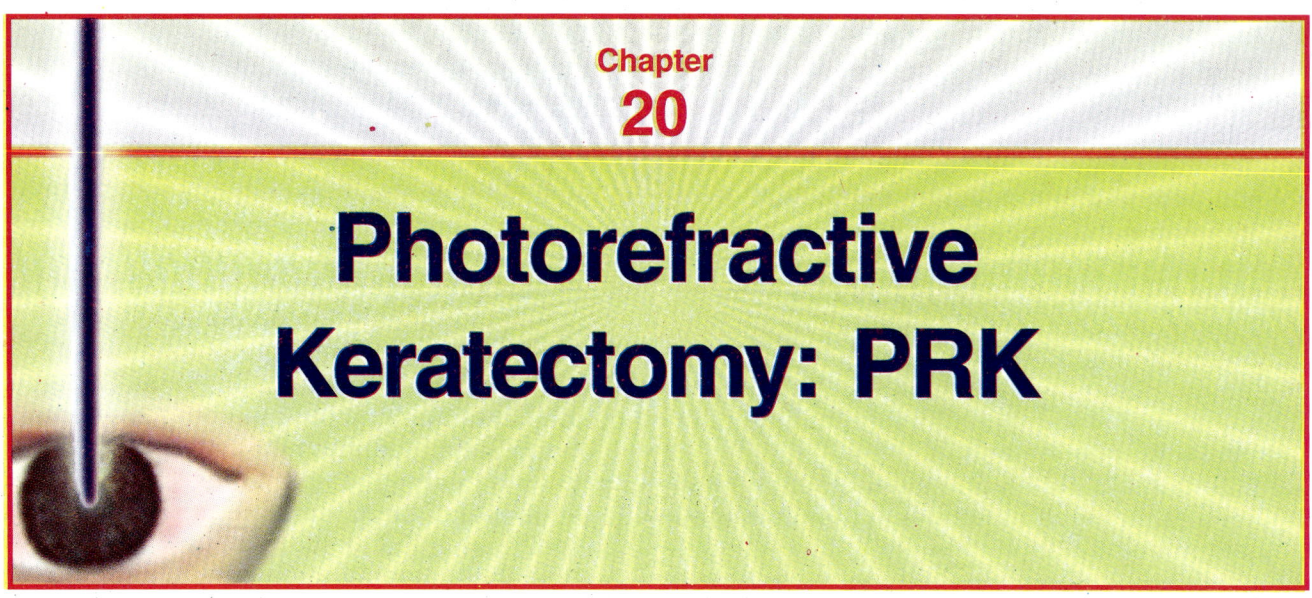

Chapter 20
Photorefractive Keratectomy: PRK

PHOTOREFRACTIVE KERATECTOMY

HISTORY OF PHOTOREFRACTIVE KERATECTOMIES

The possibility of application of the excimer lasers for corneal surgeries and refractive corrections was suggested by the pioneering work of Stephen Trokel, Srinivasan in 1983. They, alongwith John Marshall and others, further studied the refractive applications such radial incisions and wide area ablation.

Munnerlyn is associated with coining the term *'photorefractive keratectomy'*, in 1984. His painstaking experiments resulted in defining a quantitative relationship between the amount of corneal tissue to be removed for correcting a given myopic error. He demonstrated that the depth of ablation to bring about the given refractive change is directly proportional to the square of the ablation zone diameter, a smaller ablation zone producing greater change. The formula developed by him is popularly known by his name as the **Munnerlyn formula**.

$$\text{Ablation depth} = \frac{(\text{optical zone})^2 \times \text{diopters}}{3}$$

The importance of the work done by Munnerlyn was not realized for almost four years till 1988, when the *first computer generated algorithm for PRK* was published. Meanwhile other scientists kept on exploring the application of excimer laser for refractive correction.

Seiler and coworkers were the *first to use* the excimer laser *clinically*. They used it to excise the diseased corneal tissue in 1986 (*first clinical PTK*) and *to treat astigmatism* in 1987 (suggesting PARK).

The excimer laser was used to give radial incision for RK by Aron-Rosa, Marshall and Trokel, Cotliar et al and Gaster et al. Problems were associated with the *excisions* produced by the excimer laser, as it removed the tissue rather than *excised* it, unlike the conventional RK knife. The excisions get filled with epithelial plugs, which persist for months or even longer, potentially weakening the cornea. The healing is with more scarring of the excised area that causes glare more than conventional RK.

However the more effective application in the form of *wide area ablation* (PRK), as suggested earlier by Munnerlyn, was being studied by *Mcdonald et al*, since 1987 in blind and sighted human eyes. They published the results of FDA sponsored, *first PRK study performed on sighted human myopic eyes in 1991*. Subsequently innumerable clinical studies have been published on the results and different techniques of photorefractive keratectomy.

The FDA approval for PRK was granted to the Summit Laser in December 1995 and to the Visx Laser in March 1996, after the phase III trials.

PRK: DEFINITION

Photorefractive keratectomy (PRK) is a technique of laser keratomileusis utilizing the 193 nm excimer laser that changes the corneal curvature by removing tissue from a wide area of the surface of the cornea. It has been used to treat myopia ranging from mild to extreme degrees, hyperopia and astigmatism of different origin.

PRK: ABLATION TECHNIQUES

Two types of laser delivery systems are used for refractive ablation. The techniques of ablation depend upon these two types of laser systems used for PRK. The two systems are:

1. Wide/broad beam laser system
2. Scanning laser system

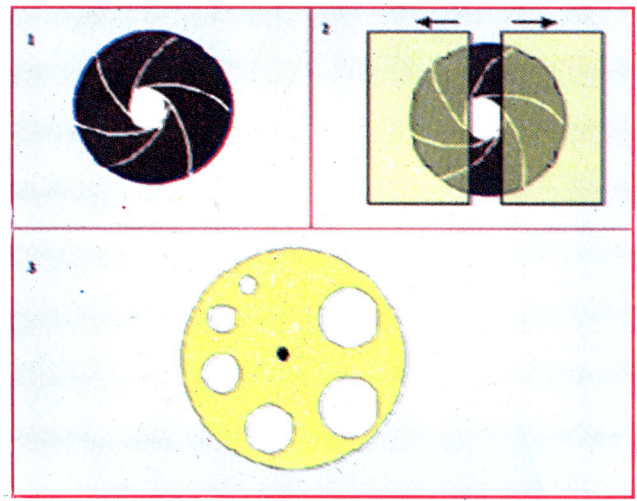

Fig. 20.1: Diagrammatic representation of an iris-aperture (1), the parallel blade shutter with iris aperture (2) and the rotating wheel apertures (3)

THE WIDE BEAM DELIVERY SYSTEMS

The earlier techniques for refractive correction were based on the *wide beam* laser systems that were available during the gestation period of the photorefractive surgeries. Modifications and refinements were centered on utilizing and adapting the wide beam delivery to suit the different types of refractive ablation profiles.

Control of the Laser Beam Shape/Profile

Control of the ablation profile with the wide laser beam delivery is achieved by one of the five devices that are inserted in the path of the incident laser beam (Figs 20.1 and 20.2). These devices are:

1. Mechanical iris diaphragm
2. Rotating wheel with different apertures
3. A moving slit
3. Combination of parallel blade shutter with an expanding aperture
5. An ablatable PMMA mask

The Mechanical Iris Diaphragm

It is a mechanical device that either contracts or expands in a controlled manner to allow a laser beam of definite diameter to reach the cornea. This is the most commonly used device for projecting the myopic ablation pattern on to the cornea.

Kruger and colleagues modified the iris aperture by '*defocusing*' the image of the aperture in an attempt to

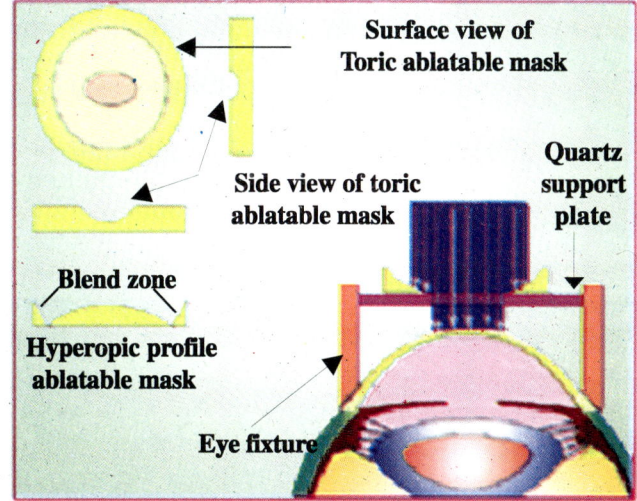

Fig. 20.2: Diagrammatic representation of the 'erodible mask' and how it works during ablation

produce a smoother ablation as the conventional contacting/expanding iris aperture tended to produce stepped up edges on the corneal surface.

Rotating Wheel with Different Apertures

This device is in the shape of a wheel with *round, slit-shaped or oval apertures* apertures of different diameter in its mid periphery, which come in the path of the laser as the device is made to rotate as per requirement. Thus laser beams of different size and shapes can be projected on to the cornea. The utility of such a device is in projecting the *multizone ablation pattern* for the treatment of very high and extreme myopia. The slit and oval apertures can be used to produce astigmatic ablation profiles.

A Moving Slit

Similarly a slit that can complete 360° of rotation around its axis can be introduced in the laser path (see chapter 7 for slit beam delivery). It is *useful for astigmatic ablation pattern*. The width of the slit is about 2 mm, though it may vary in different systems. The slit can moves a complete 360° to ablate the corneal surface.

This slit can be so oriented to give more ablation in a particular meridian to treat simple astigmatism. The *flattening of the corneal curvature is produced in the meridian perpendicular to the long axis of the slit*. For treating compound astigmatic error, the rotation of the slit can be so controlled by the computer as to allow more laser ablation along a particular meridian by keeping the slit for a longer time in that particular position.

Combination of 'Parallel Blade Shutter' with an Expanding Aperture

This mechanism, devised by Munnerlyn, is used for treatment of astigmatism associated with spherical errors. The long axis of the blades is aligned with the axis of the minus cylinder to produce more ablation along the meridian perpendicular to this long axis, as the blades gradually open in this direction (the mechanical axis of the blades). This produces a flattening of the cornea in the meridian opposite to the long axis of the blades, which is the steep meridian. The *correction of the astigmatism is greater if the blades open more slowly*, i.e. the laser beam is given more exposure time to ablate a thinner zone. The circular iris aperture is then utilized to give the remaining spherical ablation.

All these devices are under the control of the computer software, which controls their size and/ movement during ablation according to the algorithm required for a particular refractive correction.

An Ablatable PMMA Mask

The ablatable or the *erodible mask* is a device consisting of PMMA material that has the same ablation rate as the corneal tissue. It is an important accessory for the treatment of astigmatism and hypermetropia.

Its principle is that when PMMA mask is placed between the corneal surface and the excimer laser path, the laser has to first perforate the PMMA at a particular site before it can ablate the cornea. Thinner the PMMA at a given location, earlier the laser would reach the cornea to ablate it. Therefore the *profile of the ablatable mask sculpted is opposite to that of the desired contour* of the corneal surface. The thickness of the *toric mask* is like a toric contact lens, being more in the axis of the flat meridian so that the cornea under it would receive less or no ablation while the area opposite, under the thinner portion is being ablated. Similarly in case of hypermetropia, the periphery is made thinner to deliver more energy to the cornea in the periphery to produce the steepening. Thus *the mask is manufactured on an individual basis in the form of a lens conforming exactly to the refraction of the case.*

Disadvantages of the Wide-Field Ablation

1. The wide beam ablation however needs a demanding mechanism to *homogenize* the beam in order to maintain uniformity of the energy distribution throughout the large beam and produce a smooth ablation.
2. The range of algorithms is also limited and the ablation patterns not very refined to produce a variety of refractive corrections.
3. These are largely replaced by the *scanning mode* of ablation, which is capable of producing an unlimited ablation profiles more accurately (see chapter 7 for more discussion on these aspects).

PRK TECHNIQUES FOR MYOPIA

The different techniques employed for the correction of myopia are:

1. Single zone/transitionzone ablation
2. The Multipass ablation
3. The Multizone technique
   a. Single-pass multizone ablation
   b. Multipass multizone ablation
4. Tapered transition zone ablation

Single Zone/Transition Zone Ablation

The single zone technique involves ablation of the central area of the cornea using only one preset ablation zone size. The iris diaphragm opens only one time to complete the full refractive ablation. This produces an aspheric ablation profile due to **transition zone** between the ablated and non-ablated corneal surface (Fig. 20.3).

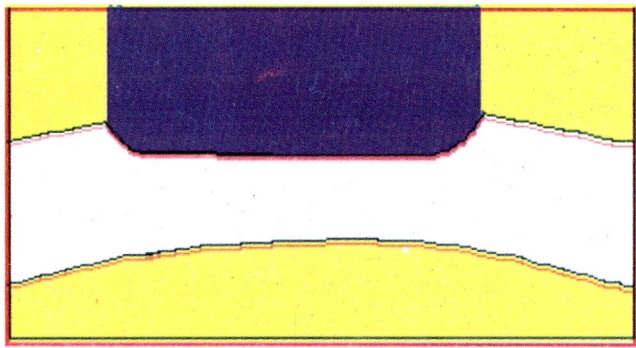

Fig. 20.3: Single zone/transition zone ablation

Ablation Zone Diameter

The effect of the ablation zone diameter on the refractive outcome and post-PRK visual disturbances has been evaluated by many studies. Munnerlyn had demonstrated through his pioneering research that a smaller ablation zone produces greater refractive change. But there are definite problems of night vision, glare and halos when the pupil size approaches or is larger than the diameter of the ablation zone, particularly under dim light condition such as night driving.

Different sizes of the ablation zones varying from 3.5 mm to 7 mm have been studied and the following conclusions have been reached.

Small Zone Ablations: Disadvantages

1. Small zone ablations (5 mm or less) are associated with high incidence of halos and night vision problems. As much as 45% of patients at 3 months and 38% at 12 months experience them with 5 mm ablation zone diameter.
2. This side effect is still higher with 4 mm and 3.5 mm zones.
3. There is increased incidence of initial overcorrections (hyparopic shift) and decreased predictability of outcome with the smaller zone ablations.
4. Even milder decentration in a case of the *small ablation zone* would cause more '*symptomatic*' vision disturbances.

Larger Zone Ablation: Advantages

1. Larger zone of ablation (6-7 mm) gives superior results.
2. The incidence of the post-PRK visual disturbance is reduced to insignificant level (5% or less at 12 month).
3. The *predictability* and *stability* of results improves and overcorrection rate decreases with large ablation zone.

Larger zone ablation: Disadvantages

Since the amount of tissue to be removed (depth of stromal ablation) is greater for an equivalent refractive change when using larger ablation zone, the incidence of associated side effects related to greater healing response, such as *corneal haze is increased.*

Multipass Ablation

1. The multipass ablation means that during the process of ablation, the *delivery of the calculated energy* is not made in a single-go but *divided into several fractions* (5–7 fractions).
2. There is a gap of about 30–60 seconds between the delivery of the successive fractions (*pass*) of the laser pulses.

Advantages of Multipass Technique

1. This approach has the advantage of allowing for correction of fixation during the 'delay' period (between each pass).
2. There is reduced surface heating, unlike that seen with the continuous delivery of a large laser beam.
3. Smother ablation due to 'averaging effect' of the multiple aperture openings.
4. The incidence of the 'steep islands' is decreased.

The multizone ablation, which divides the total-ablation into several *zones* is inherently using the multipass technique as there is a delay before switching over to the next zone (vide infra).

Multizone Technique

This technique is specially useful in treating cases of *high and extreme degree of myopia*[19-22] It can be performed in two ways.

Single-Pass Multizone Ablation

In this technique, all the zones are ablated with a single-pass of laser delivery i.e. continuously without any stopping of the laser before switching to the next zone (Fig. 20.4).

Multipass Multizone Ablation

The technique is called multipass multizone ablation technique if there is a break (delay) in the laser delivery before the ablation of the next zone begins, i.e. the laser delivery also gets divided into several *passes* (Fig. 20.5).

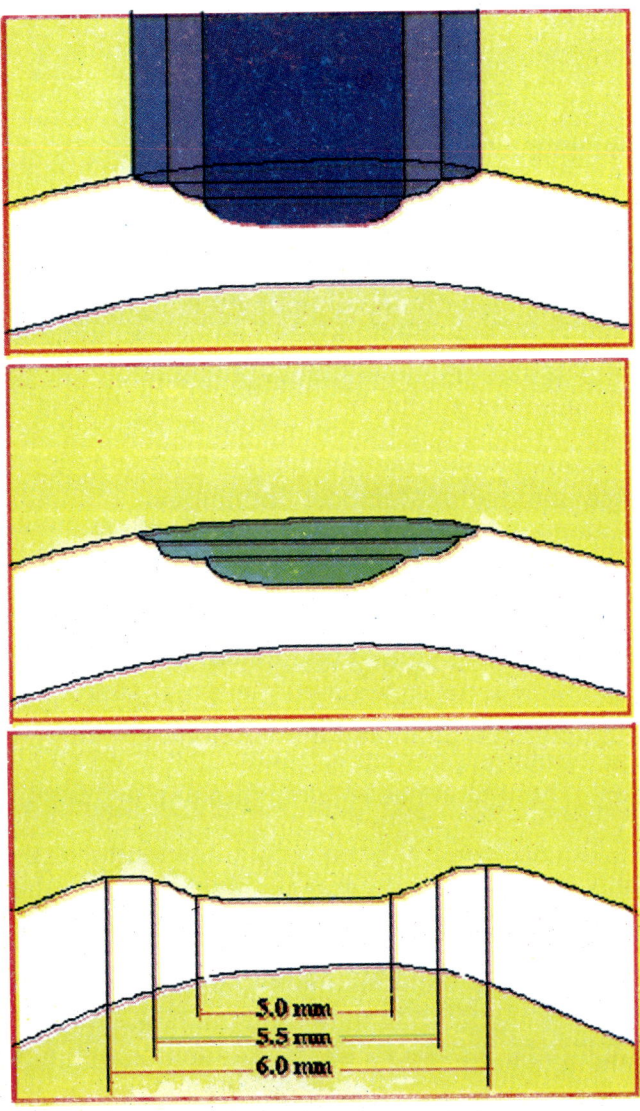

Fig. 20.4: Diagrammatic representation of multizone ablation and the corneal profile produced after such ablation

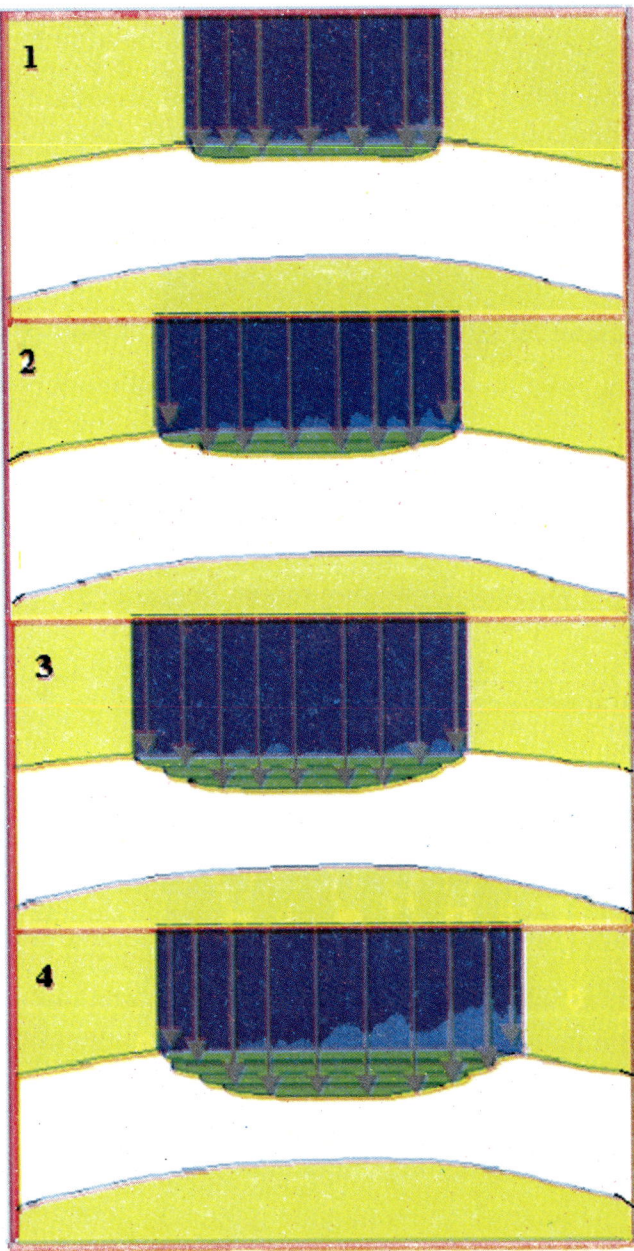

Fig. 20.5: Diagrammatic representation of the multipass–multizone ablation technique. With each pass an additional amount of corneal tissue is removed. The ablation zone diameter increases with each pass of the excimer laser

The multizone ablation essentially involves the following steps.

1. The *total correction* to be performed is *divided into several optical zones* (usually three, e.g. 5.0 mm, 5.5 mm and 6.0 mm) depending upon the algorithm available with the system.

2. The number of zones is up to 7 in case of multipass multizone technique, the zone diameter ranging from 3.5 mm to 7.0 mm.
3. The power is usually equally divided into the zones.
4. In case of the single-pass multizone ablation utilizing only 3 zones, if the calculated power to be corrected is high, the correction by the outermost zone may be kept smaller than inner zone to achieve a *tapering effect* of the ablation zone and avoid subsequent epithelial hyperplasia and *regression of effect*.
5. Sometimes the central zone is allotted the maximum power correction, up to 80% to substantially decrease the ablation depth in cases of very high myopia. In this approach the small inner zone would produce the same visual problems as seen with a small single zone ablation.

Advantages of Multipass Multizone Ablation

1. The multizone ablation approach decreases the ablation depth by about 25%. Still greater reduction in ablation depth can be achieved by allotting more refractive correction to the inner zone. The decrease in ablation depth reduces the incidence of corneal haze and regression.
2. It allows treatment of extremes of myopic errors (up to –27.0 D has been treated with this technique[19]).
3. The incidence of central steep islands is reduced to zero with multipass multizone technique as compared with 56% incidence rate with the *single zone technique* and 8% with the *single-pass multizone technique*.
4. There is less overcorrection and hyperopic shift.
5. Visual recovery is faster with better uncorrected vision.

Tapered Transition Zone Ablation

This technique involve creation of an additional 1.5 mm *'tapered transition zone'* between the central *refractive zone of about 4 mm and the peripheral part* of the ablation zone that extends to a maximum of 7 mm.

This technique is said to decrease the regression of effect and improves the stability of the refraction in cases of high myopia by taking care of the abrupt transition that induces epithelial hyperplasia (an important cause of regression post-PRK surgery).

ABLATION TECHNIQUES FOR ASTIGMATISM

For a successful treatment of the astigmatism (simple, mixed or compound), the preliminary considerations of importance are:

1. An accurate determination of the axis of astigmatism must be done.
2. The determination of the axis of astigmatism should be assisted by objective retinoscopy, computerized videokeratography, keratometry and autorefractor (see preoperative evaluation).
3. The cylindrical error should be converted to *'minus cylinder'*. This makes the ablation easy, as the axis of the cylinder can be used to ablate the opposite meridian and cause flattening thereby reducing the minus cylinder.
4. The treatment of *mixed astigmatism* may demand splitting the astigmatism into two components in such a way that they can be easily treated in a *two step* procedure. Each component is treated separately by successive ablations.
5. Treatment of the *irregular astigmatism* involves a *PTK mode of approach*, in which the area/areas appearing as low power/curvature maps on videokeratography are *masked* by a suitable agent and 50% of the high power area ablated. This is followed by the remaining correction given to the whole ablation zone to achieve the final correction.

PHOTOASTIGMATIC REFRACTIVE KERATECTOMY (PARK)

Historically, the large beam laser systems utilized one of the following techniques to achieve an astigmatic ablation.

1. The slit-scanning beam delivery.
2. An ablatable mask.
3. The revolving band/wheel with oval or slit apertures.
4. The 'parallel blade shutters' with an expanding iris aperture.
5. An *hourglass-shaped* rotating mask.
6. The scanning spot laser algorithm.

The first four devices have been already described in the beginning of this chapter.

The 'Parallel Blade Shutter' With An Expanding Iris Aperture

The 'parallel blade shutter' with an expanding iris aperture can be used in two types of techniques for correction of *myopia with astigmatism*.

1. The sequential method
2. The elliptical method

The Sequential Method

For treating myopia with astigmatism, the 'sequential' method performs ablation in two phases. First the astigmatism is corrected by opening the blade-shutter while the round iris diaphragm remains open throughout its movement. In the second treatment, the remaining spherical component is treated by using the round diaphragm to project a myopic profile while the blade-shutter remains fully open.

The Elliptical Method

This method treats both the spherical and the cylindrical components simultaneously. The gradual expansion of the blades is combined with the controlled contraction of the iris diaphragm. This *produces an elliptical ablation zone*, hence the above name of this method. *The ratio of the sphere to the cylinder determines the width of the short-axis of the elliptical zone.*

Advantages of the Elliptical Method

1. This one stage combined treatment reduces the operating time, thereby decreases the fixation losses.
2. It also decreases the chances of uneven drying of the cornea that may result in irregular ablation and irregular astigmatism.
3. Prevents any inadvertent narrowing of the short-axis of the *ellipse* that may result due to an *overtreatment* of the cylindrical component first. This is crucial because the short axis may encroach upon the pupillary zone resulting in disturbing visual symptoms.

Limitation of the Elliptical Method

It is implied by the above explanation that 'elliptical method' cannot treat cases where the cylindrical component in minus form is more than the sphere because the short-axis of the elliptical ablation zone that would be produced in this situation would lie in the pupillary area. The *sequential method* produces a circular ablation zone and *therefore* should be *preferred in these case where the cylinder is larger than the sphere.*

Hourglass-shaped Rotating Mask

This hourglass-shaped mask can be rotated in a full circle with the computer control.

1. It projects a slit shaped beam on the cornea that can be held at any desired position for a longer time to produce differential ablation..
2. The aperture of the mask also can be varied to produce the required correction as the astigmatic change is greater with a narrower beam.
3. Both these effects in combination are thus able to correct the required magnitude of the astigmatism at the given axis. Moreover the *hour glass-shaped ablatable mask* can correct both the myopic as well as the hyperopic astigmatism.

Spot Scanning Laser Delivery

The scanning laser is a more useful method of treating any type of refractive error including the astigmatism. This is because the small size laser beam can be moved around the corneal surface to obtain the desired ablation profile in a more controlled manner. It *can also treat the hyperopic astigmatism* by selectively ablating the periphery to cause steepening of the flat meridian.

ABLATION TECHNIQUES FOR HYPEROPIA

HYPEROPIC PRK

The correction of hyperopia requires the preferential ablation of the corneal mid-periphery to produce steepening of the central cornea (Fig. 20.6).

The following points summarize the essential facts relating to a hyperopic ablation.

1. Unlike the myopic PRK, for hyperopic correction the central cornea is either not ablated or minimally ablated in comparison to the peripheral part to cause a steepening effect. *The techniques of hyperopic PRK sparing the central optical zone avoids any corneal haze and opacity in this area.* The techniques that also ablate the central optical zone are associated with an increased corneal haze, which is greater than in a case of myopic PRK performing an equitable ablation.

2. An annulus of tissue is removed from the mid-periphery of the cornea.
3. The *midperipheral trough* created by the *hyperopic ablation* is blended with the central optical zone and the peripheral part of the cornea to avoid any 'abrupt step' between the adjacent zones. This is achieved through smooth transition of ablation. *This step is crucial in preventing the regression of effect* after correction because the trough fills up as more compensatory healing is induced by the abrupt edge.
4. *An accurate centration is the key* for good visual results, even more so than in cases of myopic PRK. This is because a decentred ablation would result in the loss of BCVA, inspite of the achievement of desired refractive change, due to the increase in corneal asphericity that is not amenable to optical correction by lenses.
5. The *size of the central zone must be about 6 mm.* The earlier techniques that utilized a 4 mm optical zone and 7 mm total ablation zone were associated with a high incidence of loss of BCVA (upto25% of eyes). This is due to the fact that even small decentration of the ablation becomes visually disabling because of irregular refraction and scarring and opacity in the optical zone. The symptoms of glare and haze are also much more.
6. Current techniques use an optical zone of about 6.0–6.5 mm and total area of about 9.0–9.4 mm. This is found to decrease the incidence of regression, decentration and visual disturbances and also increase the stability of refraction. The loss of 2 or more lines of BCVA was less than 2% as reported by Dauch et al (using 6.0 mm/9.0 mm zones) and zero in the study of Rogers et al, in which 6.5 mm optical zone and 9.4 mm total ablation area was used.
7. Incorporation of a larger mask that allows the visualization of the pupil improves the centration. The modern eye tracking systems are highly effective in preventing the centration problems and improving the visual results.

Both, the wide as well as the scanning laser delivery systems can be used for correction of hypermetropia.

HYPEROPIC PRK: THE TECHNIQUES

The treatment of hyperopia with the PRK technique is assisted by different devices and methods as listed below.

1. An ablatable mask.
2. An ablatable mask and the Axicon lens.
3. A non-ablatable mask.
4. Use of iris diaphragm to create a small circular beam.
5. Use of a rotating slit-beam with a non-ablatable mask.
6. The flying spot-scanning laser beam.

Ablatable Mask

The ablatable/erodible mask consisting of PMMA material, having a shape that is thicker in the center than the periphery, can be used to produce the hyperopic profile (see above and Fig. 20.2). The mask is placed into a cartridge that is inserted in the rail in the path of the laser beam to avoid decentration associated with the hand-held mask.

Ablatable Mask With An Axicon Lens

This technique treats hyperopia in two stages.

- In the first stage a suitable profile ablatable mask inserted in the rail is used to create the hypermetropic ablation of the central 6.5 mm central zone.
- Then the used mask is substituted in the rail by the Axicon lens. This specially designed lens *diverges* the large laser beam by its *prismatic* action into such *an annular configuration* that the central 6.5 mm central zone now receives no laser energy. The maximum laser is delivered to the 6.5–7.0 mm midperipheral zone with a tapering off of the laser energy extending up to 9.4 mm.
- The result is creation of the midperipheral *trough* with a smooth peripheral transition.

The Non-Ablatable Mask

These can be of two types.

1. A fixed non-ablatable mask that allows the delivery of a wide/broad laser beam to the mid-peripheral area while protecting the central zone from ablation (Fig. 20.6).
2. A rotating non-ablatable device combined with a slit-beam scanning delivery can be used to produce hyperopic ablation profile. This combination creates a ring shaped beam that spares the central 1mm of the cornea.

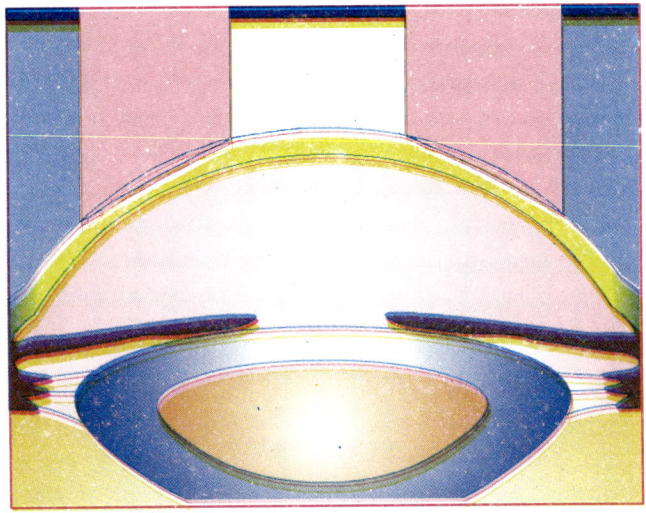

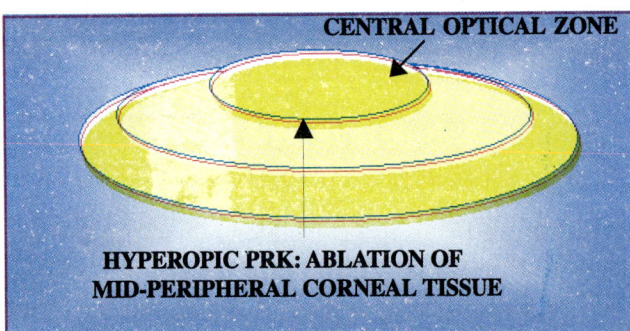

Fig. 20.6: Hyperopic PRK: The corneal profile after ablation

A Rotating Small Circular Beam

The appropriate size of an iris aperture on a wheel can be utilized to convert a broad laser beam into a small circle beam that can be moved in a circular manner to ablate the corneal midperiphery.

The Flying Spot-scanning Laser Beam

The flying spot-scanning laser is the most precise, accurate and simple method of creating the hyperopic profile by scanning the small spot of laser around the corneal surface at the desired location (see below).

THE SCANNING MODE OF ABLATION

The scanning systems deliver a thin slit (slit-scanning) or a very small diameter beam (flying spot-scanning) that is moved across the corneal surface within the given ablation zone by the computer controlled mirrors. These systems are capable of producing a wide range of ablation profiles more precisely and efficiently, added by a large number of algorithms loaded into the computer software. The control of the energy distribution within these small scanning beams is much more demanding.

The scanning system also can be used for keratomileusis of the corneal surface (PRK) but the more recent and superior techniques of LASIK and LASEK have largely replaced this method of refractive corrections except in a few limited situations. These situations are:

1. Cases of high and extreme myopia where the *residual bed thickness* (RBT) may limit the LASIK surgery.
2. Cases of hypermetropia, in which a large area (up to 9.4 mm) needs to be treated but the diameter of the flap (average 8.5 mm) limits this ablation.
3. Cases where availability of the expensive LASIK instrumentations or the surgeon's familiarity with the technique are the limiting factors.

Suggested readings

1. Trokel Sl, Srinivasan R, Braren B: Excimer laser surgery of the cornea. Am J Ophthalmol 1983; 96: 710-715.
2. Marshall J, Trokel S, Rothery S et al: Photoablative reprofiling of the cornea using an excimer laser: photorefractive keratectomy. Lasers in Ophthalmol 1986; 1: 21-48.
3. Marshall J, Trokel SI, Rothery S, Krueger R: A comparative study of Corneal incisions induced by diamond and steel knives and two ultraviolet radiations from excimer Laser. Br J ophthalmol 1986; 70:482-501.
4. Munnerlyn CR, Koons SJ, Marshall J: Photorefractive keratectomy: a technique for laser refractive surgery. J Cat Refract Surg 1988; 14: 46-52.
5. Seiler T, Bende T, Trokel S, Wollensak J : Excimer laser keratectomy for correction of astigmatism. Am J Ophthalmol 1988; 105:117-24.
6. Aron-Rosa D, Carre F et al: Keratorefractive surgery with the excimer laser. Am J Ophthalmol 1985; 100: 741-742.
7. Cotliar AM, Schubert HD et al: Excimer laser radial keratotomy. Ophthalmology 1985; 92: 206-208.
8. Gaster RN, Berns MW et al: Excimer laser interaction with the cornea (ARVO abstract). Invest Ophthalmol Vis Sci 1986; 27 (Suppl): 92.
9. McDonald MB, Beureman R, Falzoni W, et al: Refractive surgery with the excimer laser. Am J Ophthalmol 1987; 103: 469.
10. McDonald MB, Kaufman HE, Fantz JM, Shofner S et al: Excimer laser ablation of a human eye. Arch Ophthalmol 1989; 107: 641-642.

11. McDonald MB, Shofner S et al: Clinical results of central photorefractive keratectomy (PRK) with 193nm excimer laser for the treatment of myopia: the blind eye study. Invest Ophthalmol Vis Sci 1989; 30 (Suppl): 216.
12. McDonald MB, Liu JC, Byrd T J et al: Central photorefractive keratectomy for myopia. Partially sighted and normally sighted eyes. Ophthalmology 1991; 98: 1327-1337.
13. O'Brart D, Gartry DS, Lohman CP et al: Excimer laser PRK for myopia : comparison of 4.0 mm and 5.0 mm ablation zones. J Ref Corneal Surg 1994; 10 (2): 87-94.
14. O'Brart D, Corbett MC, Lohman CP: The effect of ablation zone diameter on the outcome of excimer laser PRK : A prospective randomized, double blind study. Arch Ophthalmology 1995; 113: 438-443.
15. Corbett MC, Verma S, O'Brart DP et al: Effect of ablation profile on the wound healing and visual performance 1 year after excimer laser photorefractive keratectomy. Br J Ophthalmol 1996; 80: 224-234.
16. Lohman CP, Fitzke F et al: Halos-a problem for all myopes? Ref Corneal Surg 1993; 9 (2): S72-S75
17. O'Brart D, Lohman CP Fitzke F et al: Night vision after PRK: haze and halos. Eur J Ophthalmol 1994; 4: 43-51.
18. O'Brart D, Lohman CP Fitzke F et al: Disturbances in night vision after excimer PRK. Eye 1994; 8: 46-51.
19. Carones F, Brancato R, Morico A et al: Evaluation of three different approaches to perform excimer laser PRK for myopia. Ophthalmic Surg Lasers 1996; 27 (Suppl): S458-S465.
20. Castanera J: Topographic comparison of monozone, multipass and multizone ablations for myopic PRK. Ophthalmic Surg Lasers 1996; 27 (Suppl): S471-S476.
21. Cho YS, Kim CG, Kim WB, Kim CW: Multistep PRK for high myopia. J Ref Corneal Surg 1993; 9 (Suppl): S31-S41.
22. Pop M, Aras M : Multizone / multipass PRK: six months results. J Cataract Ref Surg 1995; 21: 633-643.
23. McDonnell PJ, Moreira H, Garbus J et al: PRK to create toric ablations for correction of astigmatism. Arch Ophthalmol 1995; 109: 710-713.
24. Shimmick J, Bechtel L: Elliptical ablations for the correction of compound myopic astigmatism by photoablation with apertures. SPIE Ophthalmic Technology 1992; 1644 : 32-39.
25. Bracchato R, Carones F, Traabucchi G et al: The erodible mask in PRK and astigmatism. J Ref Corn Surg 1993; 9 (Suppl): 125-130.
26. Dausch D, Klein R, Schroder E et al: PRK to correct astigmatism with myopia or hyperopia. J Cataract Ref Surg 1994; 20 (Suppl): 252-257.
27. Maloney RK, Friedman M, Harman T et al: A prototype erodible mask delivery system for the excimer laser. Ophthalmology 1993; 100: 542-549.
28. Carones F, Venturi E, Gobbi PG et al: Hyperopia correction using an erodible mask in-the-rail excimer laser delivery system. Ophthalmic Surg and Lasers 1996; 27 (5): S531 (Abstract).
29. Dausch D, Klein R, Schroder E: Excimer laser PRK for hyperopia. J Ref Corn Surg 1993; 9(Suppl): S20-S28.
30. Dausch D, Landesz M: Laser correction of hyperopia. Aesculap-Meditec results from Germany, in Salz JJ, McDonnell PJ, McDonald MB (Eds.): Corneal Laser Surgery. St. Louis. Mosby-Yearbook 1995; pp 239-247.
31. Dausch D, Smecka Z, Klein R et al: Excimer laser PRK for hyperopia. J Cataract Ref Surg 1997; 23: 169-176.
32. Dierick HG, Missotten L: Corneal ablation profiles for correction of hyperopia for excimer laser. J Ref Surg 1996; 12: 767-773.
33. Jackson WB: Results of hyperopic PRK. American Society of Cataract and Refractive Surgery Meeting, Boston 1997.
34. Seiler T, Bende T, Matallana M et al: PRK for hyperopia (Abstract). Invest Ophthalmol Vis Sci 1990; 31 (Suppl): 246.

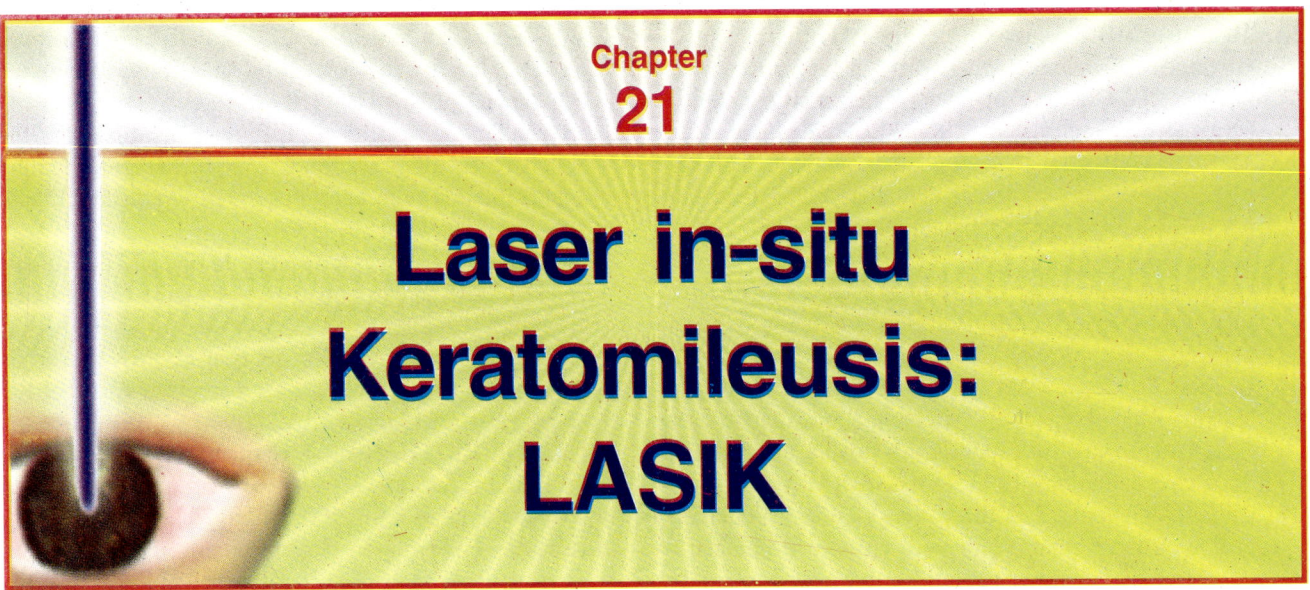

Chapter 21
Laser in-situ Keratomileusis: LASIK

WHAT IS LASER IN-SITU KERATOMILEUSIS (LASIK)?

Laser in-situ keratomileusis is the technique of altering the corneal curvature, for treating a wide range of refractive disorders, by removing complex patterns of corneal tissue from the stromal bed through the use of the argon fluoride ArF excimer laser after raising a flap of the anterior cornea.

HISTORY OF LASER IN-SITU KERATOMILEUSIS

The long experience with different types of keratomileusis since the days of Barraquer and the development of the excimer laser techniques for the correction of refractive errors has culminated in the unique combination of the two techniques in the form of in-situ keratomileusis using the excimer laser.

The passion of Jose Barraquer with his technique of changing the refraction of eye through meticulous *lathing of the removed disc* of corneal tissue (called *refractive keratoplasty*) had resulted in many refinements in this technique since the first description by him in 1949. Professor John Charamais of Athens coined the term keratomileusis for this technique of *sculpting the corneal curvature* (the literal meaning of keratomileusis is 'carving the cornea').

Although the concept of removing a plano disc from the stromal bed after creating a flap for producing a flattening effect was developed by Pureskin as early as 1966, who called this procedure **'stromectomy'**, the credit of reviving keratomileusis in-situ, i.e. on the stromal bed rather than on the corneal disc/flap goes to Ruiz in the year 1988.

By this time the mechanically operated keratome to create the corneal flap had been developed and the use and safety of the excimer laser was well established. *Pallikaris and colleagues* combined these advances to introduce the *hinged-flap technique of LASIK in 1990* and published their first report for its use in human eyes in 1991. During the same period, Buratto and co-worker were developing another technique of using the excimer laser for keratomileusis in Italy. They used the back surface of the corneal flap to perform the refractive ablation. Initially they called this procedure '*photokeratomileusis*' or PKM but published a paper in 1992, describing the technique as 'Excimer L*aser Intrastromal Keratomileusis*' or ELISK. This later technique of refractive correction could not become popular due the longer operating time and the complications associated with the removal of the corneal flap away from the eye because this can result in flap loss, desiccation and resuturing problems, etc.

The recent years have witnessed tremendous advancements in the instrumentations, algorithms of refractive correction, techniques and postoperative management with deeper understanding of the indications and safety guidelines for the LASIK procedure.

ADVANTAGES OF LASIK

1. Wide range of refractive corrections can be performed using the flying spot laser to create complex ablation profiles.
2. LASIK is to PRK what PHACO is to ECCE.
3. The postoperative pain is minimum.
4. The visual rehabilitation is rapid with useful uncorrected visual acuity restored within few hours.
5. The quality of vision is better and the refraction stabilizes more rapidly, within the second month as compared to PRK where it may not do so for months or even after a year in some cases.
6. LASIK is an outpatient procedure.
7. The patient can return to work with minimum precaution (relating to the flap adherence).
8. The surgery is short lasting taking about 10-5 minutes.
9. The hinged flap technique avoids any suturing and ensures excellent realignment of the flap.
10. The Bowman's layer is undisturbed, eliminating the theoretical possibility of any surface irregularity.
11. The epithelium is not disturbed, therefore no epithelial healing is involved and the stromal healing response is minimum. These factors make the refractive outcome more stable, undisturbed by the abnormal healing response.
12. The ablation under the flap avoids any interaction of the epithelial growth factors that induce stromal healing response. This ensures minimum or no corneal haze. The corneal haze is a nuisance in PRK, making the visual recovery a protracted process.
13. For the same reason no prolonged use of modulators of healing such as topical steroids, is required. This eliminates drug induced side effects like rise of IOP and cataracts.
14. Re-operations for any modifications of the refractive outcome are possible as the corneal flap can be re-lifted even after many months.
15. High patient acceptability.

LIMITATIONS OF LASIK SURGERY

1. High cost of the surgery is the major limiting factor. Apart from the cost of the excimer laser system itself, the costly devices for evaluation like the CVK, wavefront aberration-sensing devices, the latest devices for measuring the flap thickness intraoperatively, the microkeratome and the disposables blades, are all expensive items.
2. The surgery is machine dependant, without much intraoperative control of the surgeon. Intraoperative laser failure, microkeratome progress, the control of accurate flap thickness, etc. are out of the surgeon's control and can sometimes compromise the surgical results.
3. The surgery is technically complex and has its learning curve depending on the skills of the surgeon.
4. The technology is continuously undergoing refinements and improvements with regard to the algorithms and microkeratome design and function.
5. The technique is still not refined and well advanced for effective treatment of hyperopia and astigmatism. The larger than normal flaps and more appropriate algorithms are needed for a desirable outcome for hyperopic correction.
6. The concept of residual bed thickness is undergoing change in the light of the long term results of LASIK induced corneal ectasia.

LASIK: INSTRUMENTATION

1. The microtome with its accessories.
2. Devices for intraoperative pachymetry for measurement of the flap and residual bed thickness.
3. The Barraquer tonometer.
4. The corneal markers.
5. The lid speculum.
6. A spatula for lifting the flap.
7. The flap protector.
8. A device for monitoring the humidity and temperature of the operating room.
9. A device to evacuate the laser plume such as a merocel sponge or a surgical vacuum evacuator.

MICROKERATOME

At the heart of the LASIK technology, the microkeratome has an important and crucial role. Its role assumes significant proportion when one considers the flap related problems and creation of a smooth, uniform and homogenous corneal flap with *predictable thickness* so that the desired residual bed thickness (RBT) is maintained to avoid corneal ectasia (chapter 6). It is also required that a homogenous and even stromal bed is left behind for smooth laser ablation after the creation of the corneal flap. This demands a sharp and uninterrupted cutting of the corneal lamellae without causing any damage to the underlying stroma.

Depending on the technology used, there are three types of microkeratomes that have been developed.

1. Mechanical microkeratomes
   a. Manual
   b. Automated
      i. Electromechanical
      ii. Turbine operated
2. Water-jet microkeratomes/Hydrokeratomes
3. Laser microkeratomes

Mechanical Microkeratomes

The mechanical microkeratomes are the most commonly used ones. The place of the manual keratome designed by Barraquer has been taken by the newer automated devices. The basic components of a mechanical microkeratome are the *suction ring*, the *head*, the *handle*, the *control unit* or console and the foot pedals. The **suction ring** has grooves or the dovetail to engage the microkeratome head and the track for movement of the gear. The **head** of the microkeratome incorporates a thickness plate, the cutting blade and the gear system (Fig. 21.1).

The head is connected to the **handle** that houses the motor in case of the automated microkeratomes. The handle is also used to stabilize the microkeratome head during its pass, so that the eye globe is not subjected to the undue weight of the device. The **control unit** supplies and monitors the power for the suction pump and the motor that moves the gears and the cutting blade. These are operated through the foot pedals provided separately.

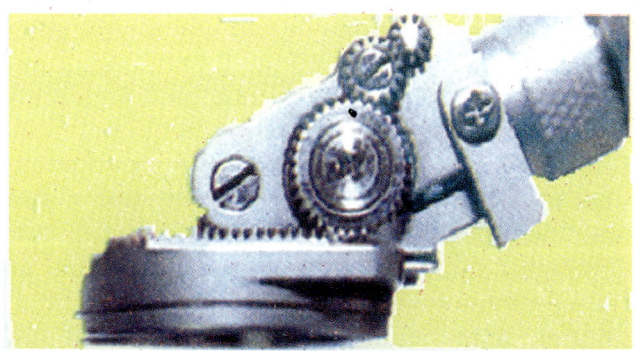

Fig. 21.1: The 'automated corneal shaper' (ACS) microkeratome with its gear engaged on the rail track of the suction ring

The head is advanced manually during the creation of the corneal flap by the **manually operated microkeratomes**, e.g. the Turbokeratome, the Microprecision's Microlemallar Keratome, the Lamallar Keratoplasty System, the Moria LSK One Disposable and the Micratome (MICRA ACRI). The oscillations to the cutting blade are powered by a gas turbine in these microkeratomes. The Moria LSK Carriazo-Barraquer microkeratome is available in manual as well as automated modes.

The **automated microkeratomes** use the gear system operated by the motor for controlled movement of the head during the cutting of the corneal flap. The gear track on the suction ring facilitates and guides smooth movement of the head and the blade during flap cutting. The **stopper mechanism** is provided to limit the complete run of the microkeratome along the gear track and to facilitate the creation of a *hinged flap*. The Solan Flapmaker Microtome has no gear system. A flexible shaft that provides the uniform motion during the pass of the microkeratome head drives it.

Some microkeratomes are made of molded plastic, e.g. the Automated Disposable Keratome and the Solan Flapmaker Disposable Microkeratome. These are **disposable** ones. Their drawback is that interface opacity may be formed due to the plastic debris.

The **suction ring** of the microkeratome has a chamber on its underside, which is applied over the eye globe. The central empty space of the suction ring allows the cornea to protrude through as the suction builds up in the vacuum chamber around it. The vacuum chamber is connected to the suction pump, which creates vacuum of about 25 mm of Hg. This vacuum created in the chamber is sufficient to raise the IOP to about 60–65 mm of Hg (Figs. 21.2 and 21.3). The suction ring serves the following functions:

1. It stabilizes the eye during creation of the corneal flap.
2. It has grooves or the dovetail rail system to engage the microkeratome head.
3. It also has the track for the gears on its upper surface to guide the head for smooth passage of the cutting blade.
4. The suction raises the IOP. This helps in creation of the corneal flap by making the cornea prominent and firm during the cutting.

The **microkeratome blade** is made of stainless steel or *sapphire* that is reusable (e.g. in Schwind Microkeratome). The blade is fitted into the blade holder of

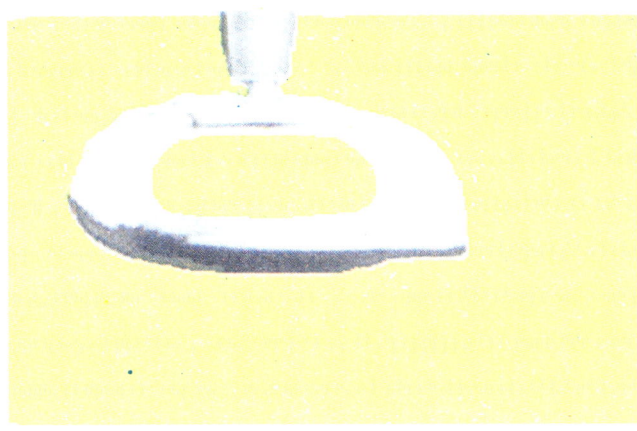

Fig. 21.2: Suction ring for the Automated Corneal Shaper (ACS)

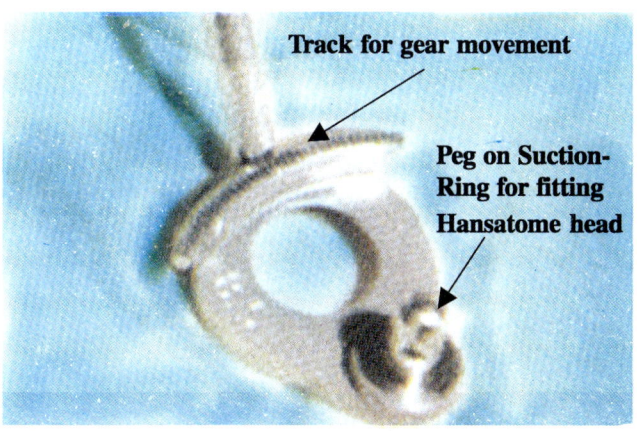

Fig. 21.3: Suction ring for the Hansatome

the head below an behind the thickness plate. The blade achieves its cutting by smooth and very fast sideways oscillations ranging from 10,000 to 14,000 rpm, depending upon the make of the microkeratome, except in case of the Schwind Microkeratome, which has slow oscillations of 1600–1800 rpm. The blade oscillations are powered by the electric motor in the automated microkeratomes and by pneumatic (gas) turbine in case of manually operated microkeratomes. There are some microkeratomes that permit a direct visualization of the cutting field, the corneal flap and its hinge due to the transparent thickness plate. The examples are the plastic microkeratomes, the Schwind Microkeratome and the Clear Corneal Molder microkeratome.

The **thickness plate** is fitted above and in front of the cutting blade in the microkeratome head. It controls the flap thickness depending upon the available space between it and the blade; a larger space between the blade and the plate would result in a thicker flap and visa versa. This is achieved either by adjusting the height of the plate or by using plates with different thicknesses. The plate consists of stainless steel or transparent plastic.

The microkeratomes that are in common use are the Chiron Automated Corneal Shaper (ACS), the Hansatome, the Nidek MK 2000 microkeratome and the Moria LSK microkeratomes.

Corneal Flap Thickness

Different makes of microkeratome are found to vary in their ability to produce a predictable thickness of the flap. The corneal flap thickness is an important consideration in calculating the safe margin for stromal ablation. The thickness of the corneal flap varies depending on the microtome used because of three reasons.

Depth Plate Setting of the Microkeratome

Different makes of the microkeratome have different plate settings (the intended flap thickness). the examples are:
- The Automated Corneal Shaper (ACS) which has 160 µ depth plate setting
- The Hansatome has two separate heads with fixed depth plates at 160 µ and 180 µ setting.
- The Nidek MK 2000 microkeratome, has has 130 µ depth plate setting.
- The Moria LSK Carriazo-Barraquer Microkeratome which has two depth plate settings at 160 µ and 180 µ.

Difference Between the Intended and Actual Flap Thickness

This difference can be due to problem with *depth plate setting* or an inherent drawback of the microkeratome.

Variability in the Flap Thickness

It has been found that some of the microkeratomes may produce different thickness flaps in different patients as well as in two eyes of the same patient. This reflects on the poor predictability and reproducibility of the cut by the microkeratome.

Some recent studies in 2002 have highlighted these facts. Shemesh G et al have found that the ACS and the Hansatome both made flaps much thinner than the expected thickness as well as showed statistically significant variation in the flaps of the two eyes of the same patient. The Nidek MK 2000 microkeratome showed no statistically significant flap thickness variation in same patient's eyes. It also made flaps of thicknesses that were close to the expected thickness. Similarly Gokmen et al found that the Hansatome made flaps varying in thicknesses from 141–209 µ and the ACS made 120–150 µ flaps, the intended thickness being 160 µ in both the cases. Spadea et al reported one case developing corneal ectasia in his both eyes. Corneal specimen taken after keratoplasty revealed the flap to be 260 µ instead of the intended 120 µ, using the Moria-manually guided MDCS.

Corneal Flap Diameter

Corneal flaps of different diameter ranging from 7 mm to 10.5 mm can be cut by different microkeratomes. Normally about 8.5 mm diameter flap if raised during myopic LASIK but hyperopic LASIK requires a larger flap of about 10.0–10.5 mm diameter to ablate the midperipheral cornea. The diameter of the corneal flap can be varied either by using different sizes of the suction ring (e.g. the Moria LSK Carriazo-Barraquer Microkeratome, Moria LSK One Disposable microkeratome, the Hansatome with 8.5 and 9.5 mm options and the Microprecision's Microlemallar Keratome) or by adjusting the height of the given suction ring (e.g. the Clear Corneal Molder microkeratome). The Universal Keratome has option for only one fixed diameter flap.

Corneal Flap Orientation

The flap orientation in two directions, i.e. a horizontal or vertical flap, with the hinge of the flap nasally or superiorly respectively, is possible by some microkeratomes (e.g. Moria LSK Carriazo-Barraquer Microkeratome) while others have only single option (e.g. superiorly hinged flap by the Hansatome).

Limitations of the Mechanical Microkeratomes

1. Complicated to use
Although the mechanical microkeratomes are the ones that are most commonly in use at present, their operation is highly demanding and complicated. It may be appropriate to say that the major part of the LASIK technology is microkeratome dependant and most of the complications are related to the flap creation.

2. High cost
The cost of these microkeratomes is very high. Even the disposable blade itself costs a few thousands of rupees.

3. Poor predictability of the flap thickness
The lack of precision, poor reproducibility of cuts and variability in flap thickness are major concerns these days, as these are directly related factors for development of corneal ectasia (see chapter 6 and above).

4. The demanding nature of maintenance
The maintenance and care of these microkeratomes is also not simple. Meticulous cleaning and special methods of sterilizations are needed to prevent debris on the parts and the gear track. These factors as well as an inappropriate assembly of the parts would lead to mechanical failures and jamming of the microkeratome pass during flap cutting.

The Maintenance of Mechanical Microkeratomes

The detachable parts of the microkeratome head and the suction ring are thoroughly cleaned of any debris by socking in hot distilled water for 15 minutes, cleaned with the special solution provided with the device using a soft bristle brush, ringed in distilled water repeatedly and then dried with microfiltered air. These steps are crucial to prevent any debris getting firmly attached on the instrument. Even the use of balanced salt solution (BSS) has been found to be associated with the deposition of salt crystal debris on the components. The handle with the motor, the control unit and the foot pedals are sterilized with the use of isopropyl alcohol cleaning using a socked applicator. Immersion of these parts into any kind of solutions must be avoided.

The Hydrokeratomes / Water-jet Microkeratomes

The Visijet Hydrokeratome and the Medjet Hydroblade Keratome utilize the water-jet technology to create a corneal flap through corneal stromal cleavage induced by the extremely high pressure of a highly collimated beam of water-jet. The pressure generated by such a water-jet is more than 1500 psi, the speed exceeds 800 miles per hour and the water-jet beam is about 36 µ thick. These properties of the water-jet enable cleavage of the stroma comparable to metal blade cutting. The water-jet beam position and the corneal cleavage is monitored by an image tracker to guide the surgeon's foot pedal control. The thickness plate controls the flap thickness as in case of the mechanical microkeratomes. The flap thickness ranging from 100 µ to 200 µ and diameter of 8–11 mm can be obtained with this technology.

The advantages of this technology are as follows:

1. Minimum tissue damage as *cleavage* rather than *cutting* is used to raise the flap.
2. Less possibility of corneal haze and irregular astigmatism as the keratocytes and the stromal lamellae are not affected much.
3. The entry into the stroma from the epithelial surface is confined to a very small area, thereby decreasing the chances of epithelial ingrowth.
4. The cleavage is accomplished at the normal intraocular pressure. Therefore the build up of suction and its associated complications are avoided.
5. The low cost and simplicity of operation are additional advantages of these Hydrokeratomes.

Laser Microkeratomes

These microkeratomes are based on the *intrastromal photodisruption* produced by ultra high frequency lasers. The precisely focused laser can create a cleavage within the stroma with microprecision through the dissolution of the tissue with photodisruption action without disturbing the corneal surface (see chapter on intrastromal PRK). Two laser microkeratomes, the Novatec Laser Microkeratome and the Femtosecond Laser Microkeratome have been developed but they are yet to find a place in clinical practice.

Advantages

1. The technique does not require the suction ring and raising of the IOP, thus avoiding the related complications.
2. The reproducibility and precision of the laser action facilitates creation of flaps of the *intended thickness* with great uniformity.

Drawbacks

1. Centration problems and increased intraoperative time as with laser ablation.
2. Problem during the *separation* of the flap.
3. Limited options regarding the flap diameter.
4. Small flap diameter in comparison to the above methods.

Suggested readings

1. Gimbel HV, Penno EE et al: Microkeratomes and laser systems, in 'LASIK Complications: Prevention and Management', Second edition, Slack Incorporated publications, 2001.
2. Schultze RL: Microkeratome update. Int Ophthalmol Clin. 2002 Fall; 42 (4): 55-65.
3. Cheng AC, Rao SK, Yu EY, Leung HT et al: Reproducibility of corneal flap thickness in laser in situ keratomileusis using the Hansatome microkeratome. Cataract Refract Surg. 2001 Nov; 27 (11): 1712.
4. Lam DS, Rao SK, Liu KY Microkeratome accuracy in LASIK. Ophthalmology. 2001 Nov; 108 (11): 1930-2.
5. Geggel HS: Microkeratome accuracy in LASIK. Ophthalmology. 2001 Nov; 108 (11): 1929-30, discussion 1931-2.
6. Schumer DJ, Bains HS: The Nidek MK-2000 microkeratome system. J Refract Surg. 2001 Mar-Apr; 17(2 Suppl): S250-1.
7. Naripthaphan P, Vongthongsri A: Evaluation of the reliability of the Nidek MK-2000 microkeratome for laser in situ keratomileusis. J Refract Surg. 2001 Mar-Apr; 17(2 Suppl): S255-8.
8. Sarkisian KA, Petrov AA: Experience with the Nidek MK-2000 microkeratome in 1,220 cases. J Refract Surg. 2001 Mar-Apr; 17(2 Suppl): S252-4.
9. Yildirim R, Aras C, Ozdamar A, Bahcecioglu H, Ozkan S: Reproducibility of corneal flap thickness in laser in situ keratomileusis using the Hansatome microkeratome. J Cataract Refract Surg. 2000 Dec; 26 (12): 1729-32.
10. Yi WM, Joo CK: Corneal flap thickness in laser in situ keratomileusis using an SCMD manual microkeratome. J Cataract Refract Surg. 1999 Aug; 25(8): 1087-92.
11. Lipshitz I, Bass R: Water-jet microkeratome—to set the record straight. J Refract Surg. 1998 Nov-Dec; 14(6): 667-9.
12. Lubatschowski H, Maatz G, Heisterkamp A, Hetzel U, Drommer W, Welling H et al: Application of ultrashort laser pulses for intrastromal refractive surgery. Graefes Arch Clin Exp Ophthalmol 2000 Jan; 238(1): 33-39.

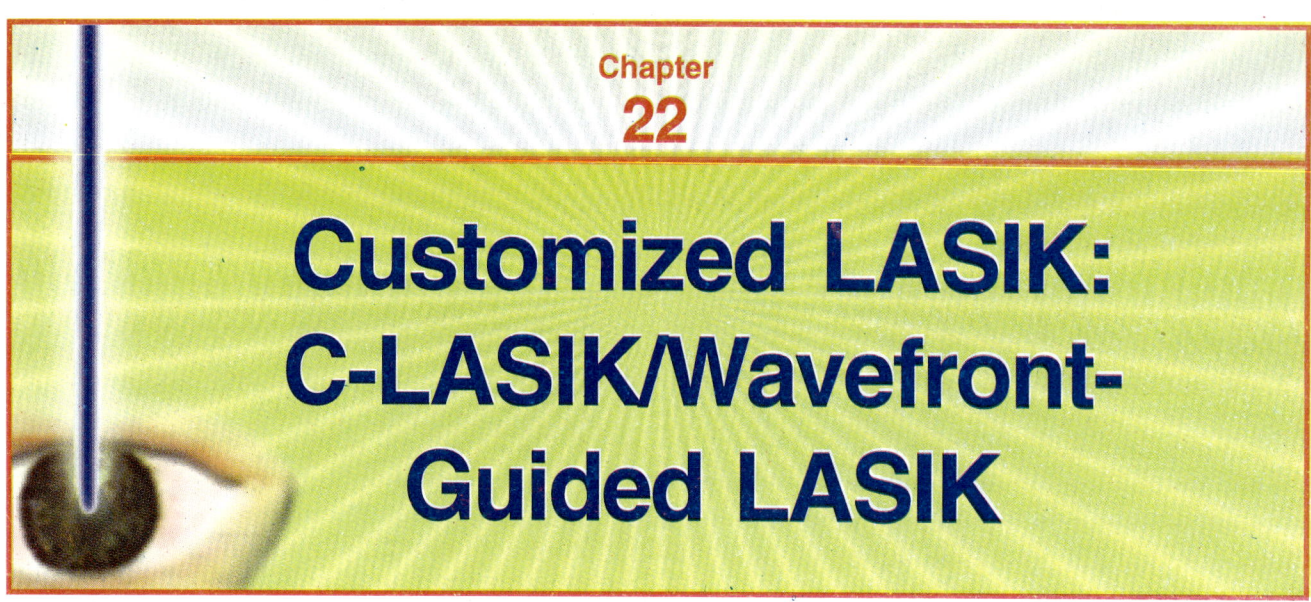

Chapter 22

Customized LASIK: C-LASIK/Wavefront-Guided LASIK

INTRODUCTION

Photorefractive surgeries utilizing the excimer laser are effective and predictable in correcting the refractive errors over a wide range. These surgeries (LASIK and PRK) focus on the correction of the *spherocylindrical errors* suffered by an individual's eye. Unfortunately there are *many other aberrations that limit the visual acuity potential* that the normal human eye is capable of achieving. These aberrations are called *higher-order optical aberrations*, which are known to the scientists for long, but no corrective modality was available to deal with them till recently. Moreover, despite the correction of the refractive error, these higher-order optical aberrations are found to significantly increase after the convention photorefractive procedures and limit visual function. Oshika and Miyata et al found significant increase in induced higher-order aberrations particularly in the eyes that suffered loss of the best-corrected visual acuity after an uneventful LASIK procedure.

The visual disability due to these aberrations increases significantly when the pupil is dilated under dim-illumination or scotopic conditions. Martinez et al found that the higher-order aberrations showed a 9-fold increase in the eyes before operation but a 100-fold increase occurred after one month of PRK procedure when the pupil was dilated from 3 mm to 7 mm. Seiler et al reported an increase of 17.65 times in these aberrations 3 months after PRK.

Optical Defects of the Eye

Although the *'schematic eye'* and the *'reduced eye'* of Donders' have made it to appear simple, the optical system of the human eye is highly complicated. This system is formed by many refracting components, e.g. the anterior corneal surface, the corneal tissue, the posterior corneal surface, the aqueous humor, the anterior lens surface, its cortex and nucleus, the posterior lens surface and the vitreous humour. Any such system involving multiple components is far from being a perfect refracting unit.

Nature has tried to bring the various components of this spectacular creation in a harmonious co-ordination, assisted by accommodation, adaptation and retinal definition and differentiation, so that a sharp focused image of an object can be formed on the retina. The ability of the eye to discern minute objects is called the *resolving power*. However the resolving power of the eye is limited by various optical defects, which decrease the efficiency of the optical system. These optical defects are listed below.

1. Lower-order optical aberrations.
2. The higher-order optical aberrations.
3. Diffraction.
4. Decentring.

Lower-Order Optical Aberrations

These aberrations include the refractive errors conventionally known to the scientists for centuries, i.e. myopia, hypermetropia and astigmatism. These refractive errors have been adequately studied. They are easily correctable by different means for improving the visual acuity, in contrast to the higher order optical defects, which are not amenable to any existing conventional mode of correction. Therefore the main concern of the ophthalmologists dealing with the optical defects of the human eye was limited, for a long time, to achieve a state of emmetropia in which the light rays could be brought to a focus on the retina.

Higher-Order Optical Aberrations

Inspite of accurate focusing of the image on the retina (emmetropia), the higher-order optical aberrations result in *degradation of the quality and sharpness of the image.* The retinal image that is so formed is not a clear point of focus but is surrounded by circles of blurred light. These are called the '*circles of diffusion*'. This decreases the efficiency of vision. The visual acuity becomes less than what is potentially achievable by the human eye due to increase in the minimum image size that can be formed on the retina as a consequence of these circles of diffusion. The average macular cone diameter is about 2 microns. Therefore a retinal image of this size should be appreciated by the eye as a distinct entity. This retinal image size corresponds to a '*visual angle*' of ½ minute of arc and a Snellen's visual acuity of 6/3. This is in contrast to the visual acuity commonly observed in clinical practice that is taken as standard for the human eye. Visual acuity of 6/6 corresponds to a visual angle of 1 minute of arc or 4 micron of retinal image size, which is larger than the cone diameter.

The higher-order optical aberrations constitute about 17% of the total optical aberrations. They are as follows:

Chromatic Aberrations

When passing through a refracting medium, the shorter wavelengths of light are retarded more than the longer wavelengths. Therefore the violet and blue rays are bent more than the rays occupying the red end of the visible spectrum. This results in the blue light being focused in front of the red light leading to *chromatic difference in magnification* of the image.

Spherical Aberrations

The periphery of a convex refracting system, like the cornea and the lens, yields more power in comparison to the power in the central part. This causes distortion of the image due to peripheral magnification in the form of barrel-distortion. This becomes significant if the pupil is dilated, as in mesopic conditions.

Coma

This type of aberration occurs due to the off-axis rays not converging at a focal plane. The rays may converge further away from the axis, giving rise to a positive coma or closer towards the axis forming negative coma-like optical aberrations. Clinically the incidence of these aberrations has been found to be significant after LASIK.

Petzval Field Curvature

This aberration makes a focal plane appear as parabolic or dome shaped in the peripheral field of vision.

Diffraction of Light

When the light waves travel through a narrow aperture, the narrow beam of light does not come to a sharp focus because the rays on the sides of the beam tend to fall apart from the main body. This forms a blurred image *surrounded by light and dark bands* and is called an 'Airy disc' (c.f. circles of diffusion where the image margin is blurred). It leads to limitation of the visual acuity. This effect becomes more significant, the smaller is the pupil size in more illuminated conditions.

Decentration

The definition of the retinal image further suffers due to the fact that the refracting surfaces of the optical system of the eye are never accurately centered, i.e. the centers of the corneal curvature and the lens surfaces are not aligned with the optical axis. Moreover the *optical axis* and the *visual axis* do not correspond in most cases.

The effect of the above-mentioned optical defects is to decrease the definition of the retinal image, which results in visual acuity less than the level of retinal potential.

NATURAL MECHANISMS TO DECREASE ABERRATIONS

Nature has provided a number of ways to deal with the different optical defects in order to obtain a sharp, clearly defined image. The optical components of the eye do not vary independently but follow a harmonious co-ordination so that an emmetropic state ensues. For example, if the axial length is longer, the corneal curvature is flatter or the lens power less.

The prolate curvature of the cornea (less power peripherally than in the center), the greater curvature and higher refractive index of the lens nucleus and the normal pupil size take care of the spherical aberrations. The location of the fovea on the side of the optical axis is said to offset the chromatic difference in magnification of the image because if the object is on the side of the optical axis, the image produced by the shorter wavelengths would be smaller than that formed by the longer wavelengths. The aberrations of image formed in the peripheral part of the retina are neutralized to a large extent by the retinal curvature.

However, these natural mechanisms are not able to take care of all the aberrations and an ideal condition of refraction is never attained. Moreover, while a desirable pupil size of 2.5–3.0 mm neutralizes the spherical aberrations, at the same time it leads to image deterioration due to diffraction.

CUSTOMIZED LASIK OR C-LASIK

The higher-order optical aberrations vary with the physiological pupil size, the state of accommodation and with age of the individual. Moreover the patients occupational conditions like illumination conditions at work and close work, anatomical variations of the corneal diameter, corneal elevation profile, pupil size and the shape of the crystalline lens, etc. have an important role in modifying the patients refraction, determining an individual's visual needs and in deciding the strategy to be followed during LASIK. The visual requirement varies among different age groups and for different occupations.

Therefore the refractive procedure must take all these factors into account on an individual basis, i.e. it should be tailor made or customized for each patient rather than using only the refraction data generated under routine conditions for LASIK. This is the basis of the customized LASIK during which the excimer laser ablation profile is planned from person to person depending on the refraction to suit the individual according to his functional and optical needs, the optical aberrations that would occur at his age in his physiological and workplace conditions and other variables.

In other words the ablation profile in customized LASIK is not based only on spherocylindrical error suffered by an individual's eye, in which a standard ablation pattern applies to all eyes with the same refractive error. But it differs in every case depending on many other variables, including the higher order optical aberrations peculiar to each eye. Thus the customization can be based on the following:

1. Patient's functional need relating to near or distant work.
2. Patient's occupational needs.
3. Anatomical characteristics of the individual's eye.
   a. Pupil size.
   b. Pupil diameter.
   c. Anterior chamber depth.
   d. Axial length.
4. Corneal topography.
   a. Power maps.
   c. Elevation/tangential maps.
5. Wavefront deformation maps.

WAVEFRONT-GUIDED LASIK

Wavefront-guided LASIK is the technology to correct the *refractive error* as well as the *higher order optical aberrations* suffered by the eye through excimer laser LASIK in order to provide the best possible visual function to that individual. It utilizes the technique of LASIK in combination with a special modified ablation algorithm that also takes into account the total higher-order aberrations while correcting the refractive error.

The technique first detects and measures the aberrations suffered by the optical system of the eye through a device called *aberrometer* using *wavefront analysis* that constructs the *wavefront deformation maps*. The data obtained from the wavefront deformation maps is used to guide the excimer laser ablation during LASIK.

The wavefront technology has been developed and introduced by Seiler and Mrochen et al in 1999 in Switzerland, to correct the higher-order optical aberrations along with the refractive correction during LASIK or PRK. There are limited numbers of published reports in this field. However the initial results are promising with many patients achieving visual acuity better than 6/6 (**supernormal vision: BCVA 6/3 or better**) and improved visual function.

Aims and Indications

1. The primary aim of wavefront-guided LASIK is to increase the visual functions such as the visual acuity and contrast sensitivity after excimer laser

refractive surgery *by decreasing the preoperative higher order aberrations.*
2. To decrease/avoid the deterioration of optical performance after conventional excimer laser refractive surgeries (PRK, LASIK), which occurs due to increase in the postoperative higher order optical aberrations specially under mesopic conditions.
3. To decrease/avoid cases of loss of BCVA after LASIK. Oshika et al in a study on 100 eyes have reported in 2002 that the higher order aberrations (spherical and coma-like) increase after LASIK. The increase in these aberrations is highly significant in the eyes that developed loss of 2 or more lines of BCVA.
4. To utilize the aberration-sensing and wavefront-guided LASIK for treating cases of grossly decentered ablation. Mrochen and Seiler et al have recently used their wavefront technology for this purpose in 2 eyes with success. They also reported that another case with 2 mm decentration could not be treated because the aberrations were too large to provide good retinal images for wavefront-sensing.

Methods of Measuring Optical Aberrations

Many devices have been developed and clinically used to detect the optical aberrations. These devices called the **aberrometers** use the same basic principle but differ in the methodology. The methods of measuring the aberrations and the ablation algorithms are undergoing continuous development and refinement to achieve the best possible results. The optical aberrations that can be measured by the available methods for correction are nomenclated in the following manner.

S_1: The tilt.
S_2: The spherocylindrical error.
S_3: The third-order optical aberrations (vertical coma).
S_4: The fourth-order spherical aberrations.
S_5: The fifth-order coma-like aberrations.
S_6: The sixth-order spherical aberrations.

Each type of optical error is converted to a '*Zernike polynomial*' according to the following equation:

$$w^2 = 1/\pi \sum (Z_n F_n)^2 = S_n$$

Where w^2 = mean-square wavefront error
Z = Zernike coefficient
F = the scaling factor

The total and the higher order aberrations can be measured separately to construct the wavefront *deformation map*, which is the sum of the Zernike polynomials.

Total Mean-Square Wavefront Error

The total mean-square wavefront error (W^2) is the sum of all the measured mean-square wavefront errors.

$$W^2 = S_1 + S_2 + S_3 + S_4 + S_5 + S_6$$

Root Mean-Square Wavefront Error (RMS)

Since the quality of vision and the best-corrected visual acuity are affected by third to sixth-order optical errors, these errors are measured and collectively denoted by a different value for the purpose of easy comparisons. It is called the '*root mean-square wavefront error*' (W_{RMS}) and represented as:

$$W_{RMS} = \leq S_3 + S_4 + S_5 + S_6$$

Aberrometers

The basic principle of the aberration detection is that the parallel light rays projected on to the retina would suffer deviations depending upon the optical aberrations. The sum total of the deviation suffered by all the rays is the *wavefront deformation*. The following methods are in clinical use for determining the optical aberrations.

1. **The Shack-Hartmann Method**
   - A *single*, highly collimated narrow laser light beam is projected on to the retina to form a point focus.
   - The light rays reflected off the retina from this point source of light are collected by an array of small lenslets placed in front of the eye.
   - The lenslets in turn focus the rays on to an array of *charge-coupled-devices* (CCD) cameras.
   - The non-aberrated parallel light rays form equidistant focal points whereas the aberrated rays do not follow this pattern. The pattern produced varies with the degree and type of the aberrations suffered by the different light rays.
   - This information provided by the CCD cameras is used by complicated computer software program to generate the wavefront deformation map in the given case. The deviation suffered by each ray, which is picked up separately, is converted to a

'Zernike Polynomial'. The shape of the wavefront constructed is the sum of a number of these Zernike Polynomials.

2. The Tscherning Aberrometer
- The pupil is dilated to 7 mm.
- This aberrometer uses a *bundle of equidistant rays* to form their point image on the retina. The bundle of rays consists of a matrix of 13 × 13 collimated beams of frequency-doubled Nd: YAG laser. The diameter of the individual beam is about 0.3 mm.
- The patient is asked to fixate on the target in the center of the laser beam grid.
- The video camera does further alignment and centration with reference to the center of the entrance pupil.
- The charged-coupled-device (CCD) camera images the pattern of spots formed by the incident laser beams on the retina.
- The computer analyzes the pattern formed by these point images on the retina.
- The wavefront deformation is then calculated as above.

3. Geometric Ray Tracing

This method involves projecting a number of point sources of light on to the retina and then tracing back the conjugate focus of each of the reflected ray. The *observed conjugate focus* is then analyzed with reference to the *ideal conjugate focus* for each ray. The difference observed is the aberration suffered by the rays. This information is then used to calculate the aberrations suffered by the wavefront.

Laser Ablation

The laser ablation during wavefront-guided LASIK differs from the one that is utilized for the conventional LASIK in the following ways.

1. In wavefront-guided LASIK the ablation profile is generated by using complex algorithms that take all the measured wavefront aberrations and the corneal topography into consideration. The measured wavefront aberrations are mathematically transferred into an ablation profile by the computer software. *The success of the wavefront-guided LASIK is dependent upon this appropriate conversion of the optical aberrations into an ablation profile for adequate correction of all the aberrations.*

2. The scanning-spot/flying-spot excimer laser is essential to perform the complex ablation. The energy distribution of the laser beam is also of importance for the desired smooth ablation profile that is so crucial for correcting the aberrations. The desired laser beam is one with a '*truncated Gaussian beam shape*'. This beam has energy profile that is a combination of a '*flat top*' laser beam and a beam with *Gaussian energy distribution*. The former has a uniform energy distribution throughout the beam for good corrective ablation. The Gaussian energy distribution, i.e. the energy profile decreasing smoothly towards the periphery like the shape of a Gaussian curve, produces a smooth ablation profile at the junction/overlapping sites of the laser spots.

3. The use of an active eye-tracker and centering device is must for wavefront-guided LASIK. Use of the same device for measuring the aberrations as well as during the laser ablation and accurate centering is crucial for an adequate correction of the aberrations and desired visual results.

4. The ablation zone diameter is kept larger, 7–8 mm, in order to minimize the visual deterioration that occurs in scotopic condition because of the higher-order aberrations. This necessitates for creation of a larger diameter flap of at least 9.0 mm.

5. A larger optical zone means that the required ablation depth for a given spherocylindrical correction would be higher. This would reduce the residual bed thickness in comparison to the standard treatment protocol and might affect the corneal integrity. Therefore the flap thickness should be less than the usual 160 μ. The flap is kept about 130 μ in case of wavefront-guided LASIK.

6. The correction of the aberrations demands higher ablation depth towards the periphery. The steep edge is known to be associated with an increased healing response. Therefore an adequate transition must be created at the edge of the ablation zone to achieve a smooth corneal surface profile. This is achieved by performing corrective ablation for the refractive error using a 6–7 mm *optical zone* that is surrounded by 1 mm transition zone. Correction of the higher-order aberration is performed using additional laser pulses, which also create the smooth transition zone in the periphery.

Limitations of Wavefront-Guided LASIK

1. The procedure technically highly demanding.
2. It requires costly additional equipments like the aberrometer, an efficient active eye-tracker and different laser system equipped with appropriate computer software.
3. The technology for accurate wavefront sensing and the algorithms for adequate correction of the measured wavefront deformation need further development and refinement to achieve the desired results.
4. The aberrations are known to change with the degree of accommodation and with age.
5. They may also change with the development of cataract and after implantation of an intraocular lens.
6. The achieved benefit of the wavefront technology therefore may not be permanent.
7. The known intraoperative and postoperative complications of the LASIK surgery are associated with this procedure also.

Suggested readings

1. Martinez CE, Applegate RA, Klyce SD et al: Effect of pupillary dilation on the corneal optical aberrations after PRK. Arch Ophthalmol 1998; 116: 1053-1062.
2. Oliver KM, Hamenger RP, Corbett MC et al: Corneal optical aberrations induced by PRK. J Ref Surg 1997; 13: 246-254.
3. Oshika T, Klyce SD, Applegate RA et al: Comparison of corneal wavefront aberrations after PRK and laser in situ keratomileusis. Am J Ophthalmol 1999; 127: 1-7.
4. Seiler T, Kaemmerer M, Mierdel P et al: Ocular optical aberrations after PRK for myopia and myopic astigmatism. Arch Ophthalmol 2000; 118: 17-21.
5. Oshika T, Miyata K, Tokunaga T, Samejima T et al: Higher-order wavefront aberrations of cornea and magnitude of refractive correction in laser in situ keratomileusis. Ophthalmology 2002; 109(6): 1154-1158.
6. Mac Rae S, Schwiegerling J, Snyder RW: Customized and low spherical aberration corneal ablation design. J Ref Surg 1999; 12: S246-S248.
7. Mrochen M, Krueger RR, Bueeler M, Seiler T: Aberration-sensing and wavefront-guided laser in situ keratomileusis: management of decentered ablation. J Ref Surg 2002; 18 (4): 418-429.
8. Mrochen M, Seiler T, Kaemmerer: Wavefront-guided LASIK: early results in three eyes. J Ref Surg 2000; 16: 116-121.
9. Knorz MC, Neuhann T: Treatment of myopia and myopic astigmatism by customized laser in situ keratomileusis based on corneal topography. Ophthalmology. 2000 Nov; 107(11): 2072-6.
10. Mac Rae S, Schwiegerling J, Snyder RW: Customized corneal ablation and super vision. J Ref Surg 2000; 16: S230-S235.
11. Arbelaez MC: Super vision: dream or reality. J Refract Surg. 2001 Mar-Apr; 17(2 Suppl): S211-8.
12. Wang JY, Silva DE: Wavefront interpretations with Zernike polynomials. Applied Optics 1980; 19: 1510-1518.
13. Mrochen M, Kaemmerer M, Riedel R, and Seiler T: Why do we have to consider the corneal curvature for the calculation of customized ablation profiles? ARVO Abstract 3669. Invest Ophthalmol Vis Sci 2000; 41 (4): S689.
14. Oshika T, Klyce SD, Applegate RA et al: Changes in corneal wavefront aberrations with aging. Invest Ophthalmol Vis Sci 1999; 40: 1351-1355.
15. Calver RI, Cox MJ, Elliot DB: Effect of aging on the monochromatic aberrations of the human eye. J Opt Soc Am A 1999; 16: 2069-2078.
16. Guirao A, Gonzalez C, Redondo M et al: Average optical performance of the human eye as a function of age in a normal population. Invest Ophthalmol Vis Sci 1999; 40: 203-213.
17. He JC, Burns SA, Marcos S: Monochromatic aberrations in the accommodated human eye. Vis Res 2000; 40: 41-48.
18. Frnkhauser F, Kaemmerer M, Mrochen M, Seiler T: The effect of accommodation, mydriasis and cycloplegia on aberrometry. ARVO abstract 2248. Invest Ophthalmol Vis Sci 2000, 41: S461.

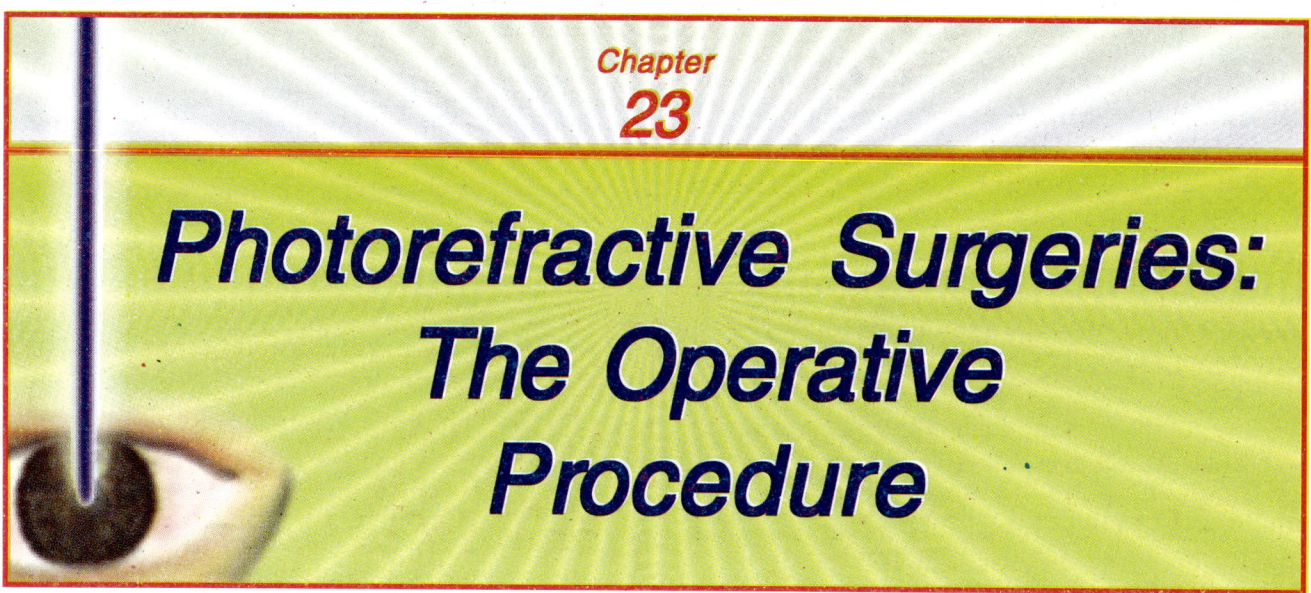

Chapter 23: Photorefractive Surgeries: The Operative Procedure

PREOPERATIVE PREPRATIONS

Sterile and Particle-Free Operation Theater

The photorefractive surgical procedures are performed in absolute sterile and particle-free conditions. Some Western literature has mentioned that the refractive surgery need not be necessarily performed in a surgical theater and a clean office environment may be sufficient. This aspect should be considered more seriously in view of the surgery being performed on an eye that is otherwise normal, the consequences of a corneal infection (though it may be rare) and the atmospheric and hygienic conditions prevailing in a particular part of the world. The surgeon must also take all conventional precautions to maintain sterility. These aspects have been already discussed in Chapter 15.

Patient Preparation

The face and eyelids are washed thoroughly with soap and water and the eye is cleaned with 5% povidone iodine. The patient wears a sterile gown and cap before entering the operating room. The name of the patient, refractive error, eye to be operated and other particulars of the patient must be put clearly on a tag that is worn by the patient. It is rechecked that an informed consent has been obtained.

The patient's apprehensions of any kind are mitigated by a friendly discussion. The patient is also made aware of the olfactory sensations produced due to ablation of the corneal tissue, clapping sounds generated by the laser pulses and the feeling of mild tapping on the eye, particularly by the wide beam acoustic waves. These steps would ensure a better patient cooperation and avoid sudden reflex reactions during ablation that could create problems in centration and proper ablation.

Premedication and Anesthesia

The PRK procedure may require peroperative use of oral or intravenous premedication, as it is a surface ablation procedure like PTK. Some surgeons use mild sedatives like 5-10 mg of oral diazepam in other cases. The procedure is performed under *preservative free* topical anesthesia using 2-4 drops of 0.5% of proparacaine (proxymetacaine hydrochloride) or 1% tetracaine (amethocaine) instilled into the eye about 10-20 minutes before surgery. To decrease patient's blinking and facilitate fixation of the eye, one drop of the anesthetic may be instilled into the fellow eye also.

In patients, who are uncooperative, who have a narrow palpebral aperture, or blepharospasm, a local lid block may be needed. It allows maximum exposure, takes care of the Bell's phenomenon and helps in self-fixation by the patient. *Using an adjustable/pediatric lid speculum and decreasing the illumination of the microscope are also useful for decreasing the blepharospasm.*

Intraoperative Centration

Ensuring exact centration during ablation is a crucial pre-requisite to avoid many postoperative problems and obtain the ideal visual results after laser refractive surgeries. Earlier, fixation devices like the *Thornton's ring* were used during PRK or the *suction ring was left without active suction during LASIK* to assist in eye fixation and centration of the ablation zone by the surgeon. *Self-fixation* of the patient at the *coaxial target* coupled with an efficient **active eye-tracker** is employed during modern day photorefractive surgeries (see Chapter 15 for other details).

PRK: PHOTOREFRACTIVE KERATECTOMY

Preparations for Laser Ablation

The eye to receive the treatment, the preoperative refractive error and correctness of the patient's particulars are reconfirmed from the clinical file. The assistant enters these particulars, the preoperative and desired refraction, the ablation zone diameter and other laser parameters into the computer of the machine. All the electrical connections are checked. The laser calibration is done by one of the methods specified by the manufacturer to ensure the desired irradiance and homogeneity of the laser beam (see Chapter 7).

Patient Preparation

The topical anesthesia may be augmented by applying a *fiber-free* cellulose sponge over the corneal surface, soaked in the anesthetic. This would make sure that the epithelial debridement is not painful. The patient is placed in the supine position without any head tilt. *The head tilt could potentially lead to misalignment of the cylindrical axis in cases of photoastigmatic keratectomy* (PARK). Avoiding the head tilt also ensure that the laser beam would be perpendicular to the cornea. The other eye is covered by a sterile disposable drape. The patient is instructed to keep the covered eye open to avoid Bell's phenomenon of the eye to be treated.

Marking of Cornea

The center of pupil is located while the patient is fixing at the coaxial target provided. The center of the graticule that represents the center of the entrance pupil is marked using a blunt tip instrument. A circular mark, about 8 mm, is applied with gentian violet around this point using a ring marker.

Epithelial Removal

The epithelium may be removed or left in situ for transepithelial ablation as discussed in Chapter 13. The edge of the removed epithelium should remain within this circular mark.

Ablation Zone Diameter

The *optic zone diameter* (the ablation zone) is crucial for the refractive ablation because of two reasons. Firstly the amount of refractive correction is inversely proportional to the ablation zone diameter, i.e. the same ablation depth produces a greater degree of refractive correction with a smaller ablation zone (see *Munnerlyn formula*, Chapter 20). In case of high refractive error the surgeon may decide to keep the ablation zone smaller. Secondly *an ablation zone that is equal or smaller than the pupil size under mesopic conditions* (about 6 mm) *is associated with troublesome glare, halos, ghost images, uniocular diplopia and night driving problems* as discussed in Chapter 20. Therefore an ablation zone of about 7 mm is found to be an ideal one to avoid these problems that would otherwise make PRK unacceptable due to visual dissatisfaction despite the achievement of desired refractive correction. This size of the ablation zone also enables the surgeon to achieve a *smoother transition zone* and decreases the incidence of potential optical aberrations.

Abrupt edge of the ablation zone without proper transition between the ablated and non-ablated cornea is found to be optically undesirable as it affects the quality of the vision. In its severe form, it may induce prismatic effect. The other optical problems that have been found to be associated with abrupt transition zone are increased incidence of spherical aberration, regression and decreased contrast sensitivity.

Laser Ablation

The laser ablation is initiated as soon as the epithelium debridement is over. This is essential to avoid corneal dehydration that would cause a change in the ablation rate. The surgeon gently holds the patient's head during the ablation to avert any gross movements by the patient and maintains the centration and alignment of the cornea with the laser beam.

The ablation may be carried on uninterrupted in case of mild to moderate corrections. In case of high refractive correction, the laser ablation may be stopped for about 10–15 seconds once or twice to allow an improved refixation by the patient. Laser ablation might have to be temporarily or altogether aborted if the surgeon finds that the centration is poor during ablation. The *active eye-tracker* automatically aborts the laser ablation in case of any gross decentration that is not correctable by the eye-tracker.

The laser ablation may be directed by the corneal topography (topography-linked PRK or *TOPOLINK*) if this facility is available with the surgeon. This technique uses elevation maps, in which the radii of curvature at various locations of the cornea of an individual's eye are converted into height values that are used by the computer software to decide the ablation profile (see Chapter 19).

Postoperative Instructions After PRK

The eye is patched or a contact lens is applied after PRK. An oral analgesic may be required for a day or two. A broad-spectrum antibiotic, teardrops and non-steroidal and low potency steroidal anti-inflammatory drops are prescribed. The eye is examined till the epithelium is regenerated completely. Antibiotic drops and bandage contact lens are discontinued after about 2 weeks. Anti-inflammatory agents and teardrops are continued to reduce corneal haze and stromal healing response. Their frequency of instillation is reduced gradually over months to once or twice daily.

It is important to remember that use of a contact lens and non-steroidal anti-inflammatory agents without concomitant use of topical steroids is associated with 'sterile stromal infiltrates, ring like opacity and even stromal melting (see Chapter 16 and complications). Teardrops are continued if one feels it necessary.

The intraocular pressure is to be monitored frequently because of prolonged use of topical steroids that are prescribed for many months for the management of corneal haze and regression. A steroid such as fluoro-methalone, which is known to be associated with low incidence of raised intraocular pressure, is prescribed.

LASIK: LASER IN-SITU KERATOMILEUSIS

The preoperative preparations are similar to these for PRK surgery except that no epithelial debridement is required. In fact the corneal surface is *not to be disturbed* to obtain the quick visual recovery that is so much expected from LASIK.

The key for successful LASIK is *creation of a good homogenous corneal flap* with uniform thickness. The microkeratome assumes an important role in this context.

Check the Instruments

The function of the *suction ring* and the microkeratome is checked beforehand. The suction should rise to about 23–25 mm of Hg after applying the thumb at the vacuum chamber and the suction ring must adhere well to the thumb.

The assembled *microkeratome head* is checked for the thickness/depth plate and the blade fitting. The *thickness plate* is checked that it is of the *desired specification* according to the intended flap thickness. In a case where deeper ablation may be needed to correct high errors, a thinner corneal flap, e.g. about 130 micron, is required and therefore a thickness plate that would leave 130 micron space between the blade and itself is to be used. Some microkeratomes have option for adjusting the thickness plate. The Hansatome has two separate heads with 160 μ and 180 μ depth plates.

The microtome head is checked for its smooth forward and backward movement and the *stopper mechanism*. The head is inserted into the dovetail of the suction ring provided to engage it. The handle of the suction ring is held in left hand and the handle of the microkeratome in the right hand while engaging the head into the dovetail. Then, by gently supporting the motor cord, the head is advanced manually on the gear track of the suction ring until the gear of the head is firmly engaged. Further smooth movement of the head is checked by pressing the foot paddle in forward position. The head should come to a gentle stop as it meets the stopper mechanism. Now the movement of the microkeratome is reversed by pressing the foot paddle in reverse position. These maneuvers also verify functioning of the foot pedal and the power supply console.

The *edge of the blade is inspected under the microscope* for its sharpness and regularity during the above movement.

Double-check the Refractive Data

The eye to be operated and the refractive error are again confirmed. All other parameters that are to be entered into the computer like the ablation zone diameter, type of ablation (myopic/hypermetropic, etc.), ablation profile, multizone components of the ablation, transition to be achieved and other relevant parameters are verified.

Laser Programming and Test Firing

It is crucial to check the functioning of the laser system before the corneal flap is made. Laser calibration and programming of the excimer laser is done as above. This will also check the functioning of the laser system before the surgery is commenced.

Apply the Lid Speculum

An adequate exposure of the cornea is must for the smooth movement of the microkeratome head while cutting the corneal flap. The appropriate size lid speculum is applied gently to separate the eyelids. One may use the *wire-speculum*, the *adjustable speculum* or a *suction speculum* depending on the availability. But the blades of the speculum should be short as longer blade provide less separation and induce more blepharospasm. A lid akinesia may be required with the help of an appropriate local block if blepharospasm is present in an anxious patient. Any secretions that are expressed after the application of the speculum are cleaned with irrigation and merocel sponge.

Although the selection of smaller size speculum and suction ring may help in cases of narrow palpabral aperture, in rare situations lateral canthotomy might have to be resorted to in order to obtain adequate exposure for a *larger diameter* corneal flap, which may be indicated in a particular case. In this case, the consent of the patient is essential after an adequate discussion about this requirement, as this proposition may not be acceptable to the patient for cosmetic or other reasons.

Mark the Cornea

Cornea is marked with a small quantity of a dye like gentian violet or methylene blue (Fig. 23.1). It serves three purposes.

1. The central circular mark (about 8 mm) helps in centration of the ablation zone.
2. The three small circular marks of about 3 mm each, placed on temporal, nasal and inferior sides of the previous mark help in accurate repositioning of the corneal flap after the ablation.
3. In case of a free corneal flap, the role of the corneal markings becomes crucial for proper alignment of the flap in its original position.

Apply the Suction Ring

The suction ring plays an important role for smooth cutting of the hinged corneal flap, as mentioned in Chapter 21. Suction ring of the appropriate size is chosen

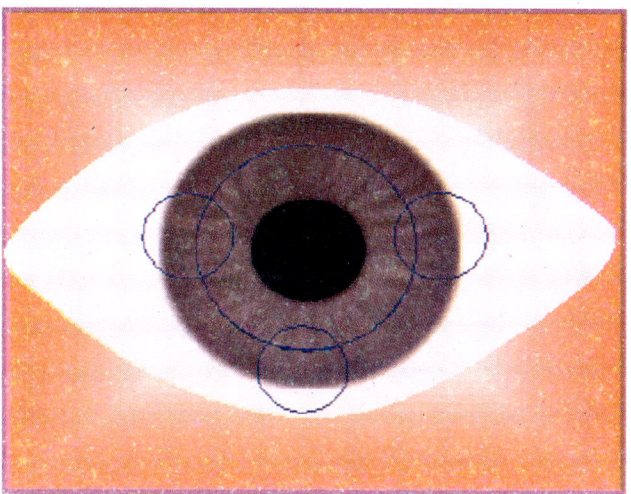

Fig. 23.1: Marking of cornea

if rings are provided separately or the size of an *adjustable ring* is manipulated to the desired diameter. For myopic ablation, usually two sizes of rings are used. The ring size is 9.5 mm in case of normal size cornea, but it is 8.5 mm if the corneal diameter is less than 10.5 mm. For hypermetropic ablation, one needs a larger corneal flap of about 10.4 mm, which demands use of a suction ring of an appropriate diameter.

The suction ring is placed gently over the globe without retropulsing it. The eye is properly positioned within the ring before the suction is activated. The eye might have to be moved under the ring by gently putting one finger over the cornea for accurate positioning. The suction ring is applied in such a way that it remains about 1 mm more on the side where the hinge of the corneal flap is intended to be. Problems in proper positioning and repeated applications may result in conjunctival hemorrhages. The handle of the ring is supported after its positioning. The vacuum is created through activating the suction pump by depressing and then releasing the foot paddle provided separately for this purpose. The foot paddle acts like an on-off switch. The suction continues until the surgeon presses the paddle again.

Confirm the Efficacy of Suction

Generation of an adequate suction to raise the intraocular pressure to a desired level is an equally important step during the creation of the corneal flap. The efficacy of suction is confirmed by measuring the intraocular pressure. The instrument used for this purpose is the *Barraquer's tonometer*. This tonometer is a small hand-held device that utilizes the applanation principle. When balanced on the cornea, its weight provides the *applanation pressure*. The cornea is dried before applying the tonometer. If the meniscus circle formed after the application of the tonometer is well within the circle etched on the tonometer tip, it indicates an IOP over 65 mm of Hg that is desirable for cutting the corneal flap.

Inadequate suction would result in less increase in the IOP, which is not suitable for making the cornea prominent and bulge forward. In this situation the corneal flap may be irregular, of incorrect size or partial or there may be no corneal flap at all.

Apply the Microkeratome

As soon as the desired intraocular pressure is achieved, the microkeratome is fitted into the grove of the suction ring and activated in the same manner as described above for checking the instrument (Fig. 23.2). The *cornea and the suction ring are moistened with distilled water* before this step to make sure that the head slides easily during the procedure (**wet cutting**). Distilled water is preferable to saline or *balanced salt solution* (BSS). Its use precludes deposition of any debris of salt crystals on the ring gear track or the head.

The surgical field is inspected to ensure that the eyelashes, lid speculum or surgical drape, etc. do not come into the way of the microkeratome head during the creation of the corneal flap. If no such obstacle or debris is in the way, the gears are properly meshed in the gear track and the surgeon is not holding the microtome with too much pressure upwards or downwards, the microkeratome would advance smoothly on activation. The surgeon stops the advancement of the microkeratome, by *releasing* the foot paddle, as soon as it meets the stopper mechanism. The movement of the microkeratome is then reversed by pressing the foot paddle in the reverse position. The paddle is released as soon as the surgeon notices the corneal flap slid out of the head on to the stromal bed as the gears reach the end of the track. The microkeratome is gently slid out of the track and removed after corneal flap is created (Fig 23.3).

Release the Suction Ring

The suction is released immediately after the creation of the flap. The suction ring may be left in place without suction to fixate the globe and maintain centration. Self-fixation by the patient, assisted by the active eye-tracker is used by modern laser systems.

Re-center the Optic Zone

After removal of the suction ring, eye centration is done again because the centration is likely to be lost during the procedures. Centration is done with reference to the pupil and not over the corneal reflection, as the anatomy and the reflection has been disturbed by the presence of the corneal flap. During the maneuver of re-centration of the eye, the corneal flap is left on the stromal bed to avoid any possibility of dehydration of the stroma that would otherwise change the ablation rate of the tissue.

Fold the Corneal Flap

The corneal flap is folded back, away from the ablation field towards its hinge, after proper centration has been done. Turning of the flap is to be done with utmost care to avoid the slightest damage to the flap or the stromal bed. A pair of fine-toothed forceps can be used to hold the flap at its margin opposite to the hinge while folding it towards the flap hinge. A *blunt spatula may also be used for this purpose but it has the potential risk of causing surface irregularity on the stromal bed during the maneuver of separating and folding the flap*. A drop of BSS is put over the folded corneal flap. It helps in keeping the flap in the folded position and adherent to the conjunctiva, by the surface tension created by the fluid. It also avoids dehydration of the flap while the stromal ablation is carried on.

Perform Intraoperative Pachymetry: Confirm the Flap Thickness

Because of high variability of the actual thickness of the corneal flap cut by the same microkeratome in different eyes, it is mandatory to perform an intraoperative pachymetry. Also, the risk of corneal ectasia induced after LASIK due to less than desired *residual bed thickness* warrants about this crucial step (see Chapter 6).

Determination of the exact flap thickness and the thickness of the stromal bed may change the plan for the amount of corneal stroma to be removed with the excimer laser. Conventionally, ultrasound pachymetry has been used for the measurement of the stromal bed and the flap thickness. The optical low coherence reflectometry (OLCR) has been found to be an appropriate alternative to ultrasonic pachymetry by Genth et al. Vinciguerra *et al* have used the 'Confoscan 2.0', which is a computerized confocal optical microscopy system, to evaluate the corneal thickness as well as intraoperative flap thickness and stromal bed. They commented that it gave precise measurement of different layers of cornea.

Ablate the Stromal Bed

The stromal ablation is done after drying it with gentle application of a merocel sponge (**dry ablation**). The lights of the room and the operating microscope are dimmed to enable the patient to see the target light well for better fixation and to reduce photophobia.

The computer software decides the ablation profile according to the data fed by the surgeon. These days, *all laser systems utilize the spot scanning laser beam to perform complex ablation profiles.* The surgeon initiates the ablation by pressing the foot switch kept in a safety housing to prevent inadvertent activation of laser delivery. The surgeon gently but steadily holds the patient's head to abort any sudden movements. The surgeon must stop the laser delivery immediately if any decentration is observed. The active eye-tracker, in the modern laser systems, assisted by patient's self-fixation, keeps the ablation zone centered. *The laser delivery is automatically discontinued if the eye-tracker is confronted with decentration that is not possible to be corrected by this device.*

An assistant keeps the **corneal flap** out of the ablation field, while the **surgeon concentrates on the tissue** ablation. If some irregularity of the stromal surface is noticed at the end of the laser ablation, a minimum (about 8–10 μ) ablation of the surface in plano-mode of phototherapeutic keratectomy (PTK) may be employed to smoothen the surface.

Remove the Ablation By-products

Evacuation of the plume of ablation by-products is done intermittently during the ablation. The surface fluid that may accumulate in the central part of the cornea is also wiped off with merocel sponge after stopping the laser delivery. Accumulation of these would otherwise lead to irregular ablation and/or steep islands. Charles K has reported statistically significant better postoperative refractive and visual results after the use of *surgical vacuum* as a plume evacuator during LASIK[12].

Replace the Corneal Flap

The corneal flap is repositioned over the stromal bed after laser ablation. Accurate repositioning of the corneal flap is greatly helped by the corneal markings (Fig. 23.4). The stromal surface is irrigated with balanced salt solution (BSS) to remove any interface debris and epithelial cells. The surface of the cornea is also irrigated and the excess fluid is removed by gently pressing the surface with merocel sponge several times *(the wet method)*. This step decreases the risk of interface debris, epithelial islands, flap folds and wrinkling of the flap. It also ensures better adhesion of the flap to the underlying stromal bed due to surface tension.

Some surgeons advocate avoiding the irrigation before repositing the flap. This is thought to provide visual rehabilitation within hours, supposedly due to minimal or no corneal edema after this *dry method* of flap repositioning. This method results in problems in flap repositioning with flap folds as well wrinkling. A high incidence of interface debris and epithelial islands is also observed subsequently.

POSTOPERATIVE MANAGEMENT FOLLOWING LASIK

Immediate Examination

The eye is examined under the slit-lamp before sending the patient home. Attention is given to proper placement of the flap, any wrinkling or fold in the flap and presence of any debris at the interface. These should be rectified inside the operating room. If everything is all right, the patient is prescribed topical antibiotic, tear substitute and anti-inflammatory agents. Before sending home, the patient must be given clear instructions about the does and don'ts after the LASIK procedure. The verbal discussion must be accompanied by written instructions.

Care of the Corneal Flap

The foremost concern is about the displacement of the corneal flap. The flap is reasonably adherent and secure immediately after its repositioning, but the forces of adhesion are not strong enough to withstand the external forces that can potentially displace the flap. Patients are therefore warned to avoid all activities that may cause trauma to the operated eye. They are advised not to rub the eyes, avoid all ocular irritants such as soap, smoke, dust and cosmetics, etc. All contact sports, swimming and scuba diving are also restricted at least for a month or so until reasonable healing of the tissue has taken place.

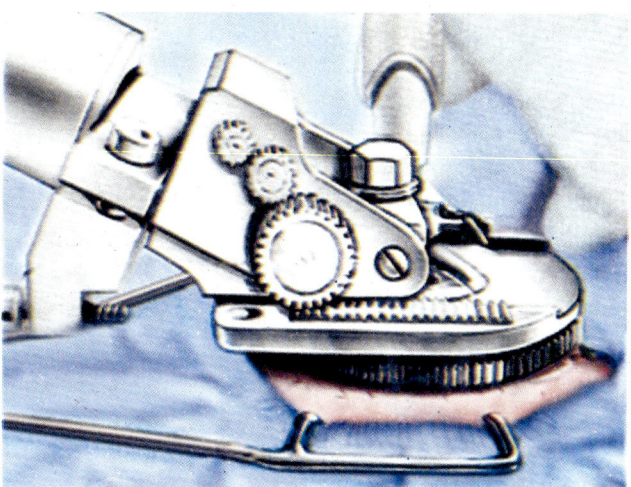

Fig. 23.2: Microkeratome in position and advancing on the gear track to create the anterior stromal flap

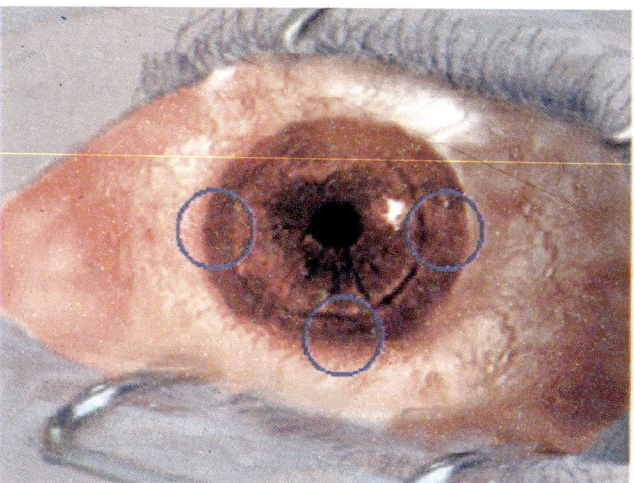

Fig. 23.4: Corneal flap has been folded back. The circular gentian violet marks help in proper repositioning of the flap

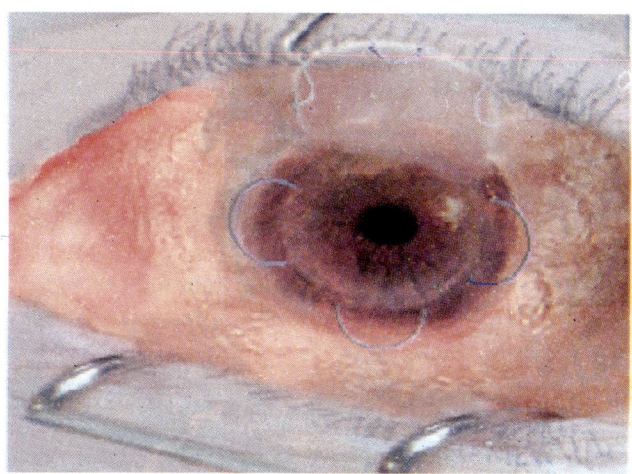

Fig. 23.3: Corneal flap with superior hinge

wound takes many months to return to normal levels. The adhesion between the corneal flap and the underlying stroma also is not complete for many months as is evident from the clinical fact that the flap can be re-lifted during *re-LASIK*. Histopathology of one case of keratectasia requiring keratoplasty has shown that the weak adhesions are due to absence of bridging collagen fibrils in the lamellar corneal wound even at sixth postoperative month (see Chapter 6). Therefore the safe period after which the risk of flap dislocation can be said to be absent is difficult to predict.

Resumption of Daily Work

The routine activities and office work can be resumed from the next day if it does not pose any risk to the eye. Returning to professional activities that may predispose to trauma, infection or irritant may be better postponed for one week or so and protective eyeglasses should be worn subsequently. *The fluctuation of vision is frequent during the early postoperative period.* The patient is forewarned about this possibility to allay any apprehension and psychological disturbances.

Postoperative Medication

The LASIK procedure does not violate the ocular surface; therefore prolonged medication with topical steroidal and non-steroidal anti-inflammatory agents is not required. These agents are used for many months to modulate the healing response after corneal surface ablation procedures such as PRK and PTK. The surface ablation is known to be associated with exaggerated keratocyte activity due to the stroma coming in contact with the epithelial growth factors (see Chapter 5 and 16). *The problem of healing of epithelium and postoperative pain are also avoided.* The postoperative medication is therefore minimum.

Topical antibiotic can be discontinued after one week, tear substitutes after about 4 weeks or even earlier and the anti-inflammatory agents after a few weeks. Early discontinuation of topical steroids avoids any risk of induced rise of the intraocular pressure. However if the surgeon feels that low potency topical steroid has to be continued for longer duration to treat or avoid regression and corneal haze in a particular case, the intraocular pressure should be monitored carefully, by the method described below. If the patient has problems of vision during mesopic condition that are intolerable, pilocarpine in low concentration may be prescribed in the evening. This problem is likely to occur in patients with large pupil diameter in dim illumination and with smaller ablation zone size.

Bandage Soft Contact Lens

Some surgeons advocate the use of a bandage soft contact lens (BSCL) socked in a broad-spectrum antibiotic for a few days. This serves different purposes.

1. The contact lens avoids any possible displacement of the flap during the early postoperative period.
2. It decreases the chance of infection by serving as a media for better continuous drug delivery.
3. It takes care of any superficial punctate keratitis (SPK) that might occur during the first few days.

Eye patching should be avoided after LASIK. It may lead to increased risk of flap displacement.

Subsequent Examinations

The patient must be examined next day for any flap related problem that is correctable. The subsequent visits are then scheduled at 1, 3, 6 and 12 months. The patient is instructed to report immediately to the operating surgeon in case of any pain, redness, excessive lacrimation or blurring of vision during the postoperative period.

During the follow up examinations the *visual functions, e.g. uncorrected visual acuity* (UCVA), *best corrected* (BCVA), *low contrast visual acuity* (LCVA) *and glare visual acuity* (GVA) are measured. Computerized videokeratography must be obtained early to assess any ablation zone decentration and central steep islands, etc. Other preoperative parameters like the keratometry, pachymetry and endothelial count are also evaluated. The surgeon should also be vigilant to pick up any of the potential complications after LASIK and treat them accordingly.

The following account summarizes the clinical findings that should be looked for during examinations at different postoperative periods.

After One-two Hours

1. Adherence of the flap.
2. Flap folds or macrowrinkles.
3. Any flap displacement.
4. Interface debris like fibers, metal fillings, glove powder particles and epithelial tags.

The fibers may originate from the sponges and poor quality eye drape. The metallic debris arises from the 'wake' of the microkeratome blade. No lifting of the flap and irrigation of the interface may be needed in case of minor interface debris in the periphery, but if it is in the visual area and potentially disturbing or consists of epithelial tags, this procedure has to be resorted to clear the debris.

Second Day

1. Make sure that the edge of the flap is covered by the epithelium.
2. Confirm the flap adherence and proper alignment and positioning. Repositioning may be required in case of flap displacement.
3. Re-evaluate for the presence of flap wrinkling. Sometimes slit-lamp retroillumination may show microstriae, which do not cause any interference with vision.
4. Rule out interface debris.
5. The epithelial surface may show superficial punctate keratitis.
6. Rule out any interface infiltrate in the periphery that may represent an early form of '*diffuse lamellar keratitis*' (DLK).
7. Infiltrate may also indicate presence of infectious or non-infectious keratitis, which must be properly investigated and managed.
8. Uncorrected visual acuity is ascertained if no epithelial complication is present.

At One Week

1. The normal finding is a clear cornea at this stage.
2. The corneal surface is examined for any remaining SPK, which is unusual at this time.
3. Refraction and best-corrected visual acuity are determined.
4. A good quality topography map can be obtained at one week.

At One Month

1. The visual functions listed above are tested.
2. Higher-order optical aberrations are measured if the facility is available. The *total mean-square wavefront error* (W^2) and the *root mean-square wavefront error* (W_{RMS}) are determined for comparison with the preoperative higher order optical aberrations.
3. Refraction starts stabilizing by this time.
4. Any under-or overcorrection is corrected by suitable lenses.
5. Appearance of corneal haze may be evident at this time.
6. Any epithelial growth also appears at one month.
7. Regression of the refraction is determined by analysis of the early and one-month refractions, keratometry change and topography.
8. Attention is given to symptoms relating to night driving and mesopic vision. Use of tinted glasses, diluted pilocarpine (about 0.5%), antireflective coating and spectacles with slight myopic correction to stimulate accommodation in the young patient may help to alleviate the problems of glare and halos.
9. The intraocular pressure is taken by applanation method, particularly in those who are prescribed topical steroids due to the postoperative requirements. *The area chosen is the peripheral cornea because the central cornea is known to give false low readings due to interface fluid and corneal edema.*
10. The examination of the optic disk should be made to rule out changes of *masked glaucoma* because of false IOP readings.

At Third Month

1. In myopes, refraction stabilizes by this time in majority of cases. If required, any corrective lenses can be finally prescribed if medical management has not helped in treating regression. Retreatment is not planned for under-or over-corrections at this time.
2. Hyperopes take longer time to achieve stability of the refraction, up to 6 months.
3. The tear-film and ocular surface is normal and tear substitutes can be withdrawn if these were prescribed.
4. Repeat refraction, keratometry and corneal topography are performed to rule out late regression and early corneal ectasia or curvature changes.
5. The patient is told to visit at sixth month and biannually thereafter. The examination is mainly focussed at any visual disturbances and any changes to suggest corneal ectasia, particularly in cases of higher correction.
6. Attention is also paid to measurement of the intraocular pressure, as was done at the one-month examination if the patient is on topical steroids for treating stromal haze or regression of refraction.
7. The higher-order optical aberrations are measured.

Suggested readings

1. Yoo SH, Azar DT. Laser in situ keratomileusis for the treatment of myopia. Int Ophthalmol Clin 1999; 39:37-44.
2. George O Waring III: Excimer laser in situ keratomileusis (LASIK). In 'Excimer Laser In Ophthalmology': Principles and Practice, ed. Charles Mc Ghee, Martin Dunitz Ltd publication 1997.
3. Gimbel HV, Penno EE et al: In 'LASIK Complications: Prevention and Management, Second edition, Slack Incorporated publications, 2001.
4. Genth U, Mrochen M, Walti R et al: Optical low coherence reflectometry for noncontact measurement of flap thickness during laser on situ keratomileusis. Ophthalmology 2002; 109: 973-978.
5. Vinciguerra P, Torres I, Camesasca FI: Application of confocal microscopy in refractive surgery. J Ref Surg 2002; 18 (3 Suppl): S378-81.
6. Erie JC, Patel SV, McLaren JW, Ramirez M et al: Effect of myopic laser in situ keratomileusis on epithelial and stromal thickness: a confocal microscopy study. Ophthalmology. 2002 Aug; 109 (8): 1447-52.
7. Alessio G, Boscia F, La Tegola MG, Sborgia C. Topography-driven photorefractive keratectomy: results of corneal interactive programmed topographic ablation software. Ophthalmology 2000; 107:1578-87.
8. Knorz MC, Neuhann T: Treatment of myopia and myopic astigmatism by customized laser in situ keratomileusis based on corneal topography. Ophthalmology 2000 Nov; 107(11): 2072-6.
9. McDonald MB, Deitz MR, Frantz JM, Kraff MC, Krueger RR, Salz JJ et al. Photorefractive keratectomy for low-to-moderate myopia and astigmatism with a small-beam, tracker-directed excimer laser. Ophthalmology 1999; 106:1481-8.
10. Seiler T, McDonnell PJ. Excimer laser photorefractive keratectomy. Surv Ophthalmol 1995; 40:89-118.
11. Carr JD, Stulting RD, Thompson KP, Waring GO 3rd Laser in situ keratomileusis: surgical technique. Ophthalmol Clin North Am. 2001 Jun; 14 (2): 285-94.
12. Charles K: Effect of intraoperative laser-plume evacuation on results of LASIK. (J Ref Surg 2002; 18 (3 Suppl): S340-2.

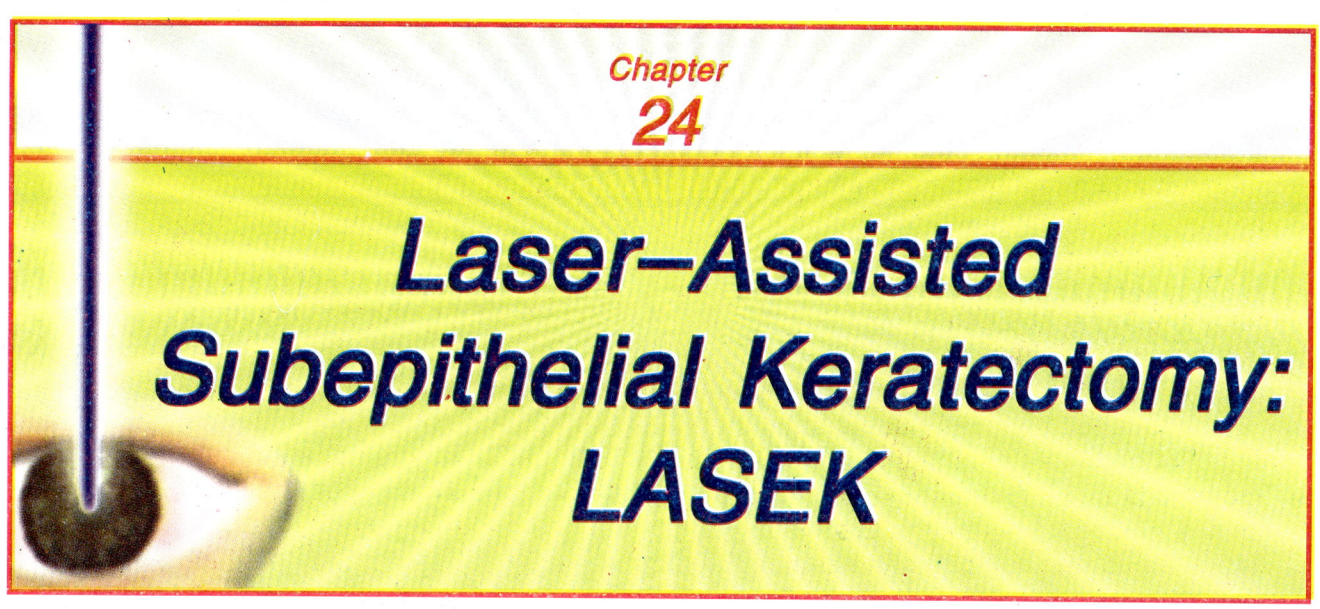

Chapter 24: Laser-Assisted Subepithelial Keratectomy: LASEK

DEFINITION AND HISTORY

Laser-assisted subepithelial keratectomy (LASEK) is a technique of excimer laser refractive ablation after *detachment of an epithelial flap assisted with ethanol* and then repositioning of this flap after the laser ablation. This procedure could be called a modification of both PRK as well as LASIK.

It is similar to PRK in so far as the ablation is done after the epithelial removal but differs from it because the epithelium is removed as a flap that can be replaced back to cover the ablated surface. On the other hand, it resembles LASIK because the procedure involves the raising of a flap under which the refractive ablation is performed. But it differs from LASIK because no deeper cutting through the corneal stroma and therefore no use of the microkeratome is required.

Massimo Camellin used the acronym LASEK in 1999 to describe his new technique called '*laser epithelial keratomileusis*'. Later in 2000, he described the surgical procedure. Now a days this acronym is used as an abbreviation for 'laser-assisted subepithelial keratectomy'. Many other eponyms have been used for this procedure like E-LASIK, Epi-LASIK, sub-epithelial PRK and excimer laser sub-epithelial ablation (ELSA).

ADVANTAGE

Laser-assisted subepithelial keratectomy combines the benefits of both PRK and LASIK and promises to avoid or decrease many of the complications associated with these procedures. Thus it is said to be a perfect blend of these two surgeries.

LASEK vs. PRK

Offers the Same Corrective Range of PRK

The range of refractive correction is higher for myopia as in case of PRK. This is because of availability of the whole stromal tissue for ablation. A safe residual stromal bed can be left after correction of high refractive error.

Provides Better Visual and Refractive Outcome

1. The visual recovery is much faster due to the intact epithelium in comparison to PRK. The epithelial flap provides a smooth refracting surface after LASEK.
2. Simultaneous LASEK can be performed in both eyes of the patient, unlike in case of PRK.
3. The predictability of correction and visual acuity results are better than after PRK (see Chapter 25).
4. No significant regression has been reported after LASEK.

Avoids the Postoperative Disadvantages of PRK

1. Photorefractive keratectomy (PRK) is associated with significant postoperative pain, longer visual

rehabilitation, corneal haze and regression of the effect. These complications are direct results or sequelae of the corneal surface ablation. There is also increased risk of the corneal infection as more ablated surface is exposed to a possible microbial insult.
2. The epithelial flap in LASEK acts as a tissue-bandage. Its effect is to minimize the postoperative pain caused by the exposed raw corneal surface. It also decreases the risk of infection.
3. Most of the clinical series have reported significantly reduced pain and corneal haze after LASEK. Prospective clinical studies by Kornilosky and Lee J B et al have compared the outcome of LASEK and PRK in two eyes of the same patient and have concurred with the above findings. In the later study (by Lee et al), 63% of the patients preferred LASEK to PRK.

Avoids the Healing Response and its Sequelae

1. The presence of the epithelial flap avoids the exposure of the stromal keratocytes to the tears, cytokines and growth factors released after epithelial injury. These factors are supposed to be responsible for the keratocyte loss as well as increases healing response and remodeling after PRK that leads to significant stromal haze and regression of the myopia.
2. A study by Rokita et al, on changes in corneal structure during the first three postoperative months after LASEK using the confocal microscope, found that the epithelial structure stabilized promptly. There was no overproduction of the collagen fibers and no scarring occurred in 50 eyes that were studied. These findings are unlike the ones that have been reported after PRK by other scientists.

LASEK vs. LASIK

Offers the Advantages of LASIK

1. The presence of the '*epithelial flap*' in LASEK offers the benefits of LASIK, which are freedom from postoperative pain, faster visual rehabilitation, less corneal haze and simultaneous treatment of both eyes of a patient.
2. In fact the visual acuity, contrast sensitivity, refractive results and corneal topography were found to be better by Scerrati et al in the LASEK group as compared to the LASIK group.
3. The postoperative medication is also minimized like in case of LASIK.

Offers Greater Correction of the Refractive Error

LASEK allows removal of greater amount of corneal stroma because the epithelial flap is only about 50 μ thick in comparison to an average 160 μ anterior stromal flap of LASIK.

Avoids the Intraoperative and Postoperative Flap Complications of LASIK

1. LASEK does not require a microkeratome, which is costly and complicated to use. Therefore it avoids the intraoperative microkeratome and *stromal flap related* complications of LASIK, which are mechanical microkeratome failures, button-holing of flap, incomplete flap, free flap, unpredictable flap thickness compromising the corneal strength or even corneal perforation.
2. LASEK avoids *interface related complications* of LASIK like interface debris, diffuse lamellar keratitis (DLK) and epithelial ingrowth.
3. The risk of late flaps complications like flap dislocation and flap melt is also not there with LASEK.

Avoids the Risk of Corneal Ectasia

1. In LASIK, the variability of the anterior stromal flap thickness results in difficulty in predicting the residual bed thickness. The predictability of the residual stromal bed is not a problem in LASEK.
2. Moreover, the stromal flap itself does not contribute to the postoperative strength of the cornea. Therefore the risk of corneal ectasia remains if the postoperative corneal thickness minus the average flap thickness, which is about 160 μ, is less than 325 μ.
3. Therefore, the risk of postoperative corneal ectasia does not exist after LASEK, if the intended correction has been planned according to the safe limit.

Intraoperative Undercorrection is Avoided

The patient might have to be deliberately undercorrected during LASIK if the stromal flap is unduly thick. This does not happen in LASEK.

Problems Related to Suction Ring and High IOP are Avoided

Application of the suction ring to raise the intraocular pressure is required during LASIK to create the stromal flap. This procedure is not required for raising the hinged epithelial flap. The suction ring can cause subconjunctival hemorrhage. Very high IOP (>60 mm Hg) generated during cutting of the flap in LASIK has the potential risk of retinal vein obstruction, glaucomatous damage, optic atrophy and retinal break in the predisposed eyes.

LASEK can be Performed in Situations where LASIK is Otherwise Contraindicated

1. *Situations where creation of the corneal flap is difficult,* for example deep set eyes, eyes with narrow palpabral fissure, too steep or too flat cornea.

2. In p*atients with epithelial basement membrane dystrophy* (EBMD), LASIK may precipitate corneal erosions. LASEK promises to treat this condition and avoid erosions by virtue of the laser ablation starting at the basement membrane level like PTK.

3. *Very high myopia* can be treated safely without the risk of corneal ectasia.

4. *Patients with thin corneas* can be treated if the planned correction leaves a safe RBT, which is a more likely possibility in comparison to LASIK.

5. *Patients with large pupils* can be treated. Laser ablation in eyes with large pupil size requires the ablation zone diameter to be larger and therefore deeper ablation, which can be performed during LASEK, as more stromal tissue is available in comparison to LASIK.

6. *Patients with glaucoma and filtering blebs* can be treated with LASEK because application of the suction ring and raising of intraocular pressure are not needed.

7. *Patients involved in contact sports* and activities where the LASIK flap is at a risk of displacement/dislocation, can be treated because adherence of the epithelial flap is strong enough in comparison to the anterior stromal flap.

Promises Better Results in "Customized Ablation"

1. The improved visual results of customized ablation, based on wavefront technology, are dependent on the complex ablation patterns requiring fine sculpting of the stroma.
2. The flap cutting through the microkeratome does not produce very fine and smooth stromal surface for ablation.
3. The microstriae and un-noticed minimum flap slippage may also nullify the benefits achieved by the customized ablation. LASEK may provide an improved flap-stromal interface to maintain the benefits of the wavefront technology.
4. Studies by Agrawal et al and Shah et al had found that the corneal surface after alcohol debridement of the epithelium was smoother as seen under the operating microscope than mechanical removal.
5. Vinciguerra and co-authors found a more regular and smooth stromal surface during LASEK using the confocal microscopy.
6. Wilson and co-authors have reported that corneal surface ablation (LASEK or PRK) may provide more accurate and better visual results using customized wavefront ablation.

LASEK: THE OPERATIVE PROCEDURE

Preoperative Preparations

LASEK surgery is performed under topical anesthesia. No strong premedication is required unlike during, PRK. All other preparations relating to patient, operative room and laser system calibration are similar to the ones needed for other photorefractive surgeries.

Creating the Hinged Epithelial Flap

Creation of the epithelial flap involves special technique and instruments. The following steps summarize the method of raising the epithelial flap.

1. The first step is '*pre-incision*' of the corneal epithelium. This is performed using a specially designed corneal *micro-trephine*. The micro-trephine has a diameter of 8.0 mm and cutting depth of about 70-80 μ with a calibrated and guarded blunt blade. It has the provision for leaving a superior hinge of uncut epithelium that extends

about 45° on either side of 12 O' clock position. The micro-trephine circumscribes the *epithelial flap* area and provides a uniform groove in the remaining 270° of the circumference for raising the flap.

2. An *alcohol solution cone* or a *holding well*, measuring 8.5 mm, is placed around the above 8.0 mm mark made by the micro-trephine. About 0.2 cc of 18-20% ethanol is filled in this cone and left for about 20-30 seconds.
3. The alcohol solution is prepared by mixing 1.0 cc of 100% alcohol with 4 cc of sterile distilled water. Alternatively 1.0 cc of dehydrated 98% ethyl alcohol can be mixed with 4.0 cc of distilled water, then passed through 0.2 µ filters. This solution can be stored for 1-2 weeks in refrigerator.
4. After a period of 20-30 seconds, the alcohol solution is absorbed from the retainer cone using a surgical sponge. The corneal surface is thoroughly washed with balanced salt solution (BSS).
5. The peripheral cornea is dried well with a merocel sponge to make the trephine mark clear.
6. A *micro-hoe* is then used to elevate the edge of the cut epithelium. This is done with a gentle digging action of the micro-hoe all along the groove made by the corneal micro-trephine.
7. Sometimes the epithelial edge does not separate easily. No force should be applied in this case to elevate the edge. Instead the alcohol retaining well is placed again over the marked area and alcohol solution applied for another 10-15 seconds.
8. Young men, post-menopausal women and those using contact lenses for long time require the *initial application* of the alcohol solution for a longer time.
9. After elevating the edge of the cut epithelium, the epithelial flap is raised using an *epithelium detachment spatula*, specially designed for this purpose. Utmost care should be taken not to damage the pliable flap while separating it from the underlying tissue. It is advisable to include the *basal lamina* with the epithelium while separating it from the Bowmen's layer.
10. The epithelial flap is folded on its hinge at the 12 O'clock position.
11. The desired refractive ablation is performed according to the planned treatment algorithm.
12. The ablated surface is washed with BSS and the epithelial flap is repositioned back using a blunt-tipped spatula. The exact alignment of the epithelial flap is not required.
13. The flap extends over the peripheral corneal epithelium due to decrease in the stromal tissue after laser ablation. This provides a good barrier action and helps in early adherence of the epithelial flap.
14. At the end of the LASEK procedure, a bandage soft contact lens (BSCL) is applied over the cornea.

Postoperative Care

The patient is prescribed broad-spectrum antibiotic drops, topical non-steroidal and steroidal anti-inflammatory agents and preservative free teardrops four times daily. The use of oral analgesics is not necessary after LASEK in most of the patients. Some patients reporting discomfort during the early postoperative period may occasionally need them.

The therapeutic contact lens is removed after 3-4 days. Topical antibiotic is stopped after about 2 weeks. Subsequently the topical low potency steroids, NSAIDs and tear substitutes are gradually tapered off on a bi-weekly basis after one month and finally withdrawn after 8-10 weeks.

The duration of the anti-inflammatory agents used depends upon the individual healing response and the early postoperative refraction. Unlike PRK, the corneal haze after LASEK appears early, is milder and clears earlier than the third month. Therefore there is no need for prolonged use of the modulating agents for the healing response. The patients who show hyperopic refraction at the second week do not require continuation of the anti-inflammatory agents for more than 8 weeks. These topical drops are given four times daily for 4 weeks, 3 times daily for next 4 weeks, twice daily for 2 weeks and once daily for next two weeks in patients who have residual myopia. Teardrops are given for a period depending upon the individual corneal surface status.

Intraoperative and Postoperative Complications

Although the LASEK procedure is relatively new, no major complications have been reported by many available published clinical series. On one hand, some of the complications related to the epithelial flap can be considered as *learning curve for the surgeon*, as their incidence has decreased significantly in the recent reports. At the same time it is too early to comment upon other effects like regression and the possible damaging effect of alcohol on the long-term functioning of the epithelial cells and keratocytes.

The various problems or complications reported with LASEK are as follows.

Alcohol Leakage

Alcohol leakage from the container may occur if not applied firmly on the cornea (in 3.6 % of eyes in series by Lee et al). No damage to the limbal cells and conjunctiva or corneal erosions occurred following the leakage.

Flap complications

The overall incidence of flap related complications reported by different clinical studies vary from 0.9–14%. The various flap complications could be:
1. Incomplete flap detachment leading to flap tear/ button hole or fragmentation of the flap.
2. Free epithelial flap.
3. Slight flap dislocation.
4. Epithelial defects.
5. Subepithelial foreign bodies.

The intraoperative flap tears and fragmentations do not affect the outcome of the surgery. These torn / fragmented epithelial flaps can be gently replaced back after the laser ablation and they heal well without any postoperative problems.

The factors that can be related to the flap complications are as follows.
1. Shallow cut of the micro-trephine.
2. Too small cut-ring.
3. Improper concentration and/or less application time.
4. Drying up of the epithelial flap.
5. Excessive irrigation of the flap.
6. Early removal of the therapeutic contact lens.

The epithelial flap of LASEK is frailer than the LASIK flap. It demands handling with utmost care and gentleness. If the flap is not easily separating, use of any force is to be avoided. Instead additional application of the alcohol solution should be utilized.

Epithelial Healing

1. No abnormality related to the epithelial healing has been reported.
2. The epithelial flap heals well within 4 days in most of the eyes and in maximum 6 days in all eyes.
3. If the epithelium shows some staining with fluorescein on the fourth day, when contact lens is removed, it is re-applied for another 1-2 more days. The frequency of teardrops instillation is increased.
4. About 2.2% of the eyes may show some epithelial defects, which heal well by the sixth day.
5. No late epithelial problems like epithelial instability as recurrent erosions or dry-eye has been reported by any study.
6. Minor *tear-film* changes may occur in about 33% eye as reported by Lee Shahinian. These patients did not have any major symptoms or problems with vision.

Postoperative Pain

1. No significant pain has been reported after LASEK. The pain score has been found to be low. Only 16% of the eyes had postoperative pain, 33.3% only slight discomfort and 50% had no pain in a case study by Kornilosky I M.
2. Most patients describe a discomfort or mild foreign body sensation during the first few postoperative days. These symptoms are relieved with frequent use of artificial teardrops.

Postoperative Haze

1. Postoperative corneal haze is minimal and it does not affect the visual acuity at any time.
2. The eyes with high refractive correction develop more corneal haze but it never exceeds a score of +1.0 and does not last longer than 3 months.
3. No late onset corneal haze has been reported even in cases of higher corrections, unlike PRK.

Contact lens Related Problems

1. Therapeutic contact lenses are used to protect the epithelial flap during the first few postoperative days.
2. Loss of the therapeutic contact lens may occur (about 2.5% cases).
3. Intolerance to contact lens has been reported in about 10% of eyes.
4. The cases of contact lens intolerance are treated with pressure patching and frequent use of lubricating agents. They respond well with this regime.

Corticosteroid Induced Glaucoma

One case of topical steroid induced glaucoma has been reported by Lee J B et al. This case responded after withdrawal of the topical steroid and use of beta-blocker.

Corneal Infection

There is no report of any postoperative infection after the LASEK procedure.

Refractive Stability

The postoperative refraction remains stable in all patients. No instability of refraction or regression has been reported by any of the clinical studies after a follow up of 6–12 months.

Retreatment rate

1. No retreatment was required in cases of low to moderate myopia.
2. The retreatment rate is about 5.5% in higher myopia (up to -12.4 D) with astigmatism.
3. Retreatment is done after about 4 months in case the patient is willing. The method of re-LASEK is similar to the initial procedure.

Viability of Epithelial Cells

Alcohol may damage the epithelial cells. Dreiss and co-workers in an experimental model using human cadaver eyes have examined this issue. They did not find any significant damage to the epithelial cells after exposure to 20% alcohol for 20–30 seconds. Majority of the cells, the basal cells in particular, were viable as confirmed by trypan blue staining. Alcohol exposure for 60 seconds resulted in most cells taking the stain, meaning that the cells were not viable.

Suggested readings

1. Massimo Camellin: M Cimberle, " LASEK May Offer the Advantage of Both LASIK and PRK," Ocular Surgery News, March 1999, p. 28.
2. Massimo Camellin: M Cimberle, " LASEK Has More Than 1 Year of Successful Experience," Ocular Surgery News, July 15, 2000, p. 14-17.
3. McCarty CA, Garrett SK, Alfred G: Assessment of subjective pain following photorefractive keratectomy. Melbourne Excimer Laser Group. J Ref Surg 1996; 12: 365-369.
4. Carones F, Fiore T, Brancato R: Mechanical vs. alcohol epithelial removal during photorefractive keratectomy. J Ref Surg 1998; 15: 556-562.
5. Shah S, Doyle SJ, Chatterjee A et al : Comparison of 18% ethanol and mechanical debridement for epithelial removal before PRK. J Ref Surg 1998; 14 (Suppl): S212-S214.
6. Agrawal VB, Haunch OE, Bassage S, Aquavella JV: Alcohol vs. mechanical epithelial debridement: effect on underlying cornea before excimer laser surgery. J Cat Ref Surg 1997; 23: 1153-1159.
7. Zhao J, Nagasaki T, Maurice DM: Role of tears in keratocyte loss after epithelial removal in mouse cornea. Invest Ophthalmol Vis Sci 2001; 42: 1743-1749.
8. Lin RT, Maloney RK: Flap complications associated with lamellar refractive surgery. Am J Ophthalmol 1999; 127: 129-136.
9. Ambrosio R Jr, Wilson SE: Complications of laser in situ keratomileusis: etiology, prevention and treatment. J Ref Surg 2001; 17: 350-379.
10. Holland SP, Srivannaboon S, Reinstein DZ: Avoiding serious corneal complications of laser assisted in situ keratomileusis and photorefractive keratectomy. Ophthalmology 2000; 107: 640-652.
11. Wong VW, Zhu CC, Rao SK, Lam DSC: Corneal perforation during laser in situ keratomileusis. (Letter). J Cat Ref Surg 2000; 26: 1103-1104.
12. Durairaj BD, Balentine J, Kouyoumdjian G et al: The predictability of corneal flap thickness and tissue laser ablation in laser in situ keratomileusis. Ophthalmology 2000; 107: 2140-2143.
13. Smith RJ, Maloney RK: Diffuse lamellar keratitis; a new syndrome in lamellar refractive surgery. Ophthalmology 1998; 105: 1721-1726.
14. Lee AG, Kohnen T, Ebner R et al: Optic neuropathy associated with laser in situ keratomileusis. J Cat Ref Surg 2000; 26: 1581-1584.
15. Wilson SE, Mohan RR, Hong J-W et al: Wound healing response after laser in situ keratomileusis and photorefractive keratectomy: elusive control of biological variability and effect on custom laser vision correction. Arc Ophthalmol 2001; 119: 889-896.
16. Dohlman CH, Gasset AR, Rose J: The effect of the absence of corneal epithelium or endothelium on the stromal keratocytes. Invest Ophthalmol Vis Sci 1968; 7: 520-534.
17. Moller-Pedersen T, Cavanagh HD, Petroll WM, Jester JV: Stromal wound healing explains refractive instability and haze development aster photorefractive keratectomy; a one year confocal microscopical study. Ophthalmology 2000; 107: 1235-1245.
18. Dastjerdi MH, Soong HK: LASEK (laser subepithelial keratomileusis). Curr Opin Ophthalmol 2002 Aug; 13(4): 261-263.

19. Anderson N, Beran R, Schneider T: Epi-LASEK for the correction of myopia and myopic astigmatism. : J Cataract Refract Surg 2002 Aug; 28(8): 1343.
20. Shahinian L: Laser-assisted subepithelial keratectomy for low to high myopia and astigmatism. J Cataract Refract Surg 2002 Aug; 28(8): 1334-1342.
21. Litwak S, Zadok D, Garcia-de Quevedo V, Robledo N, Chayet A: Laser-assisted subepithelial keratectomy versus photorefractive keratectomy for the correction of myopia. A prospective comparative study. J Cataract Refract Surg 2002 Aug; 28(8): 1330
22. Lee JB, Choe CM, Seong GJ, Gong HY, Kim EK: Laser Subepithelial Keratomileusis for Low to Moderate Myopia. 6-Month Follow-up. Jpn J Ophthalmol 2002 May-Jun; 46(3): 299-304.
23. Rouweyha RM, Chuang AZ, Mitra S, Phillips CB, Yee RW: Laser epithelial keratomileusis for myopia with the autonomous laser. J Refract Surg 2002 May-Jun; 18(3): 217-24.
24. Vinciguerra P, Torres I, Camesasca FI: Applications of confocal microscopy in refractive surgery. J Refract Surg 2002 May-Jun; 18 (3 Suppl): S378-81.
25. Vinciguerra P, Camesasca FI: Butterfly laser epithelial keratomileusis for myopia. J Refract Surg 2002 May-Jun; 18(3 Suppl): S371-3.
26. Zhou X, Wu L, Dai J, Zhu R: The epithelial-flap abnormality of laser epithelial keratomileusis. Chung Hua Yen Ko Tsa Chih 2002 Feb; 38(2): 69-71.
27. Lohmann CP, Winkler Von Mohrenfels C, Gabler B, Hermann W, Muller M: Excimer laser subepithelial ablation (ELSA) or laser epithelial keratomileusis (LASEK) - a new keratorefractive procedure for myopia. Surgical technique and first clinical results on 24 eyes and 3 months follow-up. Klin Monatsbl Augenheilkd 2002 Jan-Feb; 219(1-2): 26-32.
28. Azar DT, Ang RT, Lee JB, Kato T, Chen CC, Jain S, Gabison E, Abad JC: Laser subepithelial keratomileusis: electron microscopy and visual outcomes of flap photorefractive keratectomy. Curr Opin Ophthalmol 2001 Aug; 12(4): 323-8.
29. Kornilovsky IM: Clinical results after subepithelial photorefractive keratectomy (LASEK). J Refract Surg 2001 Mar-Apr; 17(2 Suppl): S222-3.
30. Scerrati E: Laser in situ keratomileusis vs. laser epithelial keratomileusis (LASIK vs. LASEK). J Refract Surg 2001 Mar-Apr; 17(2 Suppl): S219-21.
31. Lee JB, Seong GJ, Lee JH, Seo KY, Lee YG, Kim EK: Comparison of laser epithelial keratomileusis and photorefractive keratectomy for low to moderate myopia. J Cataract Refract Surg 2001 Apr; 17(4): 565-70.
32. Dreiss AK, Winkler Von Mohrenfels C, Gabler B, Kohnen T, Marshall J, Lohmann CP: Laser epithelial keratomileusis (LASEK): histological investigation for vitality of corneal epithelial cells after alcohol exposure. Klin Monatsbl Augenheilkd 2002 May; 219(5): 365-9.
33. Rokita-Wala I, Gierek-Ciaciura S, Mrukwa-Kominek E, Obidzinski M: Vital changes in corneal structure after LASEK during the early postoperative period. Klin Oczna 2002; 104(1): 13-8.

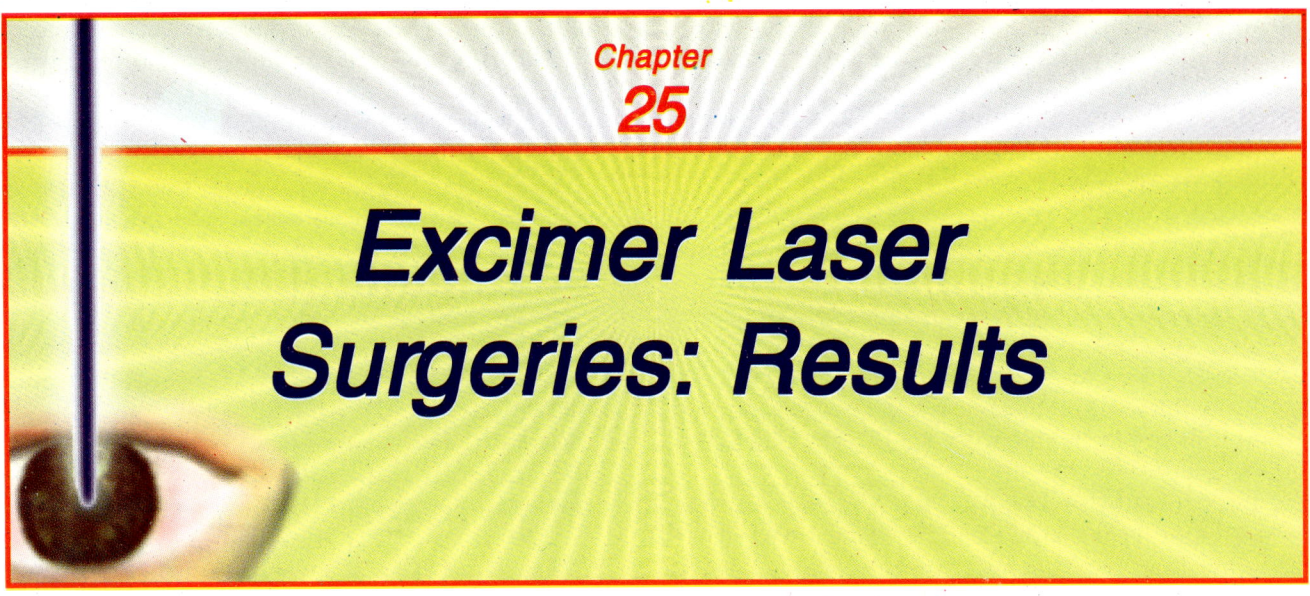

Chapter 25: Excimer Laser Surgeries: Results

EXCIMER LASER CORNEAL SURGERIES: RESULTS

The excimer laser corneal surgeries (refractive and phototherapeutic) have come as a great technological advancement during the last two decades. They have proved to be superior in terms of efficacy, predictability and safety in comparison to the other conventional surgeries in their respective fields. Like any other procedure, the excimer laser surgeries also have taken some time to come out from the gestation period, evolve, mature and get established. The development and refinement is still continuing due to a natural quest for achieving the best possible results. As a result of this ongoing development, we have witnessed in recent times newer technologies like *customized-LASIK* and *LASEK* to attain the maximum possible efficacy with least complications.

RESULTS OF PTK

Excimer laser phototherapeutic keratectomy offers highly significant advantages over other available modalities for treating superficial corneal disorders. The available clinical work from different parts of the world has shown PTK to be effective and safe method for treating the superficial corneal disorders as well for improving vision. The advantages and results of PTK have been discussed in Chapters 11 and 17.

A prospective study was conducted at Dr. Rajendra Prasad Center for Ophthalmic Science, AIIMS, New Delhi, by the author on 48 eyes with different corneal disorders to evaluate the efficacy and safety of excimer laser PTK for treating superficial corneal disorders. It was the first prospective study on PTK in India. Seventy-three percent eyes' had improvement in UCVA by 2 or more lines and in 85% eyes BCVA improved by 2 or more lines. There was a significant improvement in the corneal clarity, meaning thereby an anatomical success in treating the corneal pathology affecting vision. Corneal haze was not significant after the third month. The refraction stabilized after the third month. The induced refractive changes were significantly less in comparison to that reported by previous studies (Chapter 17).

The *major disadvantage of PTK* has been found to be the *induced refractive change, particularly hyperopic shift*. The improvements in the technology of plano-ablation such as *tapering of the ablation edge* and use of a *masking agent* as well as *pharmacological modulation* have drastically reduced this side effect. These aspects are discussed in Chapter 14 on 'treatment strategies' and also in the following chapter on PTK complications. In our study the refractive change was not problematic for the patient. It could be managed with spectacle correction. The mean change in refraction was 1.30 ± 1.44 D of spherical equivalent at the sixth postoperative month.

RESULTS OF REFRACTIVE PROCEDURES

The results of various excimer laser refractive surgeries were not satisfying during the earlier period, in so far as being below their expectations. Nevertheless, they were superior to other refractive procedures available during those days with respect to efficacy and predictability of refractive outcome, the range of correction, stability and safety. As said in the beginning of this section, *the predictability and stability of refractive results following the excimer laser refractive procedures have shown significant improvement with the development of newer techniques and algorithms.* The advancement in the laser delivery systems from wide beam to the scanning laser with advanced nomograms, the active eye-tracker and incorporation of the topography and wavefront deformation data into the treatment nomograms are other major advancements that have greatly improved the results.

PRK RESULTS

Photorefractive keratectomy (PRK) offered many advantages over radial keratotomy for the correction of myopia. It has been widely used as a refractive surgical procedure for low to extreme degrees of myopia. In addition to myopia, hypermetropia and astigmatism are also being treated with this procedure. Over one million eyes have been treated with PRK all over the world.

The refractive results of PRK depend upon several factors. These factors affecting the outcome in different clinical studies are given below.

1. The type of refractive error: myopia, hypermetropia or astigmatism
2. The degree of myopia
3. The laser system used: wide beam or scanning laser
4. The ablation zone diameter
5. The ablation algorithm: single zone, multizone or multipass multizone
6. The method of eye fixation
7. Use of active eye-tracker
8. The method of centration
9. The method of removal of ablation byproducts
10. The experience of the surgeon
11. Postoperative care

Because of so many variables, the results of different studies are difficult to compare. Therefore, one finds a wide variation in the reported visual and refractive outcomes. The number of eyes having uncorrected visual acuity of 20/40 (6/12) after PRK ranges from 27% to 98%. Similarly, the eyes within ±1.0 D refraction range from 34–100%. The eyes with loss of 2 or more lines of BCVA range from 0–22%. Results of PRK from different studies are summarized in Tables 25.1–25.4 for different refractive errors.

Initially the results of PRK were not so predictable and the effectivity was less than what can be achieved now. Moreover, the problem of glare, halos and ghost images frequently disturbed the patient and haunted the surgeon.

Review of various reports shows that the outcome is worse in the following situations.

1. *Higher attempted correction and greater ablation depth* are associated with significant haze, greater variability of outcome, poor effectivity, high incidence of regression and loss of BCVA. Therefore, the surgeons now limit the use of PRK to mild to moderate refractive errors and leave high and extreme myopia to the domain of LASIK and LASEK.
2. *Smaller diameter of the ablation zone* is associated with visual disturbances. Ablation zone diameters of 6.5 mm–7.0 mm have significantly reduced the incidence of halos and glare, etc.
3. The earlier *method of removal of ablation byproducts* (nitrogen gas blower) was associated with high incidence of irregular surface, irregular astigmatism and overcorrection due to tissue dehydration.
4. *Non-availability of a proper centration and fixation device* was associated with problems of decentration that could result in ghost images, halos, irregular astigmatism and decreased visual acuity. Use of an active eye-tracker has decreased the decentred ablation zone problem.
5. *Use of broad beam laser system* was associated with uneven ablation due to non-homogenous energy profile, higher incidence of central islands and limited ablation patterns.
6. *Use of scanning laser, laser beams with Gaussian energy distribution and tracker-assisted ablation* has significantly improved the results of PRK during the recent period. Exploitation of these advancements is particularly useful for treating different types of astigmatism. The computer-controlled algorithms are able to create complex

toric contours utilizing a small scanning-spot laser beam. A Gaussian energy profile of the laser beam ensures that the irregularities at the sites where the laser spots overlap are minimized and a smooth ablated surface is produced. Table 25.4 shows the improved results of uncorrected visual acuity with the scanning spot laser for treating hyperopia and astigmatism.

Table 25.1: Results of PRK for different degrees of myopia

Refractive Group	Investigator (year)	No. of Eyes	Follow-up months	Preoperative refraction (Diopters)	UCVA 20/40 or better (% Eyes)	Within ± 1.0 D (% Eyes)	Loss of 2 or more lines of BCVA (% Eyes)
MYOPIA Low	Seiler et al[1] (1993)	42	12	-1.25 to -3.0	97	100	0
	Amano et al[2] (1995)	11	24	-2.0 to -3.0	NR	100	0
Low to Moderate	Gartry et al[3] (1991)	176	8-18	-1.5 to -7.0	61%	50%	NR
	Levery[4] (1993)	99	12	-1.25 to -9.6	84%	93%	1%
	Salz et al[5] (1993)	71	12	-1.25 to -7.5	84	91	1.4
	FDA Study[6] Summit (1994)	576	12	-1.5 to -6.0	91	78	<1
	VISX (1994)	691	24	-1.0 to -6.0	85	79	1
	Epstein et al[7] (1994)	495	24	-1.25 to -7.5	91	87.5	0
Moderate	Talley et al[8] (1994)	85	12	-3.1 to -6.0	92	97	0
		27	12	-6.1 to -9.0	44	60	7.4
Moderate to High	Chan et al[9] (1995)	66	12	-6.2 to -11.9	75	34	0
	Siganos et al[10] (1996)	40	18	-7.0 to -13.5	NR	NR	15
	Hersh et al[11] (1998)	105	6	6.0 to -15.0	66.2	57.4	11.8
Moderate to Extreme	Goes[12] (1996)	68	12	-8.0 to -24.0	48	74	14
	Williams[13] (1996)	88	12	-6.0 to -20.0	NR	64	14

NR= Not reported

Table 25.2: Results of PRK for myopia and/or astigmatism

Refractive group	Investigator (year)	No. of eyes	Follow-up months	Preoperative cylinder (diopters)	UCVA 20/40 or better (% eyes)	Postoperative cylinder (diopter)	Loss of 2 or more lines of BCVA (% eyes)
Astigmatism	Kremer et al[14]* (1996)	28	12	-0.8 ± 0.22	89	-0.40 ± 0.33	NR
		44	12	-1.7 ± 0.42	82	-0.54 ± 0.48	NR
		20	12	-3.54 ± 0.64	90	-0.69 ± 0-.32	NR
	Brancato et al[15$] (1996)	21	6	-2.46	60	-1.56	0
	Dausch et al[16@] (1996)[16]	17	18	-2.33 ± 1.32	93	-0.44 ± 0.67	0
		11	18	- 4.75 ± 1.17	82	-0.89 ± 0.60	0
Compound Astigmatism	Stevens et al[17]* (2002)[17]	200	12	-0.5 to -5.0 Sph up to -3.5 Cylinder MSE reduced from -3.5 D to 0.0 ± 0.67 D	97	NR	0.5%
	Shah et al[18]* (2002)	6097	12	-0.75 to -13.0 Sph -0.5 to - 6.0 Cylinder	91.2	87.9 depending on degree of astigmatism	1.1 to 5.8
	Beauduin et al[19]# (2002)	93	24	-1.5 to -8.0 Sph - 0.75 to -3.0 Cylinder	64% eyes 20/20 UCVA and 92.3% ± 0.5 D cylinder within ± 0.5 D in 86.4 % eyes		

*Whole field method; $= Use of ablatable mask;   @=Use of scanning laser system;   MSE=Mean spherical equivalent; NR= Not reported; Sph= spherical;   *Use of scanning laser system;   # Use of *Gaussian energy distribution* broad beam laser

Table 25.3: Results of PRK for hyperopia with wide beam laser

Technique used: 4 mm Optical Zone, 7 mm Ablation Zone

Investigator (year)	No. of eyes	Follow-up months	Preoperative refraction (diopters)	Mean preoperative UCVA	Mean postoperative UCVA	Mean postoperative refraction	Loss of 2 or more lines of BCVA (% Eyes)
Dausch et al[20] (1995)	15	12	+2.00 to +7.50	20/60	20/30	+0.3 D	6.6
	8		Aphakia (Mean +13.10)	20/35	20/57	+1.5 D	24.5

Technique used: 6 mm Optical Zone, 9 mm Ablation Zone

Investigator (year)	No. of eyes	Follow-up months	Preoperative refraction (diopters)	UCVA 20/40 or better (% Eyes)	Within ± 1.0 D (% Eyes)	Mean postoperative refraction	Loss of 2 or more lines of BCVA (% eyes)
Dausch et al[21] (1997)	68	12	+2.0 to +8.5	97	81	+1.08 D	2
Jackson[22] (1997)	25	6	up to +4.0	88	NR	+0.27 D	NR

Table 25.4: Results of PRK for hyperopia and astigmatism with scanning beam laser

Investigator (year)	No. of eyes	Follow-up months	Preoperative refraction (diopters)	UCVA 20/40 or better (% Eyes)	UCVA 20/20 or better (% eyes)	Within ±1.0 D (% eyes)	Within ±0.5 D (% eyes)	Loss of 2 or more lines of BCVA (% eyes)
Stevens et al[23] (2002)	32	12	0.0 to +1.75 Sph up to -2.5 Cylinder	93	NR	NR	65	0
Nagy et al[24]* (2002)	62	12	up to +3.0 Sph < +1.0 Cylinder	NR	88.7	NR	82.2	1.6
	56	12	> +3.0 Sph < +1.0 Cylinder	NR	78.6	NR	76.8	5.4
	44	12	up to +3.0 Sph ≥ +1.0 Cylinder	NR	77.2	NR	68.1	9.1
	38	12	> +3.0 Sph ≥ +1.0 Cylinder	NR	60.5	NR	42.0	15.8

*Use of *Gaussian* flying spot scanning laser

RESULTS OF LASIK

As mentioned in the previous section, the results of PRK were poor for high refractive errors, particularly for high and extreme myopes. LASIK had been initially used to treat this group of patients to avoid the undesired complications associated with deeper surface-based ablation. *It is now the most commonly performed refractive surgery for an effective treatment of patients with low, moderate and high myopia with or without astigmatism, as well as hyperopia with or without astigmatism.*

PRK vs. LASIK

In general, the overall results of LASIK are superior to that of PRK in terms of efficacy, postoperative uncorrected visual acuity and stability of refraction. Table 25.5 summarizes the one-year results of a large number of studies utilizing these two procedures.

When comparing LASIK with PRK, several variables like safety/complications rate, early results, long-term stability and efficacy in different degrees of refractive errors are to be considered.

The period during which a particular study was conducted is also of importance. During the period when LASIK was being developed, the long-term results after LASIK were not as good as today (Tables 25.7 and 27.8). The intraoperative complication rate related to the microkeratome and the flap was also significantly more during that learning curve of the surgeons (see Table 26.2 under flap complications).

The immediate and early postoperative results of LASIK are better when compared with PRK. It provides quick visual recovery, significantly better-uncorrected visual acuity during the early postoperative period, causes insignificant postoperative pain and offers the advantage of simultaneous correction of both eyes.

The *incidence of postoperative haze, regression and central steep islands is found to be much less* with LASIK[70-73]. The *predictability and stability of refractive outcome is also better* with LASIK[70]. Refraction stabilizes early, within first three 3 months, when compared to PRK, where it takes 6 or more months particularly for higher degree of refractive errors.

Table 25.5: One-year results of PRK and LASIK

Procedure	UCVA 20/20 or better (% eyes)	UCVA 20/40 or better (% eyes)	Predictability within one diopter (% eyes)	Patient satisfaction (% eyes)
PRK	53 to 86	94.4 to 98.1	87 to 94.4	52
LASIK	67 to 90	97 to 100	90 to 98.7	90

Table 25.6: PRK vs. LASIK

Investigator (year)	Procedure	No. of eyes	Preoperative refraction (diopters)	Follow-up	Mean UCVA	UCVA ≥ 20/20 (% eyes)	UCVA ≥ 20/40 (% eyes)	Mean Refraction (diopters)	Within ±0.5 D (% eyes)	Within ±1.0 D (% Eyes)	Loss of ≥ 2 lines of BCVA (% Eyes)
MYOPIA and ASTIGMATISM											
Durrie et al[43] (1998)	PRK	105	Mean -9.23	1 day		0	4.5	NR	NR		
				6 month		19.1	66.2			57.4	11.8
	LASIK	115	Mean -9.3	1 day		10	68.6	NR	NR		
				6 month		26.2	55.7			40.7	3.2
Walker et al[44] (2001)	PRK	77	-2.8 ± -0.20	1 week	20/25			+ 0.23 ± 0.12			
				1 month	20/20			+ 0.19 ± 0.10			
				6 months	20/20			+ 0.02 ± 0.08			
	LASIK	76	-2.5 ± -0.22	1 week	20/20			- 0.02 ± 0.07			
				1 month	20/20			- 0.02 ± 0.19			
				6 months	20/20			0.00 ± 0.08			
Lorencova et al[45] (2001)	PRK	56	-6.0 to -9.0 -1.23±1.1 Cyli	6 month 1 year	0.86±0.35 0.81± o.31			-0.23± 1.24 -0.44± 1.26			
	LASIK	90	-6.0 to -9.0 -1.23±1.1 Cyli	6 month 1 year	0.65±0.25 0.75±0.25			-0.29± 1.19 -0.14± 0.86			
Tole et al (2001)	PRK	206	-0.5 to -6.0	6 months		65				82	1.0
	LASIK	125	-0.5 to -6.0	6 months		80				78	1.4
HYPERMETROPIA											
el-Agha et al[46] (2000)	PRK	22	+2.25 ± -1.16	1 month	-0.82 ± 0.89						
				6 month	-0.16 ± 0.37						
				1 year	-0.20 ± 0.35	47.1	100		83.3		9.0
	LASIK	26	+1.81± -0.92	1 month	+0.19 ± 0.47						
				6 month	-0.29 ± 0.51						
				1 year	-0.37 ± 0.44	54.5	100		54.5		7.6

Many studies have evaluated the results of PRK and LASIK. These studies have found that the visual and refractive outcome of the two procedures *are similar and comparable in terms of efficacy and safety for low to moderate degree of refractive errors* (myopia and hyperopia with or without astigmatism) *after about 3–6 months of surgery* (Table 25.6).

However long-term visual and refractive results of LASIK are significantly better in high-myopia[70]. Refractive stability is greater in flap-based procedures than in PRK-based procedures and yields a marked reduction in the astigmatic cylinder in patients having A-LASIK (astigmatic-LASIK)[47]. The same facts are evident when PRK results for high-intended corrections (Tables 25.1 to 25.4) are compared with those of LASIK (Tables 25.7 and 25.8). The difference is mainly due to an aggressive healing response after surface based ablation, which results in significant subepithelial haze and epithelial hyperplasia. The consequences of this adverse healing are regression and even scarring in worst situations, jeopardizing the results of PRK for higher intended corrections.

Limitations for Corrective Range of LASIK

Although LASIK had become widely popular for treating a wide range of myopic errors due to more experience and confidence gained by the surgeons, some limitations have been recognized after longer follow-ups have become possible. These limitations are due to the risk of *corneal ectasia* and *endothelial damage* as a result of higher attempted correction. Cases of corneal ectasia have been reported with corrections over -12.0 D or residual bed thickness of < 325 μ.

Moreover the recent series by Yang et al, Chitkara et al, Knorz et al and other scientists have found best results in low, moderate and high myopia not exceeding –12.0 D. therefore the surgeons now limit the myopic correction to –12.0 D. Interestingly, *Pallikaris et al found that no case of corneal ectasia developed in 2873 eyes if the attempted correction was < -8.0 D (Chapter 6).*

Astigmatic Correction With LASIK

As mentioned in the previous section, improvements in the algorithms using the flying-spot scanning laser have

Table 25.7: Results of LASIK for myopia and astigmatism

Investigator (year)	No. of eyes	Follow-up months	Preoperative refraction (diopters)	UCVA 20/40 or better (% eyes)	UCVA 20/20 or better (% eyes)	Within ±1.0 D (% eyes)	Within ±0.5 D (% eyes)	Loss of 2 or more lines of BCVA (% eyes)
Low to extreme myopia								
Salah et al[25] (1996)	88	3-8	-2.0 to -20.0	71	NR	73	NR	3.6
	40	3-8	-2.0 to -6.0	NR	NR	93	NR	NR
	29	3-8	-6.1 to -12.0	NR	NR	65	NR	NR
	19	3-8	-12.1 to -20.0	NR	NR	43	NR	NR
Gimbel et al[26] (1996)	5	1	< -10.0	100	NR	NR	NR	0
	32	1	-10.0 to -15.0	50	NR	NR	NR	15
	11	1	-15.0 to -20.0	36	NR	NR	NR	27
	5	1	> -20.0	0	NR	NR	NR	40
Gimbel et al[27] (1998)	1000	6	-1.0 to -23.0	NR	NR	87.8	61.5	1.6
Perez-Santonja[28] (1997)	143	6	-8.0 to -20.0	46	NR	60	NR	1.4
Lyle et al[29] (2001)	332	12	-10.0 to -18.0	89.5	45.8	84	NR	1.8
	208	12	-10.0 to -11.9	NR	52	86	NR	NR
	94	12	-12.0 to -14.0	NR	38	86	NR	NR
	30	12	-14.1 to -18.0	NR	23	70	NR	NR
Yang et al[30] (2002)	1285	24	-1.5 to -6.0	99.6	90.4	93.4	84.4	NR
		24	-6.12 to -12.0	93.8	68.6	86.7	79.4	NR
		24	-12.12 to -25.0	62.6	27.2	65.5	42.1	NR
Myopia with astigmatism								
Lindstrom et al[31] (1997)	10	11	-0.75 to -6.0 Sph < 1.0 Cylinder	90	NR	89	NR	NR
	109	1	-6.12 to -20.0 Sph up to +4.0 Cylinder	71	NR	63	NR	NR
Salchow et al[32] (1998)	66	6	-1.5 to -16.0 Sph 0.0 to -3.0 Astig	82.5	NR	81	NR	9.5
				96.8 within ± 1.0 D of cylinder				
Knorz et al[33] (1998)			**Astigmatism < 1.0 D**					
	8	12	-5.0 to -9.9 Sph	87.5	NR	100	NR	0
	10	12	-10.0 to -14.9 Sph	77.8	NR	60	NR	10
	19	12	-15.0 to -29.0 Sph	33.3	NR	38.9	NR	5.6
			Astigmatism 1.0 to 4.5 D					
	12	12	-5.0 to -9.9 Sph	70	NR	75	NR	0
	24	12	-10.0 to -14.9 Sph	86.4	NR	78.3	NR	4.3
	20	12	-15.0 to -29.0 Sph	40	NR	21.4	NR	7.1
Knorz et al[34]* (2000)			**Astigmatism 0.0 to -4.0 Cylinder**					
	51	3	-1.0 to -6.0 Sph	100	82.4	NR	96.1	3.9
	40	3	-6.1.0 to -12.0 Sph	95	62.5	NR	75	5
Balazsi et al[35] (2001)	1236	6	-0.5 to -7.0 Sph < 2.5 Cylinder	94.6	81.9	91.2	73	0
						86.8	73	0
Chitkara et al[42]$ (2002)	129	12	up to -13.0 Sph	92.8	71.4	89.9	79.1	1.6

*TopoLink LASIK (topography linked laser in-situ keratomileusis); $ = T-LASIK (tracker assisted LASIK)

Table 25.8: Results of LASIK for hyperopia and astigmatism

Investigator (year)	No. of eyes	Follow-up months	Preoperative refraction (diopters)	UCVA 20/40 or better (% eyes)	UCVA 20/20 or better (% eyes)	Within ±1.0 D (% eyes)	Within ±0.5 D (% eyes)	Loss of 2 or more lines of BCVA (% eyes)
Argento et al[36] (1998)	679	6	< +2.0	94.1	NR	100	NR	NR
			+2.0 to +3.0	100	NR	95.3	NR	NR
			> +3.0	87.8	NR	71.4	NR	NR
Ditzen et al[37] (1998)	43	12	+1.0 to +4.0	86.2	NR	NR	NR	NR
			+4.25 to +8.0	74.6	NR	NR	NR	NR
Goker et al[38] (1998)	54	19	+4.25 to +8.0	66.6	NR	75.9	NR	NR
Rashad et al[39] (2001)	85	12	+1.25 to +5.0	92.9	24.7	89.4	61.2	1.2
			< +3.0 Cylinder	Astigmatism reduced to mean of 0.36± 0.57 D				
Tabbra et al[40] (2001)	80	6	+0.5 to +11.5	97.5	44	84	58	NR
Salz et al[41]* (2002)	360	12	Refractive error of up to +6.0 D and astigmatism up to -6.0 D divided into three groups					
	117	12	Simple Hyperopia	93.9	NR	91.4	74	3.4
	74	12	Hyperopic Astigmatism	93.8	NR	89.2	74	3.4
	38	12	Mixed Astigmatism	94.4	NR	94.7	73.7	0

*Technique used: active eye-tracker with the LADAR Vision excimer laser system

been successful in creating complex toric ablation profiles. This has facilitated treatment of simple, compound as well as mixed astigmatism (Tables 25.7 and 25.8). Predictability of refraction within ±1.0 D has been achieved in 94–96.8% of eyes when treating up to 4.0 D of cylindrical error. Ruiz et al treated astigmatism up to 8.0 D. They were able to reduce the astigmatism to 0.35–1.31 D at one year of follow up with uncorrected visual acuity 20/40 in 94% of eyes. Salchow et al reported postoperative refraction within ±1.0 D in 96.8% eyes and Knorz et al in 96.1% eyes while treating myopia with astigmatism up to –3.0 D and –4.0 D respectively. Salz et al obtained refraction within ±1.0 D of emmetropia in 89.1% eyes with hypermetropic astigmatism and 94.7% eyes with mixed astigmatism in case of hypermetropic treatment ranging up to +6.0 D.

Hypermetropic Correction With LASIK

The result of hypermetropic LASIK had been variable during the initial period. The problems with hypermetropic LASIK had been mainly with creation of a larger flap (> 9.5 mm) to facilitate ablation of the peripheral cornea, maintaining an accurate centration during this ablation and refinement of the treatment algorithms for hypermetropic correction. The latter is one of the factors that can improve the predictability of hypermetropic LASIK. The results for treatment of low and moderate degree of hypermetropia had been satisfactory but correction of high hypermetropic errors had been associated with problems of high incidence of regression and variable corneal scarring. Tabbra et al treated 80 eyes with +0.5 to +11.5 D preoperative error. They reported uncorrected visual acuity 20/40 or better in 97.5% eyes and 20/20 0r better in 44% eyes. The postoperative refraction was within ±1.0 D in 84% and within ±0.5 D in 58% eyes. The loss of best-corrected visual acuity was not reported in this study.

RESULTS OF CUSTOMIZED ABLATION AND LASEK

Photorefractive surgeries using wavefront-guided ablation (customized-LASIK and customized-PRK) and LASEK are relatively newer procedures of refractive correction. At present only few clinical reports are available on these procedures. Large prospective studies with long-term follow up are required to make any comment on the performance of these technologies. However the initial visual and refractive results of these surgeries are promising.

Results of Customized-LASIK and Customized-PRK

Conventional LASIK and PRK procedures are found to increase the higher-order aberrations of the eye leading to loss of best-corrected, low contrast and glare visual acuity[48-51]. PRK results in an increase in the higher-order aberrations by a factor of 8-17.65 times of the preoperative aberrations.

Martinez et al[48] found that the higher-order aberrations showed a 9-fold increase in the eyes before operation but a 100-fold increase occurred one month after PRK procedure when the pupil was dilated from 3 mm to 7 mm. Seiler et al reported an increase of 17.65 times in these aberrations 3 months after PRK.

Oshika et al[52] reported 4.4± 3.3 fold increase for coma-like and 9.4± 5.2 fold increase for spherical-like aberration after LASIK surgery correcting 100 eyes with −2.0 to −13.0 D of myopic error. *This increase in induced aberrations was significantly higher in eyes that lost 2 or more lines of best-corrected visual acuity.*

Panagopoulou et al[58] found an increase in higher-order aberrations only 1.3 times after C-PRK and 1.8 times after C-LASIK. *The difference was significant when compared to the preoperative as well postoperative aberrations using the conventional PRK and LASIK procedures in the same study design.* Vongthongsri et al[59] conducted a prospective randomized study to compare the visual outcome of conventional LASIK and wavefront-guided LASIK in 22 eyes of 11 patients. One eye of the patient received wavefront-guided customized ablation and the other conventional LASIK ablation. They did not find any statistically different reduction of higher-order aberration in two eyes at 1 month of follow up.

Mrochen et al also had commented that the reduction of higher-order aberrations is though reduced, yet is not optimal with the present available algorithms.

Customized ablation based on wavefront technology has been found to provide better uncorrected and best-corrected visual acuity. It is also associated with less degradation of low contrast and glare visual acuity. It also has been able to produce superior visual acuity ("supervision")[57]. The results of wavefront-guided LASIK and PRK are shown in Table 25.9.

Table 25.9: Results of Wavefront-guided LASIK and PRK

Investigator (year)	No. of eyes	Follow-up months	Preoperative refraction (diopters)	BCVA 20/20 (% eyes)	BCVA 20/10 (% Eyes)	UCVA 20/10 or better (% eyes)	UCVA 20/20 or better (% eyes)	Within ±1.0 D (% eyes)	Within ±0.5 D (% eyes)	Postoperative aberrations	Loss of ≥ 2 lines of BCVA
Wavefront-guided LASIK											
Mrochen et al[54] (2000)	3	1	NR	100	66.3	100	NR	NR	NR	27% decrease	NR
Mrochen et al[55] (2001)	35	3	-4.8 ± 2.3 Sph -1.1± 0.9 Cylinder	16	66.3	93.5	93.5	68		1.44±0.74	0
Wavefront-guided PRK											
Nagy et al[60] (2002)	150	6	-4.02 ± 1.04 SE	Mean BCVA > 20/16		Mean BCVA > 20/20		100	98	1.4 times	0
Nagy et al[61] (2002)											
C-PRK	40	6	+2.9 ± 0.80	Mean BCVA > 20/20		Mean UCVA 20/20		NR	85	Increased	12.5
Conven PRK	40	6	+2.9 ± 0.80	Mean BCVA 20/20		Mean UCVA 20/25		NR	67.5		10

Sph = sphere; SE= spherical equivalent; C-PRK= customized PRK; Conven PRK

Results of LASEK

Laser subepithelial keratomileusis (LASEK) is again a recent photorefractive surgical technique that is still evolving. It promises to combine the advantages of LASIK (less postoperative pain, faster visual recovery, less corneal haze, early stability of refraction and simultaneous treatment of both eyes) with PRK (avoidance of microkeratome, flap and interface related complications).

Many studies have documented the benefits of LASEK for the treatment of low to high myopia with or without astigmatism. The results of LASEK have been promising in terms of visual rehabilitation, predictability and stability of refractive correction as well as regarding safety of the procedure. *However the long-term effects of alcohol, which is used for creating the epithelial flap, are a matter of speculation due to limited period of available follow up of the cases.* The results of LASEK are summarized in Table 25.10.

LASEK vs. PRK

Two studies have compared early visual rehabilitation, postoperative pain, epithelial healing time and refractive outcome of LASEK with conventional PRK for treating myopia. In these prospective studies one eye was treated with LASEK and the contralatreral eye with PRK for an equivalent degree of refractive error.

Lee et al[67] reported significantly less postoperative pain and corneal haze in the LASEK treated eyes. No significant difference was found in epithelial healing time, UCVA and refractive results between the two eyes treated with the two procedures. However 63% of the patients showed preference for LASEK.

Litwak et al[68], on the contrary found less discomfort and better visual acuity during the early postoperative period in patients treated with PRK. The visual and refractive results in 25 patients were similar at one month of follow up.

LASEK vs. LASIK

In another study Scerrati and co-authors[69] found better results in terms of BCVA, corneal topography, contrast sensitivity and refractive outcome after LASEK than LASIK in 15 patients after 6 months.

Table 25.10: Results of LASEK*

Investigator (Year)	No. of Eyes	Preoperative Refraction (Diopters)	Follow-up	UCVA 20/20 (% Eyes)	UCVA 20/30 (% Eyes)	UCVA 20/40 or better (% Eyes)	Within ±1.0 D (% Eyes)	Within ±0.5 D (% Eyes)	Postop Pain (% Eyes)	Visually Significant Haze	Loss of ≥ 2 lines of BCVA
Anderson et al[62] (2002)	343	-1.0 to -14.0 up to 4.75 Cylinder	1 week	50	70	90	NR	NR	13 (mild)	–	–
			1 month	70	92	97	92	73	–	Nil	–
			3 months	80	93	95	92	78	–	Nil	–
			6 months	84	95	98	94	85	–	Nil	0
Shahinian[63] (2002)	146	-1.25 to -14.38 (0 to 4.5 Cylinder)	1 week	NR	NR	78		NR	mild	–	0
			3 months	50	NR	95		100		Nil	0.7
			6 months	57	NR	96		100	–	Nil	0
			12 months	56	NR	96		100		Nil	0
Lee et al[64] (2002)	84	-3.25 to -7.0	1 week	NR	78.6	NR					
			6 month	NR	96.4	NR	94	50	mild	Nil	
Rouweyha et al[65] (2002)	56	-1.5 to -14.75	1 day	NR	NR	45					
			1 week	NR	NR	83					
			2 weeks	NR	N	85					
			1 month	NR	NR	89					
			6 months	73	NR	97	NR	68		7	0

* The time taken for epithelial healing varied between 3-6 days

Suggested readings

1. Seiler T, Wollensak J: Results of a prospective evaluation of photorefractive keratectomy at one year after surgery. Ger J Ophthalmol 1993; 2: 135-142.
2. Amano S, Shimizu K: Excimer laser photorefractive keratectomy for myopia: two year follow up. J Ref Surg 1995; 11(Suppl): S253-S260.
3. Gartry DS, Kerr Muir MG, Marshall J: PRK with an argon fluoride excimer laser: a clinical study. Ref Corn Surg 1991; 7(6): 420435.
4. Levery FL: Photorefractive keratectomy in 472 eyes. J Ref Surg 1993; 9: 98-100.
5. Salz JI, Maguen E, Nesburn AB et al: A two-year experience with excimer laser PRK for myopia. Ophthalmology 1993; 100: 873-882.
6. Seiler T, McDonnell PJ: Excimer laser photorefractive keratectomy. Survey Ophthalmol 1995; 40: 89-118.
7. Epstein D, Fagerholm P, Hamberg-Nystrom H et al: Four month follow up of excimer laser PRK for myopia. Refractive and visual acuity results. Ophthalmology 1994; 101: 1558-1563.
8. Talley AR, Hardten DR, Sher NA et al: results one year after using the 193 nm excimer laser for PRK in mild to moderate myopia. Am J Ophthalmol 1994; 118: 304-311.
9. Chan WK, Hang WJ, Tseng P et al: PRK for myopia of 6 to 12 diopters. J Ref Surg 1995; 11(Suppl): S286-S292.
10. Siganos DS, Pallikaris IG, Margartis VN: PRK with a transition zone for myopia from –7 to –14 diopters. J Ref Surg 1996; 12 (Suppl): S261-S263.
11. Hersh PS, Brint SF, Maloney RK et al: PRK vs. LASIK for moderate to high myopia. Ophthalmology 1998; 105(8): 1512-1522.
12. Goes FJ: PRK foe myopia of –8 to –20 diopters. J Ref Surg 1996; 12: 91 97.
13. Williams DK: Excimer laser PRK for extreme myopia. J Cataract Ref Surg 1996; 22: 910-914.
14. Kremer I, Gabbay U, Blumenthal M: One year follow up results of PRK for low, moderate and high primary astigmatism. Ophthalmology 1996; 103: 741-748.
15. Brancato R, Carones F, Venturi E et al: PRK for compound myopic astigmatism with an eye cup erodible mask delivery system. J Ref Surg 1996; 12: 501-511.
16. Dausch D, Klein R, Schroder E et al: PRK for hyperopic and mixed astigmatism. J Ref Surg 1996; 12: 684-692.
17. Stevens J, Giubilei M, Ficker L, Rosen P: Prospective study of photorefractive keratectomy for myopia using the VISX StarS2 excimer laser system. J Refract Surg 2002 Sep-Oct; 18(5): 502-8.
18. Shah S, Chatterjee A, Smith RJ: Predictability and outcomes of photoastigmatic keratectomy using the Nidek EC-5000 excimer laser. J Cataract Refract Surg 2002 Apr; 28(4): 682-8.
19. Beauduin P, Gobin L, Trau R, Tassignon MJ: PRK with InPro-Gauss excimer laser: statistical analysis of results. Bull Soc Belge Ophtalmol 2002;(284): 65-71.
20. Dausch D, Landesz M: Laser correction for hyperopia. Aesculap-Meditec results from Germany, in Salz JJ, McDonnell PJ, McDonald MB (eds): Corneal Laser Surgery. St. Louis Mosby-Yearbook 1995; 239-247.
21. Dausch D, Smecka z, Klein R et al: Excimer laser PRK for hyperopia. J Cataract Ref Surg 1997; 23: 169-176.
22. Jackson WB: Results of hyperopic PRK. American Society of Cataract and Refractive Surgery Meeting. Boston 1997.
23. Stevens JD, Ficker LA: Results of photorefractive keratectomy for hyperopia using the VISX star excimer laser system. J Refract Surg 2002 Jan-Feb; 18(1): 30-6.
24. Nagy ZZ, Munkacsy G, Popper M: Photorefractive keratectomy using the meditec MEL 70 G-scan laser for hyperopia and hyperopic astigmatism. J Refract Surg 2002 Sep-Oct; 18(5): 542-50.
25. Salah T, Warring GO, El Maghraby A et al: Excimer laser in situ keratomileusis under corneal flap for myopia of 2 to 20 diopters. Am J Ophthalmol 1996; 121: 143-155.
26. Gimbel HV, Basti S, Kave GB, Ferensowicz M: Experience during the learning curve of LASIK. J Cataract Ref Surg 1996; 22: 542-550.
27. Gimbel HV, Penno EEA, Westenbrugge JAV et al: Incidence and management of intraoperative and early postoperative complications in 1000 cases of consecutive LASIK. Ophthalmology 1998; 105: 1839-1847.
28. Perez-Santonja JJ, Bellot J et al: LASIK to correct high myopia. J Cataract Ref Surg 1997; 23: 372-385.
29. Lyle WA, Jin GJ: Laser in situ keratomileusis with the VISX Star laser for myopia over -10.0 diopters. J Cataract Refract Surg 2001 Nov; 27(11): 1812-22.
30. Yang Y, Du X, Pan Q, Xia W, Yao K: A long-term observation of laser in situ keratomileusis for myopia. Chung Hua Yen Ko Tsa Chih 2002 Mar; 38(3): 151-3
31. Lindstrom RL, Hardten DR, Chu YR: LASIK for the treatment of low, moderate and high myopia. Trans Am Ophthalmol Soc 1997; 95: 285-296.
32. Salchow DJ, Zirm ME, Stieldorf C, Parisi A: LASIK for myopia and myopic astigmatism. J Cataract Ref Surg 1998; 24 (2): 175-182.
33. Knorz MC, Wiesinger B, Liermann A et al: LASIK for moderate and high myopia and myopic astigmatism. Ophthalmology 1998; 105(5): 932-940.
34. Knorz MC, Neuhann T: Correction of myopia and astigmatism using topography-assisted laser in situ keratomileusis (TopoLink LASIK). Ophthalmologe 2000 Dec; 97(12): 827-31.
35. Balazsi G, Mullie M, Lasswell L, et al: LASIK with a scanning excimer laser for the correction of low to moderate myopia with and without astigmatism. J Cataract Refract Surg 2001 Dec; 27(12): 1942-51.

36. Argento CJ, Cocentino MJ: LASIK for hyperopia. J Cataract Ref Surg 1998; 24 (8): 1050-1058.
37. Ditzen K, Huschka H, Pieger S: LASIK for hyperopia. J Cataract Ref Surg 1998; 24 (1): 42-47.
38. Goker S, Er H, Kahvecioglu C: LASIK to correct hyperopia from +4.25 to +8.0 D. J Ref Surg 1998; 14 (1): 26-30.
39. Rashad KM: Laser in situ keratomileusis for the correction of hyperopia from +1.25 to +5.00 diopters with the Technolas Keracor 117C laser. J Refract Surg 2001 Mar-Apr; 17(2): 113-22.
40. Tabbara KF, El-Sheikh HF, Islam SM: Laser in situ keratomileusis for the correction of hyperopia from +0.50 to +11.50 diopters with the Keracor 117C laser. J Refract Surg 2001 Mar-Apr; 17(2): 123-8.
41. Salz JJ, Stevens CA; LADAR Vision LASIK Hyperopia Study Group: LASIK correction of spherical hyperopia, hyperopic astigmatism, and mixed astigmatism with the LADAR Vision excimer laser system. Ophthalmology 2002 Sep; 109(9): 1647-56; discussion 1657-8.
42. Chitkara DK, Rosen E, Gore C et al: Tracker-assisted laser in situ keratomileusis for myopia using the autonomous scanning laser: 12 month results. Ophthalmology 2002; 109 (5): 965-72.
43. Durrie DS, Gordon M, Michelson MA et al: Phototherapeutic keratectomy versus laser in situ keratomileusis for moderate to high myopia. Ophthalmology 1998; 105(8): 1512-1522.
44. Walker MB, Wilson SE: Recovery of uncorrected visual acuity after laser in situ keratomileusis or photorefractive keratectomy for low myopia. Cornea 2001 Mar; 20(2): 153-5.
45. Lorencova V, Rozsival P, Feuermannova A, Kvasnicka J: PRK and LASIK in patients with myopia ranging from -6 to -9 D. Cesk Slov Oftalmol 2001 Nov; 57(6): 395-402.
46. el-Agha MS, Johnston EW, Bowman RW, Cavanagh HD et al: Excimer laser treatment of spherical hyperopia: PRK or LASIK? Trans Am Ophthalmol Soc 2000; 98:59-66; discussion 66-9.
47. Van Gelder RN, Steger-May K, Yang SH, Rattanatam T, Pepose JS: Comparison of photorefractive keratectomy, astigmatic PRK, laser in situ keratomileusis, and astigmatic LASIK in the treatment of myopia. J Cataract Refract Surg 2002 Mar; 28(3): 462-76
48. Martinez CE, Applegate RA, Klyce SD et al: Effect of pupillary dilation on the corneal optical aberrations after PRK. Arch Ophthalmol 1998; 116: 1053-1062.
49. Seiler T, Kaemmerer M, Mierdel P et al: Ocular optical aberrations after PRK for myopia and myopic astigmatism. Arch Ophthalmol 2000; 118: 17-21
50. Oliver KM, Hamenger RP et al: Corneal optical aberrations induced by PRK. J Ref Surg 1997; 13: 246-254.
51. Oshika T, Klyce SD, Applegate RA et al: Comparison of corneal wavefront aberrations after PRK and laser in situ keratomileusis. Am J Ophthalmol 1999; 127: 1-7.
52. Oshika T, Miyata K, Tokunaga T, Samejima T et al: Higher-order wavefront aberrations of cornea and magnitude of refractive correction in laser in situ keratomileusis. Ophthalmology 2002; 109(6): 1154-1158.
53. Mac Rae S, Schwiegerling J, Snyder RW: Customized and low spherical aberration corneal ablation design. J Ref Surg 1999; 12: S246-S248.
54. Mrochen M, Seiler T, Kaemmerer: Wavefront-guided LASIK: early results in three eyes. J Ref Surg 2000; 16: 116-121.
55. Mrochen M, Kaemmerer M, Seiler T: Clinical results of wavefront-guided LASIK 3 months after surgery. J Cataract Ref Surg 2001; 27 (2): 201-207.
56. Knorz MC, Neuhann T: Treatment of myopia and myopic astigmatism by customized laser in situ keratomileusis based on corneal topography. Ophthalmology. 2000 Nov; 107(11): 2072-6.
57. Mac Rae S, Schwiegerling J et al: Customized corneal ablation and super vision. J Ref Surg 2000; 16: S230-S235.
58. Panagopoulou SI, Pallikaris IG: Wavefront customized ablations with the WASCA Asclepion workstation. J Refract Surg 2001 Sep-Oct; 17(5): S608-12.
59. Vongthongsri A, Phusitphoykai N, Naripthapan P. Comparison of wavefront-guided customized ablation vs. conventional ablation in laser in situ keratomileusis. J Refract Surg 2002 May-Jun; 18(3 Suppl): S332-5.
60. Nagy ZZ, Palagyi-Deak I, Kelemen E, Kovacs A: Wavefront-guided photorefractive keratectomy for myopia and myopic astigmatism. J Refract Surg 2002 Sep-Oct; 18(5): S615-9.
61. Nagy ZZ, Palagyi-Deak I, Kovacs A, Kelemen E, Forster W: First results with wavefront-guided photorefractive keratectomy for hyperopia. J Refract Surg; 2002 Sep-Oct; 18(5): S620-3.
62. Anderson N, Beran R, Schneider T: Epi-LASEK for the correction of myopia and myopic astigmatism. J Cataract Refract Surg 2002 Aug; 28(8): 1343.
63. Shahinian L: Laser-assisted subepithelial keratectomy for low to high myopia and astigmatism. J Cataract Refract Surg 2002 Aug; 28(8): 1334.
64. Lee JB, Choe CM, Seong GJ, Gong HY, Kim EK: Laser Subepithelial Keratomileusis for Low to Moderate Myopia. 6-Month Follow-up. Jpn J Ophthalmol 2002 May-Jun; 46(3): 299-304.
65. Rouweyha RM, Chuang AZ, Mitra S, Phillips CB, Yee RW: Laser epithelial keratomileusis for myopia with the autonomous laser. J Refract Surg 2002 May-Jun; 18(3): 217-24.
66. Claringbold TV 2nd: Laser-assisted subepithelial keratectomy for the correction of myopia. J Cataract Refract Surg 2002 Jan; 28(1): 18-22.

67. Lee JB, Seong GJ, Lee JH, Seo KY, Lee YG, Kim EK: Comparison of laser epithelial keratomileusis and photorefractive keratectomy for low to moderate myopia. J Cataract Refract Surg 2001 Apr; 27(4): 565-70.
68. Litwak S, Zadok D, Garcia-de Quevedo V, Robledo N, Chayet A: LASEK versus photorefractive keratectomy for the correction of myopia. A prospective comparative study. J Cataract Refract Surg 2002 Aug; 28(8): 1330.
69. Scerrati E: Laser in situ keratomileusis vs. laser epithelial keratomileusis (LASIK vs. LASEK). J Refract Surg 2001 Mar-Apr; 17(2 Suppl): S219-21.
70. Pallikaris IG, Siganos DS: Excimer laser in situ keratomileusis and PRK for correction of high myopia. J Cataract Ref Surg 1994; 10: 498-510.
71. El-Maghraby A, Salah T, Warring GO III et al: Randomized bilateral comparison of excimer laser in situ keratomileusis and PRK for 1.2 to 8.0 diopter of myopia. Ophthalmology 1999; 106: 447-457.
72. Wang Z, Chen J, Yang B: Comparison of LASIK and PRK to correct myopia from –1.25 to –6.0 diopters. J Ref Surg 1997; 13: 528-534.
73. Kremer I, Kaplan A, Novikov I, Blumenthal M: Patterns of late corneal scarring after PRK in high and severe myopia. Ophthalmology 1999; 106: 467-473.

Chapter 26

Complications of Excimer Laser Surgeries

Available studies have reported that the excimer laser corneal surgeries are comparatively safe procedures. Nonetheless some complications do occur following these procedures. These complications can be either reduced or avoided by careful pre-operative selection, appropriate knowledge, skill and experience about the excimer laser procedures; and appropriate post-operative care and medication. Few serious complications have been reported with some of the procedures. However, the incidence of such complications is low. Therefore these do not make the procedures unsafe or risky in general.

Many of these complications are more common with a particular excimer laser procedure than with another one because of different methodology involved. For example, the problems of postoperative pain, corneal haze and refractive instability are more of a problem with corneal surface ablation procedures like PRK and PTK. On the other hand, the problems related to microkeratome and corneal flap; and suction ring related complications are inherent in LASIK procedures (LASIK and customized-LASIK technology; Table 26.1).

Among the excimer laser refractive surgeries, regression of refractive correction, longer visual rehabilitation time and side effects related to prolonged use of postoperative medications to modify the healing response are problems mainly after PRK. No regression has been reported after LASEK. Regression is less common with LASIK procedures. In addition, prolonged postoperative medication is also not required following LASIK unlike PRK. The most commonly noticed undesired outcome after PTK is hyperopic shift, among other refractive changes.

Table 26.1: Complications of laser refractive surgeries

More common with PRK	With PRK and LASIK	With LASIK and C-LASIK
* Postoperative pain	* Overcorrection	* Microkeratome jam
* Delayed epithelial healing	* Undercorrection	* Flap complications
* Infection	* Astigmatism	* Epithelial ingrowth
* Corneal haze	* Loss of BCVA	* Diffuse lamellar keratitis/
* Regression	* Glare, halo, monocular diplopia	"Sands of Sahara" syndrome
* Central islands	* Decreased contrast	* Late flap dislocation
* Scarring	* Dry-eye symptoms	* Corneal ectasia
	* Decentered ablation	

However, there are certain problems and complications that are common to all excimer laser surgeries. These are related to the laser delivery and centration of the ablation zone.

The complications of corneal excimer laser surgeries may be divided into:

INTRAOPERATIVE COMPLICATIONS

Common to All Procedures

1. Laser failure of ablation
2. Laser mechanical failure
3. Inappropriate ablation
4. Decentration of ablation zone

With Corneal Surface Ablation (PRK, PTK)

Failure to remove the epithelium adequately

With LASIK and C-LASIK

1. Inadequate exposure
2. Inadequate suction
3. Problems in advancement of the microkeratome
4. Thin flaps
5. Buttonholes
6. Free caps
7. Incomplete flap
8. Corneal perforation
9. Lost flap
10. Flap edema
11. Mechanical damage to flap
12. Flap shrinkage
13. Interface debris
14. Flap wrinkling
15. Intraoperative bleeding

IMMEDIATE AND EARLY POSTOPERATIVE COMPLICATIONS

Common to All Procedures

1. Post operative pain
2. Bacterial keratitis
3. Transient minor complications
    a. Mucus plaques or tags
    b. Corneal edema
    c. Anterior chamber cells and flare
    d. Lid edema and blepharoptosis
4. Complications of topical medication
    a. Drug toxicity
    b. Drug hypersensitivity

With Corneal Surface Ablation (PTK, PRK)

1. Delayed epithelial healing
2. Sterile corneal infiltrates

With LASIK and C-LASIK

1. Wrinkled flap
2. Flap folds
3. Interface debris
4. Displaced flap
5. Diffuse lamellar keratitis
6. Epithelial ingrowth

INTERMEDIATE TO LONG TERM COMPLICATIONS

Common to Refractive Procedures

1. Undercorrection
2. Overcorrection
3. Induced astigmatism
4. Irregular astigmatism
5. Central islands
6. Decentred ablation
7. Regression
8. Corneal haze
9. Loss of BCVA
10. Halos and ghost images
11. Recurrent corneal microerosions
12. Recurrent corneal erosion syndrome
13. Steroid induced elevation of intra-ocular pressure

With LASIK and C-LASIK

1. Epithelial ingrowth
2. Stromal melts
3. Corneal ectasia
4. Late flap detachment

With PTK

1. Refractive changes
2. Recurrence of dystrophies
3. Graft failure
4. Corneal haze
5. Steroid induced elevation of IOP
6. Corneal hypoesthesia

7. Recurrence of corneal erosions
8. Reactivation of herpes simplex keratitis

EXCIMER LASER ABLATION: INTRAOPERATIVE COMPLICATIONS

INTRA-OPERATIVE LASER FAILURE

Complete failure of the laser to fire can occur, although it is extremely uncommon. The result is that the ablation cannot begin. This problem may be due to computer failure or an intrinsic malfunctioning of the laser system.

M*echanical failures* of an iris diaphragm or the scanning system are also extremely rare events. The mechanical failure can produce an inappropriate ablation profile or deposition of excessive energy at one point on the cornea.

Proper servicing and maintenance of the laser system can prevent these problems. Preoperative calibration of the laser beam used for testing the energy output and beam homogeneity, also ensures that the laser system is working.

Management
The procedure should be immediately cancelled in case of intrinsic *laser system malfunction.*

In case the *computer failure* has occurred before the surgery is begun, the procedure can be postponed.

If the epithelium has already been removed in case of PTK or PRK, or if the corneal flap has been made during LASIK, the cornea and the flap must be protected. An eye shield should be used in case the fault can be corrected in 2-3 minutes. Cornea is wetted with saline to prevent dehydration, if the delay is 4–6 minutes. If laser firing cannot be restarted within 5–6 minutes, the surgery should be abandoned. An eye patch is applied in case of PTK or PRK. The corneal flap is repositioned back in case of LASIK and surgery can be safely resumed at a later date by simply lifting the previous flap. As said earlier this laser system failure is an extremely rare event with the modern laser systems.

DECENTRATION OF ABLATION ZONE

An accurate centration is crucial during any excimer laser surgery. Decentration of the ablation zone is associated with far reaching implications. The methods of ablation zone centration have previously been discussed in Chapters 15 and 23.

It is important to note that the best landmark for marking the center of ablation zone is the center of the entrance pupil. This is because the corneal light reflex (*Purkinje-Sanson image*) is subject to parallax. Moreover, the light passing through the center of pupil is more effective in stimulating the photoreceptors. *The photoreceptors have been shown to actively orient themselves towards the center of pupil even in eccentric pupils*[1,2]. This is called the **Stiles-Crawford effect**.

The patient fixates at the target light, which is coaxial with the microscope light. *The eye tracker is activated after* centration of the light of the microscope. Since the laser beam has the same path as the co-axial light of the microscope, its centration follows automatically.

The following may lead to decentred ablation during refractive ablation.

1. Poor patient fixation either due to nervousness or oversedation.
2. Involuntary movements of the eye during *self-fixation* because no mechanical fixation device is used by modern surgeons.
3. Prolonged ablation, which requires increased fixation time. This is likely during higher attempted corrections.
4. Difficulty in seeing target due to blurred vision. This may occur because of high refractive error as well as due to the blurring induced by stromal ablation and lifting of flap during LASIK.
5. Improper alignment of the ablation zone due to surgeon's inexperience.
6. Misalignment of the laser optics or the centering aids in the laser delivery system.
7. Lack of an efficient active eye-tracker during the ablation.

Decentration During Phototherapeutic Keratectomy (PTK)

Corneal ablation during PTK is done by plano-mode in which the laser energy is delivered over the ablation zone uniformly. Centration of the laser beam is done in relation to the visual axis. The surgeon may decide to ablate a particular area/paracentral lesion more by maneuvering the patient's head. This is done by turning the eye-tracker off. But over treatment of a paracentral lesion may cause avoidable refractive changes because this *off-axis ablation* would result in decentration of ablation zone and iatrogenic astigmatism, which may be troublesome.

Decentration During Refractive Surgeries

Older studies on PRK have reported an incidence rate of 32% for decentration ranging 0.3–0.6 mm[3-10]. The incidence has reduced significantly with the use of an active eye-tracker system. Visually significant decentered ablation is now less common

Mulhern et al[11] reported decentration of the ablation zone to be almost twice after LASIK as compared to PRK. This may be due to the effect of the stromal flap removal resulting in loss of the pre-aligned centration or the patient's inability to maintain fixation at the target due to blurring after flap creation. Movement during creation of the flap and during removal of the suction ring may lead to the same effect.

Effects of Decentred Ablation

Decentered ablation results in shifting of the center of the ablation zone away from the pupillary axis (Colour Plate 11, Photograph 57). This means the flatter tangential curvature is shifted peripherally leaving the central optical zone with greater corneal power. In addition, irregular astigmatism also results due to this abnormal corneal ablation. This peculiar corneal curvature leads to a number of symptoms.

The symptoms arising from significant decentered ablation zone are blurred image, ghost images, monocular diplopia, decreased contrast and BCVA; and night vision problems like halos and glare. These symptoms depend upon the following factors.

Degree of Decentration with Respect to the Pupillary axis

Decentration more than 1 mm is likely to be symptomatic. Less than 0.5 mm of decentration is unlikely and less than 0.3 mm rarely to be symptomatic.

The Ablation Zone Diameter

Smaller ablation zone is more symptomatic even with lesser decentration. This is because with a small ablation zone the unablated area is more likely to encroach upon the pupillary axis. The rays passing through this untreated area result in defocused *ghost images* and *monocular diplopia.*

Degree of Attempted Ablation

Higher attempted ablation is associated with greater induced irregular astigmatism in case of decentered ablation.

Larger Pupil Diameter

Patients with larger pupil diameter would often develop visual symptoms. This is because the edge of the decentered ablation is more likely to come within the visual axis.

Prevention

Decentred ablation is best treated by preventing it. The following points are essential for preventing decentered ablation zone.

1. Proper preoperative and intraoperative instructions to the patient. The patient must be warned about sounds and smells that arise during ablation. These may startle the patient and cause reflex movements.
2. Careful stabilization of the patient's head and instructing the patient not to move during ablation as this causes the head to move.
3. Asking the patient to keep both eyes open and not to squeeze or close the fellow eye, which is under the drape. This would avoid Bell's phenomenon and any movement of the eye that is being treated.
4. Minimum sedation should be used as it hampers fixation by decreasing concentration of the patient.
5. Thornton ring may be used for fixating the eye during PRK. The suction ring may be left in place after releasing the vacuum in case of LASIK in patients who are uncooperative.
6. Most important is to be alert and stop ablation if the patient looses fixation.
7. *Use of an active eye-tracker is of great help in avoiding decentration.* It automatically aborts ablation in case of gross decentration.

Management

Postoperative computerized corneal topography is essential for detection and management of decentered ablation (Chapter 19). It is important to rule out central islands and focal scarring in a suspected case of decentered ablation. Vinciguerra et al[11a] investigated 148 cases of refractive surgery for presumed decentred ablation. They found only 3.4% eyes with true decentred ablation. The majority (72.3%) belonged to high dioptric gradient due to focal scarring. Central islands were detected in 5.4% of eyes.

Retreatment may be required in case of significant decentration causing loss of BCVA or other visual disturbances. The strategies of managing significant decentered ablations are discussed in Chapter 27.

INAPPROPRIATE ABLATION

The surgeon or the assistant may enter *incorrect data* into the computer resulting in *inappropriate ablation.* The ablation for PTK is done in *plano*-mode i.e. the refractive error entered is zero. This ensures equal ablation throughout the ablation zone through uniform distribution of laser energy over the area. For refractive surgeries the ablation pattern is decided by the complex algorithms according to the refractive data fed into the computer.

INADEQUATE/IRREGULAR REMOVAL OF THE EPITHELIUM

Inadequate removal of the epithelium may lead to irregular ablation during PTK and PRK. This can cause induced irregular astigmatism. It may also lead to formation of central steep islands if the central epithelium is not removed adequately.

The intraoperative complications related to flap and microkeratome are discussed below under 'LASIK complications'.

EXCIMER LASER ABLATION: TRANSIENT COMPLICATIONS

LID SWELLING AND PTOSIS

During the initial few postoperative days lid swelling due to edema and mild mechanical ptosis may occur. This is attributed to the inflammation caused by prostaglandin release after excimer laser surgery. The orthostatic effect of the eye patching may also contribute to these. The incidence is about 1–6% after excimer laser surgery. The ptosis may last for 1–3 months but is self-limiting. Permanent ptosis is a rare finding. The ptosis also can be taken care of by the use of NSAIDs in all postoperative cases.

Permanent mild to moderate blepharoptosis may occur in a few cases persisting beyond few months. Many factors have been implicated in the causation of ptosis after excimer laser surgery[33].

1. Effect of the corticosteroids on Muller's muscle.
2. Trauma to the Muller's directly by the lid speculum.
3. Persistent lid swelling leading to aponeurotic disinsertion.

COMPLICATIONS OF TOPICAL MEDICATIONS

Following complications may occur due to the topical medications.

Hypersensitivity to the topical medications or the preservatives used in these preparations may manifest as burning, redness of conjunctiva and lid swelling in severe cases. In mild cases, these problems are managed by withdrawal of all topical medications and substitution with alternate ones. Preservative free preparations should be used if possible. Severe cases may require addition of local and systemic antihistaminic and topical steroids if these are not being already administered.

Epithelial toxicity due to the topical preparations or the preservative can occur. This possibility should be suspected if there are persistent epithelial defects in the absence of other predisposing factors.

Antibiotics like ciprofloxacin and genticin and even topical steroids are known to be epitheliotoxic. Antibiotic known to cause less epithelial toxicity, for example chloramphenicol should be preferably used, more so if these are preservative free or have less toxic preservatives.

Other Transient Minor Complications

Mucus plaques or tags, corneal edema and anterior chamber cells and flare are some transient effects observed after excimer laser ablation. Their incidence is more in eyes that have undergone surface ablation where the epithelial defect is present for some days.

The incidence of *mucous plaques or tags* reported after PRK is about 14%. They are formed by mucous and cellular debris or even loose epithelium. Their presence is usually inconsequential for epithelization. Occasionally they may cause discomfort and increased lacrimation, when they should be removed with a sterile spatula[33].

Mild, barely discernible, anterior chamber cells and flare may be noticed after excimer laser ablation in many cases. These findings are self limiting.

In cases of PTK and PRK, mild to moderate stromal edema may be seen. It disappears after the epithelial defect is covered.

EXCIMER LASER ABLATION: IMMEDIATE POSTOPERATIVE COMPLICATIONS

PAIN

Postoperative Pain after PTK and PRK

Severe post-operative pain lasting for few days used to be a significant complication of excimer laser corneal surface ablation like PTK and PRK. The pain is most marked during the first 24–48 hours and disappears by 3–4 days. Most of the earlier studies had reported postoperative pain that required large doses of oral analgesics or even narcotics. Latter clinical studies also have reported mild to moderate pain during first 1–2 days in spite of topical and oral analgesics. The severity of pain decreases with the use of pre- and postoperative topical and systemic analgesics.

This pain is attributed to increased sensitivity of corneal nerves and to release of PGE_2 following excimer laser ablation (Beurman et al, Sher and Fantz et al Sher and Bark et al). A rapid and sustained rise in corneal PGE_2 levels, a potent sensitizer of pain fibers have been demonstrated after excimer laser corneal surgery. This response is *much more than after mechanical keratectomy*. McDonald postulated that the spike in PGE_2 could be partially related to the mechanism of corneal tissue removal. Treatment with topical diclofenac significantly decreases the levels of PGE_2 and pain in the postoperative days.

Postoperative Pain after LASIK

Pain is not a problem following LASIK procedure. Significant postoperative pain that requires analgesics is uncommon after LASIK. The patients may experience some discomfort or foreign body sensation during the first 24–48 hours after an uncomplicated surgery. Occasionally an epithelial abrasion caused inadvertently or areas of loose epithelium can result in watering, photophobia and pain. This is more likely after retreatments where the flap is re-lifted. Severe pain should warn about other causes like a shifted/displaced flap and keratitis etc.

DELAYED EPITHELIAL HEALING

Epithelial Healing after PTK and PRK

As noted previously, most studies have reported complete re-epithelization of the corneal surface in 3–5 days. Delayed healing beyond 7 days is uncommon. Many local factors may contribute to delayed re-epithelization such as:

1. Epithelial toxicity from topical medications (local anesthetics, aminoglycosides, ciprofloxacin, Corticosteroids) or their preservatives.
2. Bad ocular surface associated with corneal disorders in case of PTK.
3. Undetected/mild dry eye.
4. Undetected case of autoimmune disorders, collagen vascular disease or diabetes mellitus.

Contrary to belief, Gimbel and co-authors[13] did not find statistically significant difference in re-epithelization between manual and laser epithelial debridement groups, though the former method produced a larger epithelial defect intraoperatively.

Prevention

The area of epithelial debridement should be minimum, just sufficient for laser ablation. The methods for limiting the debridement area have been described in Chapter 13.

Management

Patching of the eye or judicious use of a bandage contact lens and preservative free teardrops, etc. should help in early epithelization of the ablated surface. Lateral tarsorrhaphy is rarely needed. Use of topical sodium hyaluronate and growth factors have also been advocated by some authors to expedite epithelial healing.

Epithelial Complications after LASIK

The faster visual recovery after LASIK is because the epithelium is not disturbed. Although minor staining with fluorescein at the flap edge is a common finding during first 24–48 hours after LASIK, the presence of punctate staining or bigger epithelial defects is an unwelcome finding. A number of factors may be responsible for the epithelial defects following LASIK. Excessive use of preoperative drops, improper maneuvers during the surgery and trauma due to careless instrumentation can lead to the epithelial defects. Basement membrane dystrophy or previous history of recurrent erosions may be found in many patients. These patients my even develop sloughing of epithelium associated with prolonged wound healing time[161].

The reported incidence rate of epithelial defects after LASIK is about 5%. The patients with persistent epithelial defects are at higher risk of epithelial ingrowth. It is more so if the epithelial defect was present during surgery or if it is located near the flap edge. They are also at a higher risk for developing diffuse lamellar keratitis (DLK).

Breil et al[13a] have described superficial punctate keratitis following LASIK as "LASIK-induced neurotrophic epitheliopathy". It is supposed to result from loss of innervations due to cutting of the corneal nerves during flap creation.

Prevention

1. This complication can be prevented by limiting the use of preoperative drops, gentle handling of the corneal flap and excluding patients with suspicion of epithelial basement membrane dystrophy.
2. PRK may be considered for the second eye if significant loose epithelium was encountered in case of first eye and for patients of suspected basement membrane dystrophy.

Management

1. Carefully smoothen the epithelium into position.
2. Excess tags need to be removed.
3. A contact lens may be placed in select cases with severe epithelial disruption.
4. Moisture chambers may be used in patients following LASIK for few days.

STERILE CORNEAL INFILTRATES

Sterile Corneal Infiltrates After PRK

There are only few reports about sterile corneal infiltrates in the literature after surface photoablation of the cornea. The sterile corneal infiltrates fall into two categories.

Peripheral Non-Infectious Infiltrates

These are non-sight threatening rare complications. They are frequently associated with blepharitis, which in many cases may be mild and remain unnoticed or may even be present in the other eye. The causative agent is thought to be staphylococcal toxin.

The infiltrates are small and usually near the limbus but often separated from it by a clear zone (Colour Plate 11, Photograph 58). They are frequently multiple. These infiltrates respond within 24 hours to topical steroids given four times a day. An appropriate topical antibiotic should also be used more frequently. If no response is seen in 24 hours the sterile peripheral infiltrates are treated intensively on lines of bacterial keratitis.

Associated with NSAID and Bandage Soft Contact Lens Use

Neil Sher et al[14] reported high incidence of sterile infiltrates (9%) in 240 of their patients treated over a period of three years. They noted an *association with the use of* **contact lens and topical NSAID** *without the concurrent use of topical steroids*. It was suggested that *this combination* without topical steroids causes cyclo-oxygenage inhibition leading to increased amount of arachidonic acid and increased formation of leukotrienes, which are potent chemotactants for polymorphonuclear leucocytes.

In a survey report of 17 surgeons in Canada, *Teal et al*[15] reported 30 such cases after PRK, presenting with pain, redness and lacrimation on the 2nd post-operative day. The infiltrates most frequently were in the shape of a paracentral immune ring placed inferiorly. They also found an association with combination of contact lens and NSAIDS in these cases.

Sterile Corneal Infiltrates After PTK

Teichmann et al[16] described a case after PTK in which he noted a Wessely-type incomplete dense white ring at the margin of the ablated zone on the fourth day. The patient was using bandage contact lens. The authors suggested that it could be an *antigen antibody reaction* involving the heat shock protein (HSP) produced locally at the margin of the ablated zone and the *pre-existing circulating antibody against bacterial antigens (HSPs)*.

Sterile Corneal Infiltrates After LASIK

Sterile corneal (interface) infiltrates of varying degree are not an uncommon finding after LASIK. These can be the result of interface debris. Sterile infiltrates after lasik are important in so far as they are to be differentiated from infectious keratitis and also because they may be the harbinger of the more serious DLK. This later peculiar entity of sterile inflammatory infiltrates is also called *Sands of Sahara syndrome*. It has its own implications and has been described under LASIK complications (vide infra).

MICROBIAL KERATITIS

Risk Factors for Microbial Keratitis

Local or environmental predisposing factors are to be blamed. Blepharitis, adnexal infection, acne rosacea and *use of bandage soft contact lenses* are important risk factors. As such bacterial keratitis is a risk in any surgical procedure that removes the epithelial barrier.

Prevention and Management of Microbial Keratitis

The use of broad spectrum antibiotics pre- and post-operatively, 5% povidone iodine solution for preparing the eye and *avoiding the use of bandage contact lenses* are essential preventive measures. *Gallo et al have also underscored the use of BSCL due to increased risk of sterile as well as non-sterile corneal infiltrates. They recommend that in case its use is unavoidable, the eye should be examined daily till healing of the epithelium.* Aggressive management is to be instituted in case this dreaded complication is suspected.

Incidence of Microbial Keratitis Following PTK and PRK

The occurrence of microbial keratitis following corneal surface ablation with excimer laser is a *rare* but *serious sight threatening complication*. Very few cases of microbial keratitis have been reported in the literature. In a survey article, *Seiler and McDonnell*[17] reported 6 documented cases of microbial keratitis, *all associated with the use of bandage contact lens* in the postoperative period. Four out of the six cases occurred in one series of PRK due to *Aspergilus* present in the air. Four cases of fungal keratitis were reported by *Faschinger et al*[18] in a series of 161 case of PRK.

al-Rajhi and Wagoner et al[18] reported 3 cases of bacterial keratitis occurring in a prospective study of 258 consecutive PTK procedures. All the cases of bacterial keratitis occurred in the patients of climatic droplet keratopathy. Two of the cases were polybacterial and Gram-positive species were predominant. The final visual outcome ranged from 20/125 to 20/400. *Maloney et al*[32] reported one case of bacterial keratitis in their series of 232 patients of PTK.

Microbial Keratitis Following LASIK

Infective keratitis following LASIK, like in case of PRK and PTK is a rare but devastating complication. It must be avoided at all costs by following intra- and post-operative utmost sterile measures and managing it on an emergency basis in case this complication occurs. The risk factors as discussed in the previous section must be identified and preventive measures taken or surgery deferred in such cases.

Different case reports have identified a varied group of organisms, including bacteria (mostly Gram-positive), fungi, atypical mycobacteria and herpes virus from cases of infectious keratitis, though some cases were found to be culture negative [21-25]. The infection is usually acquired intraoperatively, but may also be caused by postoperative contamination.

Majority of the patients present within 72 hours of the surgery with an acute onset symptoms of pain, redness photophobia, lacrimation and decreased vision. The examination may show subtle corneal infiltrates/ interface haze to frank ulceration; circumcilliary or more sever congestion and even abscess formation at the interface. Early cases may be difficult to diagnose *but the dictum is that all suspected cases must be treated as infective keratitis even if they are culture negative.*

Cases of microbial keratitis after LASIK must be treated with aggressive topical fortified antibiotic therapy. Scraping of the infiltrate / interface material for microbiological evaluation should precede the antibiotic therapy. This therapy should be combined with irrigation of stromal bed with antibiotic solution after lifting the flap.

The course of infectious keratitis is variable depending on the pathogen. The keratitis heals with scarring. Many case reports have shown a favorable outcome with intensive management of bacterial keratitis with best spectacle-corrected visual acuity of 20/40 or better in majority of the patients.

Incidence of Microbial Keratitis Following LASIK

Many case reports have appeared on microbial keratitis following LASIK[21-31, 162, 163]. However incidence of this serious vision threatening complication following LASIK is very low considering millions of surgeries that have been performed till today all over the world. *Narottma Pushker* et al[29], in a literature review, have found 41 eyes to have microbial keratitis after LASIK.

Qun Peng et al[26] reported 5 case of fungal keratitis during early postoperative period after LASIK. All the cases were caused by *Candida albicans*, all resolved with antifungal treatment with good visual recovery. An association of moist and warm climate was proposed with the occurrence of fungal keratitis.

Since differentiation of inflammatory from the infectious keratitis, which is a serious vision threatening complication, may not be easy, the same authors recommended that in addition to the topical steroids, cases of suspected grade I and II diffuse lamellar keratitis (DLK) should be covered with antibiotics. Lifting of the flap, culture of scrapings and irrigation must be done after 24 hours if Grade III DLK does not show improvement and immediately in case of grade IV DLK.

Fulcher et al[28] reported 7 cases of atypical mycobacterium keratitis developing 7 to 24 weeks after (LASIK). *Although mycobacterial keratitis after LASIK is a diagnostic and management challenge, the outcomes can be satisfying with judicious use of antibacterial agents guided by culture–sensitivity reports*. In this report, the keratitis resolved in all patients with treatment that included clarithromycin, based on susceptibilities. Six of seven patients recovered best-corrected visual acuity (BCVA), while one patient lost one line of BCVA.

REACTIVATION OF HERPES SIMPLEX KERATITIS

Perry et al[30] reported one case of herpes simplex reactivation following LASIK in a case that underwent LASIK after penetrating keratoplasty for herpes simplex keratitis. Corneal perforation occurred subsequently. *Davidorf et al*[31] also found reactivation of herpes simplex keratitis after LASIK. These reports emphasize that cases with history of this infection or those having reduced corneal sensation should be excluded for the purpose of refractive surgery. This issue relating to PTK has been addressed to in the concerned section.

EXCIMER LASER ABLATION: INTERMEDIATE TO LONG TERM COMPLICATIONS

CORNEAL HAZE

Corneal Haze After PRK

Every cornea exhibits some form of haze following excimer laser photoablation. The corneal haze is a major problem after surface ablation like PRK and PTK. Haze is visually significant when it exceeds 1.5 to 2 grade as assessed by the slit-lamp examination according to the method given by Gartry et al (Colour Plate 11, Photograph 59). Haze at this level leads to loss of one Snellen's line of best-corrected visual acuity. Visually significant corneal haze is found in 3-11% of the patients undergoing moderate photoablation. Its incidence increases to 10-40% in patients with higher depth of ablation[33, 38, 69].

Early Haze

Development of subepithelial corneal haze is a major setback for photorefractive surgeries. It is one of the main factors responsible for *loss of BCVA* and *regression* after PRK[35, 41]. The haze appears many weeks after PRK. It is most intense during second and third months and then clears over next 6-12 months. Cases have been reported to last for more than 2 years. The genesis, evaluation and pharmacological modulation of corneal haze have been previously mentioned under respective heads (Chapters 5 and 16).

It occurs with more severity and may last longer (for up to 12-18 months) in cases of higher myopia with greater attempted correction[37]. Other factor contributing to greater level of corneal haze are male patients, non-compliance with postoperative steroid medication, history of significant haze in the first treated eye and intraoperative dehydration. It is also more severe with smaller ablation zone. The exposure to ultraviolet-B radiation has been found to increase the haze in animals[40].

Late Haze

Development of corneal haze may occur after many months, although the cornea in these cases had been previously clear[39, 40]. Incidence of this late onset haze is low (about 0.6%).

Management of Haze

The early onset haze responds well to intensive topical steroid therapy along with the NSAIDs[43, 44, 69]. Other pharmacological agents like mitomycin-C also had been tried for the management of haze and regression[47]. Rarely superficial keratectomy or superficial PTK may be required to treat the persistent subepithelial haze. This is more so in cases of late onset haze, which are not responsive to the steroid therapy[45, 46].

Recently Kang et al[47], in an animal model have reported the efficacy of 0.5% *topical zinc sulfate* in reducing haze after PRK. This agent was found to decrease apoptosis of the keratocytes that results in compensatory over-proliferation of keratocytes leading to abnormal healing response.

Corneal Haze After LASIK

The incidence of corneal haze is much less after LASIK as compared to PRK[48-51]. The haze is not visually significant and hardly requires prolonged steroid therapy unlike in case of PRK. This is because the stromal keratocytes are not exposed to the factors responsible for exaggerated healing response (see Chapter 5).

Other possibilities like epithelial ingrowth and interface debris may simulate haze in cases of LASIK. The latter and certain toxic materials introduced from the cul-de-sac and irrigating fluids may cause interface haze due to inflammation. Interface haze caused by these factors responds well to low dose of topical steroid therapy.

Iskander et al have suggested a minimal PTK smoothening of the stromal bed at the end of hyperopic ablation to prevent/minimize crystalline haze that occurs after hyperopic LASIK[52].

STEROID INDUCED RISE OF INTRAOCULAR PRESSURE

This is a not so uncommon complication, particularly if one happens to be a steroid responder. This is because *the topical steroids have to be used for long time, may be for 6 months or longer, to modulate stromal healing response and to avoid corneal haze* in cases of PRK and PTK.

Moderate rise of pressure has been reported in 8-24% of cases with the use of potent topical steroids. Increase in the IOP beyond 30 mm Hg is less frequently seen. It occurs in 1.0 to 8% eyes [56-58]. But such an eventuality is likely to occur with the use of the potent topical steroids. Gartry et al[69] reported an IOP of more than 40 mm Hg in 2% eyes, which were on intensive topical steroid therapy for management of corneal haze and regression. The occurrence of this complication is less common with fluorometholone. A moderate rise of IOP has been reported with topical fluorometholone also in 1.7–10.0% eyes [53-55]. **Therefore preoperative as well frequent postoperative evaluation of the intraocular pressure is crucial.**

Method of Evaluating the IOP

The applanation tonometry with Goldmann tonometer has been found to underestimate the intraocular pressure after excimer laser corneal ablation. There are case reports where the patient developed glaucomatous changes, although the IOP readings with this method were normal on serial follow-ups[63-66]. There was also no history or suspicion of preoperative glaucoma.

The cause of the underestimation of IOP by Goldmann tonometer is the decrease in corneal thickness and the corneal curvature. It is known that applanation reading is low with thinner corneas[59,60]. The applanation reading has also been found to vary with corneal curvature[61]. A difference of 1.0 D leads to difference of 0.34 mm Hg in the pressure recording within corneal power range of 40–49 D.

There are reports of this phenomenon of IOP underestimation *in LASIK patients* also. The *interface edema has also been implicated as one of the factors responsible for the pressure underestimation*[63-66].

It has been observed that the *pressure recording in the peripheral area of the cornea* that is not affected by laser ablation and away from the corneal flap *is more accurate using the applanation method*[61]. Therefore the available unablated peripheral cornea should be used for monitoring the postoperative IOP after excimer laser surgery in *all cases who have to be put on prolonged topical therapy.*

Wang et al[67] evaluated the reliability of IOP measurements by Goldmann applanation tonometry and pneumotonometry (PT) after hyperopic LASIK. Postoperative measurements of IOP from the central as well peripheral corneal areas made by either method were significantly lower ($P < 0.001$) than central IOP measured preoperatively. This is due to the fact that hyperopic ablation removes tissue from the peripheral cornea. There were no significant differences between central and peripheral IOP measurements using either method.

Lee et al [68] have reported that the Orbscan II may help in predicting actual IOP values after LASIK and avoid the misinterpretation of high IOPs as normal IOPs. They found that using a noncontact tonometer (NCT CT-60, Topcon), the pressure readings were falsely lower. The postoperative IOP results were corrected with the Orbscan II program. After compensation with Orbscan II, there were no statistically significant differences between the preoperative and postoperative IOPs.

Management

Mild elevation of pressure responds to steroid withdrawal but pressure > 30 mm Hg requires short course of treatment with anti-glaucoma drugs. With proper monitoring and medical management, any field defects or disk cupping should not occur. Such an occurrence indicates total ignorance and mismanagement on the part of the surgeon or non-follow up on the part of the patient.

CORNEAL HYPOESTHESIA

Following the initial heightened pain response, there is a transient decrease in corneal sensitivity (about 50%) during the first post-operative month. Sensitivity returns to normal levels by 3 months in all cases except in the eyes receiving deeper ablation[70-72].

The loss of corneal sensitivity correlates histologically with removal of subepithelial nerve plexus following excimer laser ablation. Regeneration of the subepithelial plexus takes place at one month, which is initially morphologically disorganized. Further regeneration continues up to 4 months. Occasionally the stromal nerves may show prolonged abnormalities for 12 months or even longer. In a rabbit model, *Ishikawa et al*[73] demonstrated that the difference in epithelial re-innervations depend on the method employed for removal of epithelium. The relative density of intra-epithelial innervations was significantly greater in eyes with laser epithelial removal compared with manual removal. Corneal sensitivity was better in the laser treated eyes throughout the study period. Manual removal therefore hampers a quicker recovery route to normal corneal sensitivity.

Matsui et al[74] compared the effect of PRK and LASIK on corneal sensations. They reported that the *loss of corneal sensations was significantly greater following LASIK than after PRK*. The recovery of sensation was within 3 months in either case.

CORNEAL SCARRING

Corneal scar is rare but visually devastating complication after surface ablation. It can be a consequence of different complications following PTK or PRK. The exaggerated healing response in the form of subepithelial haze may culminate in corneal scarring[74]. The poor epithelization of the surface is rare. It occurs only in a badly managed case or in an eye neglected by the patient. Bacterial keratitis may also heal with scarring of the cornea.

In a study conducted by Seiler and co-workers, the incidence of scar tissue due to subepithelial haze was 1% in eyes that underwent correction of < -6.0 D and 17% in eyes where correction exceeded –6.0 D[38].

COMPLICATIONS AFTER PTK

Phototherapeutic keratectomy (PTK) has been found to be a relatively safe procedure by all the clinical studies and the incidence of vision threatening complications is rare (Chapter 11).

The complications following PTK are listed below.
1. Postoperative pain
2. Delayed epithelial healing
3. Sterile stromal infiltrates
4. Microbial keratitis
5. Corneal haze and scar
6. Corneal hypoesthesia
7. Steroid induced rise of IOP
8. Reactivation of herpes keratitis
9. PTK induced refractive changes
10. Recurrence of corneal dystrophies and degenerations
11. Graft failure

The first seven complications have been discussed in the preceding section. However these post-PTK problems are minor and rarely disturbing when compared to the complications and results of keratoplasty. *The only undesired effect that is a common occurrence after PTK is hyperopic shift.*

CORNEAL HAZE

This complication needs to be discussed again in the context of PTK for a number of reasons. First in cases of PTK, corneal haze should be differentiated from a partially treated corneal opacity. Secondly corneal haze is not disturbing in cases of corneal disorders. The reason is that the corneal disorders themselves are associated with decrease in corneal clarity. There is improvement in corneal clarity following PTK even in the presence of corneal haze. Moreover persistent corneal haze is an uncommon finding. It responds well to topical anti-inflammatory agents. Our own clinical results in 48 eyes with different corneal pathologies showed significant improvement in corneal clarity and no clinically significant haze after third postoperative month. The incidence of visually significant corneal haze has been reported from 3% to 40% by different studies depending upon the depth of ablation and other factors (vide supra).

REACTIVATION OF HERPES SIMPLEX KERATITIS

Reactivation of herpetic keratitis has been reported after PTK in cases of herpetic keratitis scars as well as other cases of corneal scars (*Pepose*[75], *Fagerholm*[76]). A past history of herpetic disease is not always elicited. Decrease of corneal sensation and presence of an unexplained sub-epithelial scarring should alert the surgeon of this possibility.

Campos et al[77] and *Hersh et al*[78] used prophylactic oral acyclovir 200 mg four times daily in such cases, started one day before PTK and continued for 10 days. No recurrence occurred during the follow-up period up to 15 months.

Talamo et al[79] pre-treated a patient of herpetic scar for several days with trifluorothymadine. No reactivation of herpes simplex keratitis was noticed in spite of the use of fluoromethalone post operatively.

PTK INDUCED REFRACTIVE CHANGES

Although any types of refractive errors can occur after PTK, *hyperopic shift is the most commonly observed and most undesirable after effect of excimer laser PTK* (see Chapter 17, discussion).

Hyperopic Shift

The ablation in PTK is done in plano-mode. Nonetheless, removal of the corneal tissue from the central part of the cornea causes flattening of the corneal curvature leading to hyperopic shift. Many studies have reported induced hyperopia after PTK. Hyperopic shift up to 8.0 D after PTK was encountered by the initial clinical studies. The degree of hyperopia depends upon:

1. The technique of ablation
2. The depth of ablation

Chamon et al[80] found hyperopia of approx. 6.3 D at 6 months with the **standard taper technique** and approx. 2.0 D using the **modified taper technique**. The later technique treats the edge of the ablated zone with a 2 mm diameter beam by moving the patient's head in circular fashion.

Gartry et al[58] found mean hyperopic shift of +2.85 D in 5 of their patients in whom refraction was possible.

Neel Sher et al[81] reported significant hyperopic shift in 50% of the eyes treated for corneal scars.

In the study by *Campos et al*[77], hyperopic shift occurred in 13 of 18 patients. Two had a myopic shift. In one eye refraction was unaltered and in 2 eyes post operative refraction was not possible due to irregular corneal surface.

Hersh et al[78] reported mean hyperopic shift of +5.40 D of spherical equivalent in 8 of 12 eyes treated with excimer laser PTK for different corneal pathologies. Three eyes exhibited mean *myopic shift* of –1.6 D of spherical equivalent. This was attributable to *off-axis peripheral ablation*.

The various mechanisms postulated for the occurrence of the hyperopic shift are given below.

Wide Beam Systems

In wide beam systems the corneal flattening occurs due to:

1. *Attenuation of laser energy* towards the periphery leading to less ablation in the periphery.
2. *Increasing oblique angle* of the wide beam toward the periphery. The beam is incident at 90 degree angle in the central part and delivers full energy but the effect decreases with oblique beam.

Applicable to Both the Beam Systems

1. *Shielding effect* due to the accumulation of the by products in the periphery caused by centrifugal spray of *the plume*.
2. *Shielding effect* caused by a less viscous masking fluid running off towards the periphery and accumulating there while exposing the central part to more ablation.
3. *Epithelial hyperplasia* occurring at the sharp transition edge between the ablated and the non ablated zones. It is known that the hyperplasia is more, the more is the edge sharpness. The epithelial hyperplasia at the edge causes flattening effect of the central ablated zone.
4. *Centrifugal contraction of* the unablated peripheral corneal lamellae leading to central flattening of the cornea.
5. *Flattening of the tear meniscus* at the periphery of the ablated zone.

Countering the Hyperopic Shift

1. *Intraoperative removal of the ablation byproducts*
   The shielding effect can be done away by appropriate use of a suitable masking agent and gentle *intraoperative removal of the ablation byproducts* with a cellulose sponge.
2. *Tapering the edge*
   Tapering the edge of the ablation zone intraoperatively helps in reducing the hyperopic shift by

reducing the corneal flattening effect at the time of ablation as well as by minimizing the epithelial hyperplasia later.

3. *Pharmacological modulation*
Topical steroids and NSAIDs have been shown to modify the healing response and stromal remodeling. Their long-term use is beneficial for controlling the corneal haze as well for modifying the hyperopic shift.

Myopic Shift

A myopic shift was found in 22 of the 67 eyes treated with Summit excimer laser by FDA sponsored phase II and phase III clinical trials. This change was attributed to paracentral ablations causing corneal steepening.

Campos et al and Hersh et al have also reported a myopic change in some of their patients.

Astigmatism

Although studies, including the FDA trials and our own study on 48 patients, have shown that there is a reduction in the corneal cylinder power, yet iatrogenically induced astigmatism particularly irregular astigmatism does occur in some cases due to the following reasons.

1. Overlapping zone ablation: 2 mm or 3 mm diameter beam ablating over 6 mm zone. The area where the beam overlap are uneven.
2. Scanning mode of ablation: the small beam edges overlap or the entire 6 mm zone may not get ablated uniformly due to unequal distribution of the laser beam over the entire area.
3. Inappropriate use of the masking agent
4. Paraxial ablation (isolated, focal)
5. Decentration of the ablation zone

The refractive changes are unavoidable to a certain extent but can be minimized by employing appropriate strategies for ablation such as:

1. Keeping the ablation depth minimum and avoiding over treatment.
    It is obvious that PTK is done in plano-mode, therefore removal of corneal tissue from the central area would lead to flattening of corneal curvature to a degree proportional to the amount of tissue removed. Recurrent erosion syndrome, where the

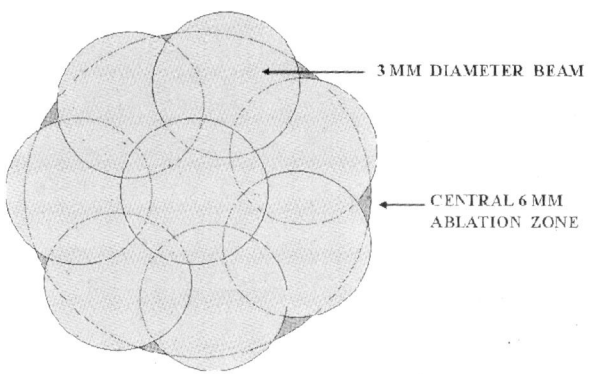

OVERLAPPING ZONE ABLATION

Fig. 26.1: *Creation of such patterns during full treatment would produce an irregular surface*

ablation is minimum (5-7 micron), would cause minimum refractive change. This is achieved by frequent intraoperative assessment of lesion to be removed.

2. Employing the 'Taper technique' to avoid sharp edge at the periphery of ablated zone
3. Using the 'partial ablation' concept
4. Avoiding treatment of visually insignificant lesions
5. Avoiding treatment in the paraxial zone
6. Ensuring proper centration of the laser beam and use of the eye-tracker
7. Frequent use of a masking agent
8. Pharmacological modulation

The number 2 to 7 strategies have been discussed in Chapter 14 and pharmacological modulation has been described under postoperative management.

RECURRENCE OF CORNEAL DYSTROPHIES AND DEGENERATIONS

Recurrences of corneal dystrophy occurring after lamellar or penetrating keratoplasty are well known in literature. Not many long-term studies are available to evaluate the recurrence rate of corneal dystrophies after successful excimer laser PTK.

Christopher J Rapuano[82] reported recurrence of granular dystrophies in 2 of the 6 treated eyes after 15 and 39 months after PTK. One out of 5 cases of Salzmann's Nodule had recurrence after two years.

Rene Dinh and Rapuano et al[83] found that clinically significant recurrence of dystrophies occurred in 17 of the 43 eyes treated by PTK after a mean follow-up of 19.5 months (1.1 to 71.2 months). The recurrence rate was highest in Reis-Bucklers dystrophy (47% after a mean follow up of 25.6 months), followed by basement membrane dystrophy (42%). Epithelial membrane basement dystrophy reoccurred earliest (mean 7.9 months). This is because they are diffuse disorders and the conventional PTK procedure treats only the 6 mm optical zone. The pancorneal ablation should be more appropriate for treating these disorders. Recurrence of Granular dystrophy was seen in 23% eyes after PTK after 28 to 48 months (mean 36.3 months) while the recurrence time reported by others after penetrating keratoplasty is 13 to 36 months in almost all grafts. The recurrence of lattice dystrophy after PTK was 14% after 6 months while it has been reported as high as 75% after primary keratoplasty and 68% in re-grafts. The mean recurrence interval could not be ascertained as these are known to reoccur after an average of 9 years (3-26 years) after penetrating keratoplasty.

The authors concluded "though corneal dystrophies are likely to recur even after PTK, re-treatment with PTK is easier and possible as long as the corneal thickness remains more than 250 micron".

GRAFT FAILURE

PTK has been utilized to correct iatrogenic refractive error, mainly astigmatism in cases of penetrating keratoplasty. There have been reports of graft rejection or failure following such treatment in some cases. This is attributed to the inflammation and large epithelial defect produced after photoablation.

Other researchers have not reported this complication. *Campos et al[84]* treated 12 eyes, *John et al* 3 eyes and *Rapuano et al[85]* 4 eyes for post keratoplasty refractive errors. They did not find any case of graft rejection or failure. *Christine et al[86]* had similar experience from a small series of post keratoplasty PTK except for the occurrence of significant corneal haze after few months.

Nonetheless, it is prudent to take preventive measures for this group while performing PTK. Potent topical steroids should be started few days prior to the procedure and stopped for initial few days after surgery. They should be restarted after complete re-epithelization has occurred.. One should not hesitate to use full doses of systemic steroids in high-risk cases. Any suspicion of this complication should warrant the use of high dose intravenous and topical steroids.

INTERMEDIATE TO LONG TERM COMPLICATIONS AFTER PHOTOREFRACTIVE SURGERIES

1. Undercorrection
2. Overcorrection
3. Induced astigmatism
4. Irregular astigmatism
5. Central islands
6. Loss of BCVA
7. Regression
8. Corneal haze
9. Halos and ghost images
10. Recurrent corneal erosion syndrome
11. Recurrent corneal micro-erosions
12. Steroid induced elevation of intra-ocular pressure

OVERCORRECTION AND UNDERCORRECTION

The currently available literature shows that excimer laser refractive surgeries have proved to be one of the most accurate refractive procedures among all such procedures that have been in practice till date. But their techniques and algorithms are yet to be refined to achieve perfection and provide an emmetropic state of refraction. The predictability of refractive correction within 1.0 D ranges from 87–94.4% on an average for PRK and 90–98.7% for LASIK (Table 25.5). For higher corrections, the predictability is still less. *Condon et al[88] reported that undercorrection occurred more commonly after LASIK while Wilson found overcorrection to be more common[89].*

Primary undercorrection has to be differentiated from *regression* and *central steep islands*, which also presents with myopic refraction after excimer laser refractive surgery. The reasons for *primary* overcorrection and undercorrection could be one or combination of the following.

Intraoperative Hydration Changes

Dehydration of the stroma results in increased ablation rate and overcorrection. This can occur due to longer time taken for epithelium removal during PRK or delay in starting ablation after creating the flap during LASIK.

The opposite effect and undercorrection would result in case of stromal hydration due to application of the fluid to the stroma before ablation.

Inadequate Removal of the Epithelium

Undercorrection after PRK can result because of inadequate epithelial debridement because the remaining epithelium would consume some of the calculated laser pulses.

Natural Variation in Healing

The healing response of an individual eye may vary. It has been found that there are three types of refractive responses after PRK. Type I healers have refraction within 1.0 D. Type II healers (inadequate responders) remain overcorrected and type III healers show undercorrection > -1.0 D (see Chapter 5).

Age of the Patient

It has been found that older patients show overcorrection because they do not have a strong healing response[87].

Inaccurate Refraction

Inaccurate preoperative determination of refraction, particularly inadequate cycloplegia in an accommodative patient or improper determination of the cylindrical axis can result in induced postoperative refractive errors. These aspects have been discussed in Chapter 19.

Refractive Instability

The preoperative myopia or the induced curvature change due to contact lens (CL) wear may not have stabilized. Warpage due to CL wear also should be ruled out by serial refraction and computerized topography.

Errors of Feeding the Refractive Data

A wrong input of the preoperative refraction into the computer of the laser system, though inadvertent, is another common avoidable cause of primary over- or undercorrection.

Management

1. Overcorrections may be treated by abrupt withdrawal of the postoperative steroid therapy after PRK. This is supposed to stimulate wound-healing response and induce regression.
2. If the overcorrection persists, scrapping the epithelium may stimulate a stronger healing response[90]. But one must be cautious because this may result in increased haze/ subepithelial opacity.
3. Management of undercorrection is heavily dependent on presence of haze, which aggravates it or even leads to regression of the refractive effect. Initial treatment is with intensive topical steroids[44].
4. Loewenstein et al[46] have advocated scrapping of epithelium for myopic undercorrection also.
5. *Specifically designed contact lenses*, which cause less stagnation of tear-fluid over the apex of flat ablation zone, are useful alternatives for treating under- and overcorrection.
6. Retreatment is indicated, at least after 6 months, when refraction has stabilized. PRK enhancement may be done for myopic undercorrection and regression. But LASIK offers a better treatment strategy for both undercorrection and overcorrection with superior results. Retreatment and enhancement strategies are dealt with in Chapter 27.

INDUCED/RESIDUAL ASTIGMATISM

Induced astigmatism is less common than primary undercorrection and overcorrection, but can be more troublesome for the patient particularly in case of an irregular astigmatism.

Several causes such as decentred ablation, asymmetrical healing after PRK and a non-homogenized laser beam may be responsible for induced astigmatism *after spherical corrections*.

Residual astigmatism can result from inaccurate refraction and determination of the cylindrical axis, imperfectness of the treatment algorithm/technique, CL induced corneal warpage and *rotational ocular shift/drift* during ablation. Moreover, treatment of primary astigmatism may be incomplete or there may even be a worsening in astigmatism or a shift in the previous axis.

After LASIK, flap folds or wrinkles are the commonest cause of irregular astigmatism. This type is amenable to the corrective procedure described for flap folds (vide infra). Cases detected later can be managed by a PTK smoothening after lifting the flap. Other causes include interface debris and epithelial ingrowths and wound margin ulcerations. These are discussed under complications of LASIK. Another important cause of irregular astigmatism post-LASIK is the damaged/blunt blade, which results in an irregular stromal bed before ablation.

Significant induced astigmatism and irregular astigmatism are major cause of decreased UCVA and loss of BCVA respectively.

CENTRAL STEEP ISLANDS

Definition and Incidence Rate

Central steep island is an area of > 3.0 D increased corneal power within an otherwise flat, centered ablation zone. It is a well-defined small area, which is usually central and oval or circular in shape (colour plate 12, photograph 60). Earlier different authors had defined a central island in different ways. Lin[93] defined it as an area steeper than 1.5 D and larger than 2.5 mm. Kruger et al[101] considered an abnormality steeper than 3.0 D and larger than 1.5 mm to be a central steep island.

The incidence of central islands varied from 0-30% in different PRK studies during the initial period. Hersh et al[91] and Salz et al[92] found none or only few cases of central island while Lin[93] and Levin et al[94] reported 25–29% incidence rate. The later authors found the overall incidence of the central steep topographical abnormality in 67% of their cases out of which 26% had elevation > 3.0 D. These differences might be due to the difference in the techniques of surgery, different methodology used for the detection, different definition adopted and the period after surgery when evaluated for central islands. Effective CVK systems were not available during the initial days of photorefractive surgeries. Moreover the islands may be missed if CVK is performed after some months because the central islands have a natural tendency to self-resolve.

The high incidence of central islands during the early period was mainly a result of wide beam ablation techniques and the method employed for ablation plume evacuation. The incidence of central islands has significantly decreased with the scanning laser beam with uniform energy distribution. *Central islands are rare with the flying spot laser[99]. In addition, the modern systems have modified software that delivers additional pulses to the central area. This strategy further minimizes the incidence of central steep islands.*

Possible Causes for Central Islands

The different explanations offered to explain the genesis of central islands are as follows[95-98].

Poor Homogenization of the Wide/Broad Laser Beam

The poorly homogenized beam might have "cold spots" that cause less ablation.

Pooling of Fluid Centrally

There may be regional difference in hydration of the cornea. The fluid may accumulate centrally, where more flattening is taking place leading to decreased ablation. Centripetal displacement of fluid may be caused by the acoustic shock waves generated by wide laser beam.

Accumulation of Ablation Plume Centrally

The ablation by-products, if not removed effectively, tend to accumulate centrally, thereby causing undercorrection in that region and development of central islands.

Focal Epithelial Hyperplasia

The deeply ablated central part of the cornea suffers from focal epithelial hyperplasia, which manifests as increased corneal power. This theory does not explain the early occurrence of central islands, much before the epithelization is complete.

Presentation

The patient presents with undercorrection within first few months or even as early as within the first postoperative week[98]. The visual symptoms due to central islands, during the early postoperative months, include decrease in BCVA, monocular diplopia, glare and ghost images. The visual rehabilitation time is prolonged. The number of eyes with central islands that suffered loss of more than two lines of BCVA had been as much as 32% in comparison to 0–8% without them.

The diagnosis of a central island is made with the use of modern computerized videokeratography (CVK). This modality differentiates a case of central island from that of primary undercorrection, focal regression and decentred ablation that also would produce similar symptoms.

Time Course of Central Islands

Central islands have been found to resolve spontaneously. This may take about 6 months in some cases. No long-term visual or refractive disability occurs in the majority of cases[93, 100].

Though central steep islands are rare after LASIK, they do not resolve spontaneously as readily as the ones following PRK[89].

Prevention of Central Islands

Central steep islands are best prevented by the use of spot scanning laser beam, with delivery of additional pulses to the central part of ablation zone.

Treatment of Persistent Central Islands

As mentioned earlier, these topographic abnormalities are self-resolving. Occasionally persisting central islands following PRK and LASIK would require treatment after about 6 months. The following may be utilized to manage a case of *persistent central island with visual symptoms*.

1. A hard contact lens may be prescribed.
2. Patient with central island and residual refractive myopia may be treated with PRK after epithelium debridement. Retreatment through the intact epithelium has been found to increase the incidence of this topographical abnormality.
3. A PTK technique may be employed with the use of a masking agent to shield the area surrounding the island.
4. The same PTK approach can be employed in cases of LASIK after lifting the flap.

DECREASE IN VISUAL FUNCTIONS

Previously photorefractive surgeries were mainly performed for correction of spherocylindrical errors and improving UCVA. The results of these refractive surgeries were mainly compared in terms of predictability of refractive correction, the postoperative UCVA and any loss of BCVA. *However, visual acuity in itself is a poor predictor of an individual's visual performance under different illumination conditions as well as for certain specific perceptual tasks.* After the introduction of wavefront technology, more concern has been generated about the other visual functions like low contrast visual acuity (LCVA), glare visual acuity (GVA) and improvement in the BCVA better than 20/20.

Loss of BCVA

Excimer laser refractive surgeries had been found to result in loss of best-corrected visual acuity (BCVA). Although LogMAR visual acuity gives a better idea, Snellen's visual acuity continues to be used in majority of clinical studies. Review of the clinical reports shows that the loss of more than two lines of BCVA ranges from 0–14% of the eyes in case of PRK and 0–9% after LASIK depending upon the degree of attempted correction and type of refractive error. *Cases of high and extreme myopia and high hypermetropia and astigmatism are associated with the highest of these figures* (Table 25.1–25.8).

The possible reasons for loss of best-corrected visual acuity are as follows.

1. Higher corrections require longer ablation time that may lead to loss of fixation with consequent decentered ablation.
2. Theoretically the chances of induced astigmatism are increased due to increased ablation time and more demanding algorithms.
3. The incidence of central islands become more due to use of higher energy with subsequent more acoustic and surface waves, and increased requirement for intraoperative removal of ablation by-products and surface fluid.
4. Association of significant subepithelial haze and scarring with higher attempted corrections after PRK.
4. Decrease in the *"effective optical zone"* with high myopic treatments. Holladay et al[144] studied the topography changes in corneal asphericity in cases of –1.5 to –18.0 D myopic corrections. They found that the effective optical zone decreased progressively, though in a non-linear manner, with increase in attempted correction. This decrease in *effective zone* was associated with poor visual outcome in > -12.0 D corrections. The results are as summarized in Table 26.2.

Table 26.2: Change in effective zone diameter with increase in the attempted correction

Myopia	Intended optical zone	Effective optical zone after treatment
-1.50 D	6 mm	6.0 mm
-5.00 D	6 mm	5.4 mm
-10.0 D	6 mm	4.6 mm
-12.0 D	6 mm	4.3 mm
-15.0 D	6 mm	3.8 mm
-18.0 D	6 mm	3.2 mm

The causes of loss of BCVA following photorefractive surgeries[4, 55, 56, 58, 102, 143-178] are listed below.

1. Corneal haze and scar after PRK.
2. Irregular astigmatism.
3. Central islands.
4. Decentration of the ablation zone.
5. Corneal infective keratitis.
6. Increase in higher order aberrations after photorefractive surgeries (Chapter 25).
7. Induced optical aberration due to LASIK flap[143].
8. Decrease in *effective zone diameter* with high correction[144].

9. Diffuse lamellar keratitis (DLK) after LASIK.
10. Flap complications in case of LASIK.
11. Inadvertent corneal perforation during LASIK.
13. LASIK induced optic neuropathy[185-191].
14. LASIK induced corneal ectasia.

Time Course and Management of Loss of BCVA

Visual loss recovers after about 6 months following PRK and earlier after LASIK as corneal haze and central islands resolve with time and medical management. Decentred ablation and astigmatism can be taken care of by repeat procedure and appropriately fitted contact lenses. Recovery in other cases is also good with proper management except in the last two situations. Flaps related complications and infective keratitis should be avoided using all possible preventive measures. Timely detection and appropriate management can avert visual loss due to these reasons and DLK also.

Low Contrast and Glare Visual Acuity

Only limited numbers of studies have reported on contrast visual acuity following photorefractive keratectomy (PRK)[103-107] and LASIK[108-112].

Time Course of Decreased Contrast Acuity

The contrast visual acuity decreases during the first few months following photorefractive surgeries. It returns to the preoperative level after about 3–6 months following PRK for low myopic correction[104, 105] but takes longer than 6 months tome in case of high myopes[104]. Similar observation about higher loss of contrast visual acuity with greater attempted correction was made by Nakamura et al[111] following LASIK. Most of the available clinical studies reported earlier recovery of contrast visual acuity (1–3 months) after LASIK[108, 109, 112].

There is a large variation in the reported time taken for recovery of contrast visual acuity (CVA), varying from 1–12 months. This difference in recovery time is mainly due to the difference in the contrast sensitivity unit/*spatial frequency* used by different authors. Perez-Santonja et al[108] used spatial frequencies at 3 cpd (cycles per degree) and 6 cpd. They reported that contrast sensitivity took 3 months to recover to the preoperative level following LASIK. Mutyala et al[108] found that recovery took place after 1 month when contrast sensitivity was tested in the relatively higher-contrast region (at 6, 12 and 18 cpd).

Contrast visual acuity in the low-contrast region (1.3–3.4 cpd) is affected more and takes longer, at least 6 months, to return to the preoperative level[110]. Nakamura et al also found higher loss of CVA in low-contrast region than in intermediate-contrast region.

In contrast, Stevens et al found that the CVA remained significantly reduced even after 12 months of follow up when the Pelli-Robson chart was used for assessment following PRK for myopia[106] and hyperopia[107].

Factors leading to loss of CVA

Decreased Corneal Clarity Corneal haze and opacities following the refractive procedure, particularly PRK with deeper ablation can cause loss of contrast visual acuity.

Optical Factors Optical factors such as surface irregularity, *induced aberrations* (spherical, coma and distortions) due to corneal asphericity. These aberrations are aggravated in dim illumination. Therefore CVA under low levels of illumination is affected more severely.

Poor Quality of Ablated Surface It results in light scattering and reduced CVA.

Interface Opacities These may be subtle amount of debris, inflammatory residua and epithelial cells that may not actually decrease Snellen's visual acuity.

Neural Factors Some studies have shown decrease in the retinal nerve fibers following LASIK. But this is not likely to be a cause for reduced CVA as there is recovery in this visual function, though the retinal nerve fiber layer may not recover.

Glare Visual Acuity

Only few studies have measured glare visual acuity (GVA) following refractive surgeries[113-121]. GVA is also reduced like contrast visual acuity. The main factors leading to loss of GVA are small ablation zone, corneal haze and disparity between the ablation zone and pupil diameter. Seiler et al[115] found loss of GVA in up to 19% of eyes after PRK. The loss of glare visual acuity showed a correlation with the attempted correction[114]. This was related to *reduction of effective optical zone* with higher correction. Moreover the eyes with clear corneas also suffered from this loss[114, 115]. This was attributed to spherical aberrations and reduced optical homogeneity of the postoperative cornea.

GLARE, HALOS WITH OR WITHOUT STARBURST AND GHOST IMAGES

These visual disturbances during night or dim illumination were the most disturbing problems during the early period of photorefractive surgeries. Their incidence was 10–80% in the earlier clinical studies[58, 116-121]. The following factors are responsible for these phenomena.

Ablation Zone Diameter vs. Pupil Size

The main cause for the above visual symptoms used to be a small ablation zone that was smaller than the entrance pupil under conditions of decreased illumination (see Chapter 20, techniques for PRK: effect of ablation zone diameter). Young myopic patients, who had larger pupillary diameter, were the main suffers.

Glare and halos occur due to light refraction through the uncorrected peripheral zone that falls within the larger pupil. In addition the rays passing through this zone are not focused on the retina and result in ghost image.

The problem of glare and halos has markedly decreased with the newer treatment protocols employing larger ablation zones. Table 26.3 shows effect of ablation zone diameter on the incidence of halos and glare.

Table 26.3: Effect of ablation zone diameter on incidence of glare and halos

Ablation zone diameter	Incidence of night glare/ halos (% of eyes)
4.0 mm	75-80%
4.5 mm	35-40%
5.0 mm	20%
6.0 mm	5%
7.0 mm	0.5%

Light Scattering

Light scattering may be caused by corneal haze, surface irregularity or induced spherical aberrations. The result is glare disability and/ or starburst effect.

Management of Glare and Halos

1. These visual disturbances are best managed through prevention of their occurrence. Pupillary diameter of the patient must be carefully measured under scotopic conditions and the ablation zone be kept larger than the pupil diameter.
2. If haze is responsible for the symptoms, it should be managed with topical steroids. The symptoms mostly abate over time. This may happen due to the resolution of the underlying cause such as haze or anatomical irregularity or may be due to patient's adaptation in other cases.
3. In case of disparity between ablation zone diameter and pupillary size, enlargement of the ablation zone may be attempted if the postoperative refraction shows residual myopia.
4. If the patient is emmetropic or overcorrected, ablation zone enlargement is not advised. The patient is managed with low concentration of pilocarpine (0.5%) to keep the pupil in a slightly constricted state.

REGRESSION

Definition

Regression is defined as a *decrease in the refractive correction following photorefractive surgery after attainment of desired correction* in the immediate postoperative period. It is a change in the postoperative manifest and cycloplegic refraction towards the original refractive error, i.e. *a myopic shift after myopic ablation or a hyperopic shift after hyperopic ablation*.

Regression should be differentiated from primary under correction, myopic refraction due to central steep islands and the natural progression in case of myopia.

Early Regression

Early regression occurs within 6 months of the refractive surgery.

Late Regression

Late regression is defined as a drift of the refraction towards the pre operative refractive state after 6 months to 1 year. In this case the postoperative refraction had been more or less stable before the occurrence of late regression.

Long-term Regression

This has been described after one year of PRK. Epstein et al[122] observed regression till 18 months and Kim et al[123] reported regression of effect up to 3 years following PRK. Seiler et al[38] found regression in 20% eyes during second year following PRK.

Factors Associated with Regression

Most studies have found that regression is significantly related to the degree of corneal haze, depth of ablation (attempted correction) and non-compliance of topical steroid therapy following surgery. Pang et al[126] have reported an association with patient's age also, with younger patients showing greater regression. This is related to a more aggressive healing response in them.

Refractive Error

Patients of high and extreme myopia, hyperopia and high astigmatism are more prone to develop regression. Stevens JD[124] reported regression > 0.5 D in 32% eyes with high myopia. Williams[125] reported regression in 14% eyes with –6.0 to –10.0 D correction, in 20% eyes with –10.0 to –15.0 D and 33.3% eyes with > -15 D of correction. Pang et al[126] found regression -1.0 D in 1.17% eyes with moderate myopia (-4.0 D to –7.9 D) and in 6.3% eyes with high myopia (-8.0 D).

Ditzen et al[127] also have found greater regression with higher myopic correction. They reported mean regression of up to –5.0 D in eyes with pre operative error more than –15.5 D as compared to mean 1.0 D regression in eyes with < -6.0 D of myopic correction. The regression rate was twice as high in the high myopia group than that in the low myopia group.

Daush et al[128] reported that the *tapered transition zone* technique for myopic correction resulted in less regression in comparison to the conventional PRK technique (see Chapter 20: PRK techniques). Seiler et al[38] reported re-operation rate ranging from 0 – 40% depending on the degree of pre operative myopia (0% in eyes with less than –3.0 D and 40% in eyes with more than 9.1 D correction).

High myopes may regress so dramatically that the postoperative refraction may reach the pre- operative value.

Refractive Procedures and Techniques

PRK: Regression used to be a significant problem with PRK during the early period (vide supra). The high incidence of regression was mainly due to smaller ablation zone diameter and wide beam laser systems. The incidence has decreased with techniques using larger zone diameter and scanning laser systems with algorithms producing smooth transitions of ablation zone periphery.

LASIK: Regression is less common following LASIK as compared to PRK[89, 129]. Refraction stability is found to be better after LASIK[48]. The overall regression rate following LASIK is about 5% to 17%[130-132]. The incidence of regression is higher with hyperopic LASIK and high myopic corrections.

Ablation Zone Diameter

Small ablation zone diameter is associated with greater incidence of regression. O'Brart et al[133] found greater regression in eyes treated with smaller ablation zone (4 mm) than in the second eye of the same patient treated with 5 mm zone. Utilization of ablation zone diameter 6 mm or more has resulted in significant reduction in the regression rate (Chapter 20)

Individual's Response

If one eye of the patient had suffered from regression, then the second eye is also more prone to develop the same complication[134]. Some individuals may develop marked regression. Grant R. Snibson[135] has reported such a tendency in some patients to develop marked regression so as to revert back to their pre operative refractive error.

Mechanisms of Regression in case of PRK

Epithelial Hyperplasia

The epithelial hyperplasia occurs in response to the depth of ablation. It tries to cover the changed surface curvature produced by ablation. *Epithelial hyperplasia occurs proportionately to the depth of ablation and the abruptness of ablation zone edge.* Smaller ablation zone and deeper ablations are associated with greater degree of epithelial hyperplasia and subsequent higher incidence of regression.

Stromal Remodeling

Synthesis of new collagen, stromal remodeling and increase in thickness are stimulated by excimer laser ablation (see Chapter 5). This stromal healing response is found to be greater with higher depth of ablation. The stromal remodeling has been implicated in regression of the refractive effect.

Corneal Haze

A definite association has been shown between the degree of corneal haze and myopic regression. Both of these changes are found to occur together in many cases. Regression and haze increase with the attempted correction/higher ablation depth. Topical corticosteroids, which control the corneal haze has been found to reduce/revert regression after myopic correction.

Beam Profile

Older, wide beam laser systems were said to cause early regression due to the hot centers within the beam. The hot spot of laser beam caused abrupt edge within the ablation zone and stimulated epithelial hyperplasia resulting in myopic regression.

Wide Beam Lasers

Wide beam lasers have high fluence. These laser beams were thought to cause greater acoustic shockwaves, which led to increased stimulation of keratocytes. This resulted in an increased stromal remodeling and regression.

Laser Systems

It has been reported that Summit Technology Excimed UV200 (Waltham, MA) Laser System produced over correction followed by early regression. Other wide beam systems, e.g. the VisX 20/20, Summit Omnimed and Apogee Lasers use large ablation zones (6 mm or more). These systems are found to produce less overcorrection and regression.

Forward Shift of the Corneal Curvature

Recently, studies have reported forward shift of the anterior as well as posterior surface of the cornea. Miyata et al[136] found significant forward corneal shift following PRK. The mean forward shift in the posterior corneal curvature was 36.6 ± 25.3 µ at 1 week and 55.1±46.1µ at one year. The shift was maximum between 1 and 6 month and stabilized thereafter. No progressive shift occurred after 1 year to suggest true ectasia. *A statistically significant correlation was noticed with myopic regression and the forward shift of the corneal curvature.* They also reported that this change was more prominent in corneas with less preoperative corneal thickness and higher myopia requiring greater ablation.

Mechanisms of Regression in case of LASIK

Regression following LASIK has different mechanisms than the ones responsible for PRK regression. Corneal haze and stromal remodeling do not seem to play any significant role for development of regression after LASIK.

Forward Shift of the Corneal Curvature

The main cause appears to be corneal curvature change following high correction. Baek et al[198] reported LASIK induced mean 40.9±24.8 µ forward shift of cornea in 196 eyes 1 month after surgery. A positive correlation with thinner corneas, higher intraocular pressure and greater laser ablation was noticed in this study.

Increase in Central Corneal Thickness

Chayet et al[137] reported that early regression after LASIK in high myopes was due to increase in corneal thickness associated central corneal steepening. They found that the mean regression, increase in corneal power and increase in corneal thickness were symmetric in magnitude and time course throughout one-year of follow-up. Increase in central corneal thickness is related to epithelial hyperplasia.

Early Corneal Ectatic Change

Regression after LASIK might represent early cases of corneal ectasia that would become evident after longer follow-up (Chapter 6). Seitz et al[199] found the increase in posterior corneal power and the curvature change to be significantly greater in eyes with residual bed thickness < 250 micron. Similar observations were made by Wang et al[197] also.

Management of Regression

The management of regression following PRK significantly depends on the degree of corneal hage. Regression associated with haze responds well with aggressive and prolonged therapy with topical steroids. Retreatment in refractory cases is deferred for 6 months till refraction becomes stable. Pop et al[138] found the outcome to be good after retreatment in cases with minimum haze in comparison to the cases with significant corneal haze. They advised a waiting period of 12 months in the latter cases to obtain best results, so that haze subsides naturally. Comaish et al[139] have opined that regression following PRK can be best treated with LASIK because PRK is less successful for retreatment. This is so because the factors operating for development of regression after *primary PRK* would again lead to regression following retreatment.

However retreatment of regression with LASIK may be limited by the *residual bed thickness*. LASEK may offer an alternative for retreating cases of regression that are left with thinner corneas (Chapter 24).

RECURRENT CORNEAL EROSION/ MICROEROSIONS AND DRY EYE

McGhee et al[140] have reported symptoms of discomfort, mild pain on waking up and feeling of stickiness of the eyelid in 1.3% of 306 eyes one-year following PRK. Epithelial microcysts were found in 2.9% eyes at 3 month and in 1.6% eyes at one year.

Hovanesian et al[141] compared the symptoms of microerosions in 231 eyes that underwent PRK and 550 post-LASIK eyes. They reported that these problems were significantly more common, more severe and more prolonged after PRK. However *dry eye* symptoms were more common in LASIK patients (48% vs. 43%).

True recurrent corneal erosion syndrome (RCES) is reported more often after LASIK than after PRK. Many studies have reported occurrence of this complication following LASIK. Ti et al[142] found that the reason may be an *undiagnosed case of epithelial basement membrane dystrophy* (EBMD) or *epithelial trauma* during the surgery. They also suggested that cases that show loose epithelium after completion of LASIK are potential candidates for RCES subsequently.

PRK, like PTK, is a surface ablation procedure. Therefore it is supposed to be beneficial for the undiagnosed cases of EBMD. However 1.2–2.5% incidence of RCES has been reported by different PRK studies[140].

COMPLICATIONS OF LASIK

INTRAOPERATIVE COMPLICATIONS

1. Inadequate exposure
2. Inadequate suction
3. Microkeratome and flap complications
   - Incomplete pass/ incomplete flap
   - Thin flaps and buttonholes
   - Free cap
   - Corneal perforation
   - Shifted flap
   - Wrinkled flap
   - Flap edema, shrinkage and stretching
   - Interface debris
   - Intraoperative bleeding
   - Epithelial complications
   - Intraoperative decentration

EARLY POSTOPERATIVE COMPLICATIONS (24-48 Hours)

1. Pain
2. Epithelial complications
3. Infections
4. Diffuse lamellar keratitis
5. Interface debris
6. Wrinkles and folds
7. Shifted and dislodged flaps

LATE POSTOPERATIVE COMPLICATIONS

1. Epithelial ingrowth
2. Stromal melts
3. Overcorrection/ undercorrection
4. Regression
5. Haze
6. Central islands
7. Irregular astigmatism
8. Small optical zone
9. Decentration
10. Keratectasia

INTRAOPERATIVE COMPLICATIONS

The intraoperative complications of LASIK are mainly related to the microkeratome and the corneal flap[145-150, 153,154]. These complications have significantly reduced over time as the surgeons have become more familiar with the technique, and with improvement in the microkeratomes themselves (Table 26.4).

INADEQUATE EXPOSURE

Adequate exposure of the cornea is an important prerequisite to avoid many of the flap related complications in LASIK. The exposure may be insufficient because of deep-set eyes or small palpebral fissure. Poor draping technique and improperly chosen lid speculum may also lead to inadequate exposure. Occasionally previous surgery or trauma to the orbit or lids may be its cause.

Adequate exposure results in difficulty in placing the suction ring, which leads to failure in achieving adequate suction before the flap cutting. It can also directly interfere with microkeratome pass.

Table 26.4: Incidence of intraoperative flap complications of LASIK (% of eyes)

Investigator (period)	No. of eyes	Total rate	Insufficient suction	Incomplete pass	Button-hole	Free cap	Irregular/thin flap	Shifted flaps	Flap shrinkage	Complications with hansatome ACS
Gimbel et al[146] (1996-1999)	4015	2.988	0.45	0.58	0.17	0.20	0.37	0.82	0.08	NR	NR
Jacobs et al[148] (1998-2000)	84711	0.302	0.034	0.099	0.070	0.012	0.087	0	0	0.16	6.38

NR= not reported

Prevention and Management

This complication can be prevented by.

1. Careful draping techniques to maximize exposure.
2. Use of speculum with good spring or locking mechanism.
3. Proper head position to achieve central eye position.
4. Assistant should provide downward pressure on speculum during microkeratome pass.
5. If the exposure is still inadequate inspite of the above measures, lateral canthotomy may be necessary in rare circumstances.

INADEQUATE SUCTION

As mentioned above, inadequate exposure can result in difficulty in placing the suction ring that leads to inadequate *build-up* of the suction. Small corneal diameter resulting in conjunctival tenting and blockage of the suction port may also be responsible for inadequate *build-up* of the suction. Inadvertent movement of suction ring, drape or speculum during the procedure can lead to *loss of suction*.

The result can be an incomplete, irregular or thin flap or button holing of the flap.

Prevention and Management

1. Attention should be paid to techniques that optimize exposure and proper placement of suction ring.
2. Suction ring should be placed firmly against globe so that it is well seated before suction is turned on.
3. Any manipulation of the suction ring, drapes or speculum must be avoided.
4. If any manipulation is made, IOP should be re-measured with Barraquer tonometer.

When inadequate suction is noticed by IOP pressure measurement, the measures to be taken are:

1. Suction is released.
2. Head position, drapes and speculum are readjusted.
3. The suction ring is repositioned after the above adjustments.
4. If available and appropriate. a smaller ring may be used in case the above measures are unsuccessful.

INCOMPLETE PASS/ INCOMPLETE FLAP

Incomplete pass of the microkeratome is due to either *mechanical obstacles* or *electrical failure*.

Mechanical obstructions may be external or *internal obstruction* in the form of debris of precipitated crystals of salt and loose epithelium, etc. inside the gear system or on the gear track of the suction ring. *External obstruction* to the microkeratome movement is commonly due to poor exposure, obstruction by drapes, lid, eyelashes or speculum and presence of conjunctival fold on the gear track. Improper cleaning and assembly of the microkeratome can lead to jamming. The gear system may itself be faulty.

Occasionally the movement may be aborted automatically or by the surgeon due to loss of adequate suction during the pass.

Incomplete pass of the microkeratome results in premature stopping of the flap cutting before the desired hinge location is reached. If the cut has not passed the ablation zone, laser ablation cannot be continued. Presence of the hinge in the optical zone leads to optical aberrations due to abnormal healing and scarring after the reposition of the incomplete flap.

Prevention

1. A meticulous cleaning method for the microkeratome, as described in chapter 21, should be followed. A careful assembly and inspection of microkeratome and suction ring should be done prior to each use.
2. The microkeratome must be tested through a complete 'forward and reverse cycle' prior to each use to ensure it's functioning. With the ACS 'reverse and forward' and 'stop-and-start' are to be avoided.
3. Proper and adequate exposure must be ensured before starting the procedure. Lateral canthotomy might be needed in rare cases.
4. Excess use of BSS fluid is to be avoided as it forms crystals that may lead to motor head dysfunction in subsequent cases. Ideally distilled water should be used.
5. The electrical connections are checked for continuity and any other fault.

Management

1. If the hinge is not in the ablation zone, ablation can be carried on after shielding its central part with a sponge.
2. In case the flap hinge is inside the ablation area, it is safe to replace the flap and postpone the procedure. The flap is recut with the same depth plate during the subsequent surgery.

THIN FLAPS/IRREGULAR FLAPS AND BUTTONHOLES

A **thin flap** is created when the microkeratome blade cuts through or above the Bowman's layer, which gives a shiny reflection when the stromal surface is examined under the microscope.

An **irregular flap** can present with either a notch or as a bisected or bi-leveled flap. A **buttonhole flap** is a bi-leveled flap in which the microkeratome blade cuts at two different levels by passing more superficially through the Bowman's layer or the epithelium. If the second level of cutting is through the Bowman's layer but spares the epithelium, then it is a *partial thickness buttonhole*. Flap buttonhole is *full thickness* if the epithelium also has been transected by the cut (Colour Plate 12, Photograph 62). The incidence of thin flap is about 0.3–0.7% and buttonholes is about 0.2–0.5%. The incidence of an irregular flap is lower than that of a thin flap.

Causes of Buttonhole and Thin/Irregular Flaps

1. *Inadequate suction* during the flap creation is often responsible for thin flaps and buttonholes. Situations mentioned in the preceding section, that might lead to inadequate suction should forewarn the surgeon about the possibility of these impending complications.
2. *Abnormal corneal curvature* (<41.0 D or >46.0 D) plays an important role because these complications can occur in spite of the IOP being > 60 mm Hg. Corneas that are excessively *steep, irregular* (e.g. following previous PRK and penetrating keratoplasty) or have *high astigmatism* are prone to develop these complications.

   Corneas *steeper* than normal are said to buckle centrally under applanation by the microkeratome footplate like a tennis ball. This results in a bi-leveled cutting with either a thin section of the central part or a buttonhole. Another explanation given is that the footplate with the cutting blade moves upwards due to an increased resistance offered by the higher corneal curvature.

   In case of *flat corneas*, the tissue may be below the cutting plane in certain location resulting in partial or full thickness buttonhole and thin or irregular flaps.
3. *Microkeratome related* problems such as *torque induced by the weight of the microkeratome* assembly, *poor blade quality* and *improper blade positioning* also might be the cause. *Lack of synchronization* between the forward movement of the head and the oscillatory movement of the blade can result in displacement of the uncut corneal tissue. Cutting through this tissue would then result in the above flap abnormalities of the corneal flap.

Laser ablation has to be aborted because these flap abnormalities carry the risk of irregular astigmatism and epithelial ingrowth after LASIK. If Lasik is performed at a later date, the flap will have to be recut.

Prevention

1. Build-up of an adequate suction and IOP > 60 mm Hg (even above 80 mm Hg) should be ensured for safe flap creation before the microkeratome pass.

2. *A new blade should be used for each patient.* The blade must be examined under the microscope for manufacturing defect or any preoperative damage particularly if it is being reused. The microkeratome should not be placed on a hard surface after assembly to avoid damage to the cutting edge of the blade.
3. In patients with keratometry readings outside the normal limits, deeper depth flap should be considered if the corneal thickness and required ablation permit. A larger suction ring is desirable in case of flat cornea to prevent small flaps and other abnormality.
4. In case of LASIK after penetrating keratoplasty (PK) and previous radial keratotomy (RK), the cornea should be examined for any epithelial plugs or inadequate healing of the keratotomy incisions.
5. The microkeratome should be properly cleaned, assembled and checked prior to each use
6. To ensure proper microkeratome pass, gentle upward support is given to the handle of the Automated Corneal shaper (ACS). A firm downward pressure is applied on the suction ring in case of the Hansatome.

Management

1. Ideally ablation should be abandoned in all cases of abnormal flaps and surgery postponed for 8-12 weeks. The flap is replaced meticulously while carefully managing the epithelial edges. Its adherence is verified. During surgery at a later date, a thicker flap, about 20-60 µ more than the previous should be cut using a *different microkeratome* and *new blade*.
2. In case of a thin flap, *some surgeons proceed with the ablation if the thin area is not in the visual axis*.
3. Other surgeons have used PRK procedure after scraping the epithelium of the repositioned flap. This approach may result in subepithelial haze and scar, particularly in high myopes.
4. Immediate transepithelial PRK after replacing the defective flap has been found to avoid irregular astigmatism and late scarring after photorefractive surgery in these cases of initial irregular cut. Jain et al[155] used this approach in 7 patients of flap abnormality. Six patients had 20/20 and one 20/30 UCVA at 6 month following this treatment.

FREE CAP

Unintended complete cutting of the flap through the hinge area leads to a free cap. Most of the times this complication is a result of *failure of the stopper mechanism* of the keratome during the pass. Loss of suction during pass and a larger and flat cornea (mean keratometry <41.00) are the other causes of a free cap. The incidence of this complication has decreased from about 4.9% to below 1% with improvement in the microkeratomes.

The only problem with a free cap is that it may be lost. Refractive ablation can proceed in case of a complete free cap.

Prevention

The entire microkeratome assembly and the stopper mechanism should be carefully checked prior to each use

Management

1. One can continue the ablation if the cut stromal surface is not less the intended ablation zone.
2. The free cap is retrieved and placed in an antidessication chamber or kept covered in the microkeratome while the ablation is done.
3. Repositioning of the free cap is helped by the regular reflection at the epithelial surface and the preoperative corneal marks. The cap is replaced with stromal side down. It is better to wait for 3–5 minutes before adherence is tested after cap replacement.
4. Sutures are not necessary in most cases. A bandage contact lens is then applied for a few days.
5. If sutures are required, X-shaped, 50% deep 10–0 nylon sutures may be applied at 4 places in, 2 in horizontal and 2 in vertical meridians.

CORNEAL PERFORATION

Corneal perforation is a rare but sight threatening and medico-legally serious complication of the LASIK procedure. Its possibility must be discussed with the patient before obtaining a written consent. Faulty microkeratome assembly like failure to place the depth plate or improper seating the depth plate into the microkeratome is the cause of this avoidable complication[156, 157].

Prevention

This eventuality is to be avoided by careful assembly and inspection of the microkeratome prior to each use.

Management

1. The management depends upon the depth and extent of the cut. A small perforation without any tissue loss and damage to other intraocular structures can be repaired and subsequently treated with systemic and local antibiotics.
2. Severe cases may require corneal transplantation and IOL implantation may be needed if the lens also has been damaged.

INTRAOPERATIVELY SHIFTED/ WRINKLED FLAPS

Microstriae representing only wrinkles in the Bowman's layer of the flap may occur as normal findings on slit-lamp retroillumination. On fluorescein staining they are seen as negatively staining lines. They do not cause any interference to the vision. They possibly form due to rough handling and stretching of the flap while repositioning[146].

Macrofolds in contrast are full thickness folds of the flap. The flap folds can result due to *shifted flap* caused by movement of the eye while doing the 'striae test' or the squeezing of the eye by the patient when drapes and speculum are being removed. *Improper flap repositioning* also causes them. For example *uneven smoothening* during centrifugal movement may cause *radial folds* and during centripetal movement *circumferential folds*. Excessive drying of the flap during the ablation is another possible cause.

Flap folds or wrinkles can lead to irregular astigmatism and visual disturbance resulting in loss of best-corrected visual acuity, particularly the ones that are located in the visual axis. The incidence of significant flap folds is about 0.2–1.5%. It is more in case of thinner and larger flaps and also in cases requiring higher correction[151, 152, 158]. In the latter situation, greater central flattening with decreased support of the stroma leads to a redundant flap, which is less likely to flatten (*the tenting effect*).

Prevention

1. Intraoperative flap displacement can be avoided by asking the patient to fixate on the fixation target while doing the striae test and to avoid squeezing when drapes and speculum are being removed. Care is also essential on the part of the surgeon during their removal.
2. The flap should be protected with a damp sponge during the ablation.
3. The re-positioning of the flap must be done with a delicate touch using a wet sponge. Flap smoothing is begun at the hinge with subsequent motions away from the flap center. The corneal marks placed in the beginning of surgery are important landmarks for an accurate flap replacement. An even 'peripheral gutter' between the flap edge and the peripheral epithelium should be the end point.
4. No fluid should be left under the flap to avoid flap displacement and subsequent folds.

Management

1. The wrinkles may disappear by simple stroking maneuver in the central part of flap using a moist merocel sponge. The edge wrinkles are then smoothened by placing gentle traction with a dry sponge.
2. Use of hypotonic saline (60–80%) or deionized water to hydrate the flap also has been recommended to facilitate flattening of the flap and smoothening the folds.
3. If the folds still remain, the flap should be immediately refloated and properly positioned with gentle manipulation.
4. Suturing of the flap edge with 10–0 nylon suture after stretching the flap may be rarely required.

SHIFTED/WRINKLED FLAPS DURING INITIAL DAYS

Wrinkled or displaced flaps on the next postoperative may be found in about 0.82–1.2% of eyes after LASIK. Several factors like exophthalmos, lagophthalmos, stromal hydration due to excessive irrigation with poor flap adherence and poor blinking, etc. may predispose to flap wrinkling. An association of increased flap wrinkling and highly myopic eyes has been found.

The causes for early postoperative shifted flap include squeezing or rubbing the eyelids, poor intraoperative adherence of the flap, abnormality that may cause poor wetting/ drying such as poor blinking, exophthalmos and lagophthalmos and postoperative trauma. *Trauma may lead to flap displacement even months later*[159, 160] *as the flap is still vulnerable due to incomplete adhesions (see Chapter 6 also)*. Larger diameter and thin flaps, flaps with a small hinge and free caps are more prone for displacement.

Prevention

1. Adherence of the flap must be ensured by the *striae test* at the end of surgery.
2. After the flap repositioning, it may be wise to wait for few minutes before removing the speculum.
3. Superiorly hinged flap avoids upper flap edge displacement caused by squeezing and blinking.
4. A contact lens may be applied during early postoperative period.
5. The patient should be instructed to avoid any contributing cause mentioned above.
6. Attention should be paid to lid abnormalities, etc. and preventive measures should be taken.
7. Wearing of moist chamber during the first 24 hours and subsequently every night for one-two week has been advocated to avoid the risk of shifted flaps.

Management

1. Flap wrinkles may be managed as described previously
2. Shifted flaps are treated by lifting it followed by adequate scrapping and irrigating the interface before carefully repositioning the flap.
3. A contact lens (or sutures) is applied to maintain the position of the flap.

INTERFACE DEBRIS

Interface debris may occur due to fibers, metal fillings, glove powder particles and epithelial tags. The fibers may originate from the sponges and poor quality eye drape. The metallic debris arises from the 'wake' or shattering of the microkeratome blade. Oily secretions from meibomian glands, particles from the cannula, syringe or bottle, tiny air bubbles and *central interface opacification of unknown origin* are some other causes of interface debris. Epithelial ingrowth may also present initially as interface debris[149, 151].

The interface debris may cause visual disturbance if located centrally due to interface irregularity resulting in irregular astigmatism (Colour Plate 12, Photograph 63). It can also leads to an inflammatory reaction and even stromal melt if left unattended.

Prevention

1. Use of 'scrub suits' by the surgeon and scrub covers by the patients, use of powder free gloves and moistening the sponge and any gauge material near the surgical field should take care of the *lint debris*.
2. Adequate cleaning of the microkeratome prior to use, irrigation and intermittent wiping of the cul-de-sac to remove mucous and debris from the microkeratome blade also should be practiced.
3. Cleaning of reusable cannulas, use of disposable syringes and avoiding use of excess fluid in the surgical field should prevent debris from these sources.

Management

1. Certain substances such as metal filings and minute mucous or lipid particles in the interface usually do not cause any inflammation and may be left untreated.
2. Minor interface debris in the periphery also does not require any treatment.
3. But *interface debris in the visual area* or *debris consisting of epithelial tags and potentially disturbing materials such as talk and fibers* needs refloating of the flap and sufficient irrigation to clear the debris.
4. Edge irrigation may be used to clear peripheral debris in some cases.

DIFFUSE LAMELLAR KERATITIS

Diffuse lamellar keratitis (DLK) is an early, non-infectious complication that occurs after *primary LASIK* or LASIK retreatment. It presents as acute inflammatory interface infiltrates, for which no definite single cause can be held responsible. DLK is potentially sight threatening if not recognized and managed early. *Most cases develop within 24–72 hours of an uncomplicated LASIK, though late onset cases have been described in the literature*[172].

This entity was known by a number of synonyms like Sands of Sahara (SOS) syndrome, shifting sands, Sterile interface keratitis, lamellar keratitis, diffuse interface, keratitis (DIK), nonspecific diffuse interstitial keratitis (NSDIK) and interface keratitis interface inflammation after LASIK. The use of so many names for the same clinical entity reflects upon the lack of a definite clinico-pathological consensus about the disorder in the past.

This complication was first noticed by Fraenkel et al[164] as central focal interface opacities. The term DLK was given by Smith and Maloney[165] in 1998. Kaufman and co-authors[166] used the term "sand of the Sahara Syndrome" for the peculiar interface inflammation. Later Maddox et al[167] reported four such cases as shifting Sands of Sahara. Later many reports followed describing this post-LASIK complication. The first widely accepted grading system was proposed by Linbarger et al. It was based on the clinical appearance, symptoms and the management of DLK (vide infra).

Most cases studies have reported occurrence of DLK in an epidemic manner *(epidemic DLK)*, i.e. a large number of cases occurring in that particular series). These are associated with common *endogenous agent* that triggers the inflammation. However Wilson et al[168] have described occurrence of *"sporadic DLK"*. They suggested that these sporadic cases occur mostly as a result of *exogenous factors* such as minor trauma and epithelial injuries after LASIK. Sometimes Betadine may be the inciting factor for inflammation.

Etiology of DLK

Great speculations about the causation of DLK have been made but no single definite cause has been attributed regarding the development of DLK. However certain facts are well accepted for the development of DLK. These are:

1. Diffuse lamellar keratitis is non-infectious.
2. A strong association has been noticed between epithelial defects and DLK. Overlying epithelial defects during LASIK are associated with a higher incidence of DLK[170]. An epithelial defect due to traumatic abrasion or other reasons during postoperative period is also associated with development of late DLK[171].
3. A strong association has been found with the intraoperative use of "Celluvisc" (1% carboxymethylcellulose sodium). Some authors had recommended the use of a lubricating agent during LASIK to prevent epithelial defects and subsequent development of DLK. Samuel et al[169] reported that 80% of their cases developed DLK after the use of Celluvisc while no case of DLK occurred previously with the use of artificial tear with low concentration (0.5%). Their interpretation was that Celluvisc is more viscous and was difficult to remove with irrigation from the interface. Contamination of the interface with this agent possibly triggered the inflammatory reaction leading to development of DLK in such a high number of cases (24 of 30 eyes).
4. The etiology is multifactorial. Large number of factors have been held responsible for the etiopathogenesis of this entity. The common consensus is that these factors incite an *inflammatory response through an immunological mechanism* that causes an acute accumulation of polymorphonuclear cells in the interface that results in different manifestations.

Buhren et al[175] studied the characteristics of cellular infiltrates, the activity of inflammation and other remnants of cellular activity in flap and stroma of stage 1-4 DLK using *confocal microscopy* to correlate these findings with clinical presentation. This study was done because the etiopathogenesis of DLK remains uncertain in the absence of histopathological reports.

In stage 1 and 2 DLK, their findings showed the cells to be mostly mononuclear, having cellular characteristics of lymphocytes and monocytes with some cells with lobed nuclei, presumed to be granulocytes.

Stage 3 showed minimal and stage 4 no active inflammation. The predominant finding was presence of spindle shaped refractile bodies representing decay of inflammatory cells. Increasing number of keratocytes with their cell processes was noticed, that represented keratocyte activation, which was maximum in stage 4 DLK. In addition Descemet's membrane folds, microfolds in the interface and dense scarring was evident in case of stage 4 DLK. These findings correlated well with the clinical findings and the previously proposed pathoanatomy of DLK.

The various agents thought to be responsible for triggering the inflammatory response are:

Endogenous Factors

1. Meibomian gland secretions
2. Bacterial components from eye lid margins
3. Transected corneal epithelial cells
4. Overlying epithelial defects
5. Additional tear film debris
6. Red blood cells (RBCs)

Exogenous Factors

1. Contaminants from instruments and sterilizers
2. Bacterial endotoxin
3. NSAID eye drops caught under the flap

4. Lubricant or dust from microkeratome
5. Particulate matter from the drapes, gown, or gloves
6. Balanced salt solution (BSS)
7. Benzalkonium chloride
8. Bacterial exotoxin
9. Povidone-iodine
10. Soaps and disinfectants on sterilized equipments
11. Excimer laser energy
12. "Celluvisc" (1% carboxymethylcellulose sodium)

Classification of Diffuse Lamellar Keratitis

Linebarger Classification

Linebarger et al have classified DLK into 4 stages. There classification is based on clinical appearance of the lamellar inflammation, its severity and resulting visual symptoms, and therapy guidelines according to the intensity of inflammation. The four stages are as follows.

Stage 1 DLK

Stage 1 is the earliest form of DLK with minimum accumulation of inflammatory cells in the periphery of the interface. Fine, white cells are distributed in a wave like fashion at the periphery of the flap. The visual axis is not involved and no loss of BCVA. Therefore this stage can be easily missed. The incidence of stage 1 DLK is about 2–4%.

Treatment of stage 1 DLK is with aggressive topical therapy with prednisolone acetate 1% every hour while awake. The patient is carefully followed for 24-48 hours.

Stage 2 DLK

Stage 2 DLK is characterized with more diffuse infiltrates involving the central part of the interface and stroma also. The cells produce granular or wave like appearance. Clumping of the inflammatory cells gives the typical *sands of Sahara* appearance. The unaided visual acuity may decrease and the patient may have photophobia and irritation. However there is no loss of BCVA. The conjunctiva is also not hyperemic and there is no anterior chamber reaction in stage 2 also. The incidence of stage 2 DLK is about 0.5%.

Treatment of stage 2 DLK is initially as for stage 1. If there is no satisfactory response in terms of decrease of inflammatory cells, oral prednisolone 60–80 mg daily is recommended, particularly if stage 2 DLK appears on the first postoperative day or there is a history of atopic or allergic disease. The patient is also given prophylactic topical antibiotics. The patient must be followed up daily for improvement.

Stage 3 DLK

The cellular infiltrate is dense and the inflammatory cells show increased clumping in the visual axis. The cellular infiltrate has now lost its wave like appearance. The eye is inflamed and there is clouding of vision and loss of BCVA of more than one line. The incidence of stage 3 DLK is about 0.2%.

Treatment of stage 3 DLK is much more aggressive. The previous treatment, if already started is continued or the medical management is started as in stage 2 for a fresh case. In addition, an immediate surgical intervention is needed. The flap is lifted from the stromal bed and the interface is thoroughly irrigated with sterile distilled water using a merocel sponge. This is done to wash out the infiltrates and any potential agents that might be responsible for the inflammatory reaction.

Stage 4 DLK

Stage 4 DLK is the worst form of this complication, representing an almost *no return stage* and associated with sight threatening sequelae. Apart from dense cellular infiltrates, there is a release of *proteolytic enzymes* such as collagenage. These enzymes lead to variable degree of *stromal damage and melting*. Subsequently irreversible change like scarring and folds in the visual axis, irregular astigmatism, hyperopia a severe decrease in BCVA occurs.

Treatment of stage 4 DLK is as for stage 3 if the case is detected early as a result of serial follow-up. However if permanent scarring has resulted, no definitive late stage treatment has been found to be effective, although some improvement may occur over next 6–12 months.

Leu and Hersh[176] have described a case that developed recurrent episodes of DLK following LASIK for many months. This case showed no significant or only partial improvement with the above regime during the successive episodes. This case successfully responded to PTK mode of ablation after relifting the flap.

Johnson's Classification

Recently Johnson et al[174] have proposed a new classification of DLK for the purpose of evaluating the incidence, association and visual outcome in 36 eyes of 2711 patients of LASIK, which developed DLK. The eye were divided into two broad groups:

Type I DLK: Center sparing DLK
Type II DLK: Centre involving DLK

These two types were further subdivided into A and B categories.
  Subgroup A: Sporadic-DLK, not diagnosed in other patients treated on the same day.
  Subgroup B: Cluster-DLK, which affected many other patients treated on the same day at the same center.

Thus IA would be center sparing DLK occurring sporadically and IB, center-sparing DLK occurring in other patients simultaneously. Similarly II A means DLK involving the visual zone and occurring sporadically, II B involving the center but occurring in cluster. They concluded that DLK involving the center of cornea and occurring in cluster had lesser association with epithelial defects and was most seriously vision threatening. The incidence, visual outcome and other relevant associations are summarized in Table 26.5.

EPITHELIAL IMPLANTATION AND INGROWTH

Epithelial implantation in the interface may occur during the LASIK surgery. Loose epithelium or epithelial injury, over manipulation of flap and faulty irrigation procedure are some of the causes of epithelial implantation during LASIK. Its management has been discussed earlier under interface debris.

Epithelial ingrowth in contrast appears later, within first few weeks of surgery. There are certain situations where epithelial ingrowth is seen more often these are:

1. After flap complications.
2. After re-LASIK.
3. After hyperopic LASIK.
4. After LASIK with smaller diameter flap.

Flap complications predispose to epithelial seedling[146]. Irregular epithelial borders at the flap edge facilitate epithelial ingrowth after repeat LASIK[179-181]. Smaller flaps and hyperopic-LASIK are associated with an increased risk due to possibility of the cut edge getting ablated[52,182].

The incidence of epithelial ingrowth has been reported from 1.5% by Stulting et al[181]. Gimbel et al[145] found 3.5% incidence rate. Incidence of epithelial ingrowth following hyperopic-LASIK is very high[182] (31.4%). Up to 31% incidence after re-LASIK has been reported[179-181].

Risk Factors for Epithelial Ingrowth

Poor flap adhesion, epithelial abrasions, buttonholes and other abnormalities of flap, flap misalignment leaving potential space for epithelial cell migration, specially if an epithelial defect is present; irregularities of the flap margin or stromal bed and inadvertent ablation of the cut edge/ flap hinge are risk factors for epithelial seedling or ingrowth later[177-184].

Helena et al[184] described the following mechanisms that can predispose to ingrowth of the epithelial cells into the interface.

1. Mechanical dragging of the cells by the microkeratome blade.
2. Backflow of the cells during irrigation that may carry the floating cells.
3. Outgrowth of cells from the epithelial plugs in case of previous incisional keratotomy.
4. The keratotomy incision site providing route for epithelial ingrowth.

Presentation of Epithelial Ingrowth

Luckily most cases of epithelial ingrowth do not result in major consequences or require any treatment. This is

Table 26.5: Classification of DLK by Johnson et al[174]

Type of DLK	No. of Eyes	Mean Time for Diagnosis	Mean Time for Resolution	Association with Epithelial defect	Loss of more than 2 lines of BCVA
Type I		1.8 days		55.4% eyes	
A	18		3.6 days		0
B	3		2.7 days		0
Type II		1.1 days		20.0% eyes	
A	10		9.3 days		0
B	5		10.2 days	40% eyes	

because of two reasons. First, the epithelial cells do not have much proliferative potential. Secondly, majority of the cases are mild and remain confined to the flap edge. These appear as *isolated small nests of cells or small cysts or pearls at the flap edge*.

However some cases do progress, resulting in extension to the visual axis and cause irregular astigmatism. Occasionally the growth may produce stromal melt due to necrosis at the flap edge. *These ingrowths are seen in continuity with the flap edge forming a "peninsula"*.

Prevention of Epithelial Ingrowth

Certain preventive measures are crucial for avoiding this complication. Manipulation and possible epithelial injuries and defects must be avoided through careful handling of the instruments and the flap. Any flap folds/striae should be properly managed. Meticulous cleaning and removal of the debris from the interface and stromal bed, which may include epithelial cells, is to be achieved by careful irrigation. Large zone ablation must be avoided in case of small cuts and the flap should be protected during ablation. The flap diameter must be sufficiently larger than the ablation area in case of hyperopic-LASIK.

Management

Most cases of isolated nests of cells do not need any intervention. They would disappear after a variable period without any sequelae. However cases of *contiguous epithelial growth with the flap edge require definite treatment* to prevent future problems. The stromal bed and undersurface of the flap are scrapped with the Paton spatula and thoroughly irrigated after lifting the flap. Meticulous care must be taken to remove all epithelial tags before replacing the flap.

Castillo et al[183] have recommended *use of minimum laser spots in PTK mode on the stromal bed and flap undersurface to avoid recurrences of epithelial ingrowth*. The same authors have also advocated application of 50% alcohol for the same purpose. However the later approach may result in undesired effects on the stromal keratocytes.

LASIK-INDUCED OPTIC NEUROPATHY

LASIK-induced optic neuropathy is another very rare but serious complication after LASIK. Six cases of LASIK-induced neuropathy have been described till date. *The term "LASIK-induced neuropathy include a heterogeneous group of cases because different causative factors are involved in each case report*. The following discussion would make this point very clear.

1. This term was first used by Cameron et al[185] when he reported *one case* with arcuate field defects, increased cupping, thinning of the neuroretinal rim in both eyes after few months following LASIK. The author ruled out steroid-induced glaucoma as the IOP was reported to be normal, though the patient was on this therapy for interface haze after LASIK.

2. Najman et al[63] had previously reported *one case*, who developed end-stage glaucoma despite normal recoding of the IOP. They found that this discrepancy was due to a false IOP reading by applanation tonometry, using the central cornea where interface edema interfered with an accurate measurement of IOP. Similar observations were made by other scientists also[64-66] (see under "rise of intraocular pressure).

3. Lee et al[186] reported *four cases* of "LASIK-induced optic neuropathy" within 1-3 days following surgery. Two cases clinically appeared like *anterior ischemic neuropathy* and the other two resembled cases of *retrobulbar neuritis*. The authors reported certain risk factors that could have had a role in development of these complications. These risk factors were small crowded disk, hypertension, factor V Leiden heterozygocity, older age and a tilted disk. They also suggested that there might be other theoretically higher risk factors like optic nerve head drusen, vasculopathies, and previous optic neuropathy.

4. Luna et al[188,189] pointed towards an *ischemic cause*, possibly precipitated by use of the suction ring creating very high IOP. In an animal model they demonstrated that the electroretinogram (ERG) amplitude showed dramatic decrease during the *suction procedure* and recovered on its immediate release. They suggested that this change could be due to a transient interruption of the intraocular blood supply during the period *when IOP was high*. Earlier also they had reported transient loss of vision in some of their patients immediately following LASIK.

5. Namrata et al[187] opined that intermittent fluctuations in the IOP is more dangerous than a

constantly raised pressure. This can happen on repeated unsuccessful application of the suction ring. This problem had occurred during the case reported by Cameron et al.

Microkeratome such as the *hydrokeratome* and *laser keratome,* which do not require a suction ring, may avoid the potential danger posed by the rise of IOP during LASIK in susceptible patients. In addition every patients must be carefully screened for all the mentioned risk factors that my predispose the eye to this complication. The IOP must be measured using the available peripheral clear cornea to avoid underestimation of the IOP during follow-up.

STROMAL MELTS

Stromal melting is a very rare but serious complication following LASIK. Melting of the stroma or keratolysis may occur in the following situations:

1. Epithelial ingrowth.
2. DLK stage 4.
3. Other inflammatory conditions.

Deprivation of nutrients, specially glucose, to the stroma from the aqueous humor as a result of mechanical barrier created by the epithelial ingrowth may be responsible for the stromal melting. The proteolytic enzymes released in stage 4 DLK may result in melting if the insult is significant. Cytokines mediated damage may be an additional mechanism leading to keratolysis[192].

Prevention and Management

Melting of the flap is prevented by its early recognition of the inflammatory process and other condition that could potentially led to keratolysis.

This disorder should be promptly and efficiently managed by appropriate measures.

LASIK-INDUCED CORNEAL ECTASIA/ KERATECTASIA

Initially LASIK came in a big way as a treatment of choice for the correction of high and extreme myopia. The reason was that results of PRK were not found to be good due to poor predictability, high regression rate, significant corneal haze and subepithelial scars in these group of myopes. However the risk posed by deeper ablation of the stroma after raising a corneal flap was not recognized for some years due to limited follow-up.

Gradually cases of corneal ectasia due to reduced stromal bed thickness following LASIK started surfacing up. The surgeons have become more and more concerned about the safe limit of maximum correction and the *minimum residual bed thickness* (RBT) below which corneal ectasia would not occur.

A great controversy prevails regarding the minimum stromal bed thickness above which the corneal integrity would not be endangered. For more than a decade the consensus was that 250 μ of remaining stromal bed would be a safe limit for excimer laser surgeries. No case of any structural weakening was reported following excimer laser procedures as the surgeons respected this sacrosanct figure.

Even many of the LASIK surgeons agreed that 250 μ of residual stroma was a safe limit[193-196]. *However following longer follow-up of LASIK cases, newer facts have come to the notice of excimer laser surgeons.* In light of these facts the concepts about the maximum correction and the minimum residual bed thickness have changed. The issues concerning methods of measuring the central corneal thickness, great variability in predictability of flap thickness cut by different microkeratomes and the value of intraoperative assessment of the flap and stromal bed thickness also have been reviewed with more concern and seriousness during the recent period (see Chapter 6 for a detailed discussion on this issue). The following facts would summarize the current opinion regarding corneal ectasia.

1. No case of corneal ectasia has been reported following PRK or PTK.
2. Corneal ectasia following LASIK is a serious, potentially blinding complication.
3. Incidence of this complication is rare. Thirty-seven cases of corneal ectasia following Lasik have been reported in the literature till April 2002, though over a million eyes have undergone this sugary.
4. The main cause of corneal ectasia is low residual bed thickness after LASIK.
5. Corneal ectasia has been reported in eyes with RBT >250 μ and correction < -12.0 D also [201,207]. Pallikaris et al[201], after reviewing 2873 cases of LASIK, found 0.66% incidence of corneal ectasia. They reported that no case with < – 8.0 D correction and > 325 μ RBT developed corneal ectasia.
6. Since cases of corneal ectasia have been reported even with RBT >250 μ also, additional factors

like IOP[195, 197], older age[201, 203] and inherent predisposition to develop keratectasia[204] also have been thought to contribute to the development of corneal ectasia. Rao et al[200] reported a case, who developed corneal ectasia in both eyes following LASIK. The RBT was 314 μ in one eye and 330 μ in the other one.

7. Other factor that may be responsible for this complication are borderline cases of *thinning corneal disorders without definite topographical evidence of the disease*. These include forme fruste cases of keratoconus, unrecognized cases of pellucid marginal degeneration and collagen vascular diseases etc. These cases may lead to dramatic development of corneal protrusion within the first week following LASIK[200, 205].

8. The *common pathological factor* in the above situations is a *biomechanical weakening* of the cornea.

9. Different microkeratomes are found to cut flaps, which can highly variable than the intended cut[212] (see Chapter 6 also). Therefore intraoperative assessment of the flap and stromal bed thickness is crucial before proceeding for refractive ablation.

10. The method of measuring central corneal thickness (CCT) is also crucial. Many studies have found that Orbscan gives statistically significant different readings as compared to ultrasonic pachymetry (see chapter 6). Chakrabarty et al[208] found an average 28 μ higher in normal eyes and 13 μ lower reading in post-LASIK eyes. In a study conducted by Francesco et al[209], the mean difference was found to be 143.1 μ in corneas with haze. The cause of error with the Orbscan is attributed to the *"optical acquisition process"* by this method.

11. Mohamed et al[210] reported that *Orbscan II pachymetry measurements correlated with the ultrasound measurements in clear corneas*. But it also underestimated the corneal thickness in the presence of corneal haze, a finding similar to that reported by Francesco et al.

Prevention of Corneal Ectasia

The key to manage corneal ectasia is its prevention. All precautionary measures must be taken to prevent post-LASIK corneal ectasia. The essential steps are:

1. Careful selection of cases.
2. Accurate measurement of the CCT.
3. Exclusion of cases at risk of developing corneal ectasia (Chapter 6).
4. Intraoperative assessment of the flap and stromal bed thickness by the best available methods. Vinciguerra et al[211] have found *confocal microscopy* to be comparable to ultrasonic pachymetry for this purpose during LASIK
5. Regular follow-up to detect the earliest case of corneal ectasia.

Management of Corneal Ectasia

The different modalities that may be used to treat a case of corneal ectasia are:

1. **Rigid gas permeable (RGP) contact lenses**: These are the first line of management of a case of corneal ectasia[193, 200].
2. **Epikeratoplasty and keratoplasty**: Epikeratoplasty may be required in severe cases of corneal protrusion[193]. Severe cases with ectasia and corneal scarring keratoplasty[193, 214].
3. **INTACS**: Siganos et al[213] used intracorneal ring segments for the management of 3 eyes with corneal ectasia. The patients achieved 20/20 to 20/25 UCVA at 6 month of follow-up. The results remained stable till the last follow-up (9 month).

Suggested readings

1. Enoch JM, Laties AM: An analysis of retinal receptor orientation. II. Prediction for psychophysiological tests. Invest Ophthalmol Vis Sci 1971; 10: 959.
2. Bonds AB, MacLeod DIA: A displaced Stiles-Crawford effect associated with an eccentric pupil. Invest Ophthalmol Vis Sci 1978; 10: 754.
3. Weber SK, McGhee CNJ, Bruce IG: Decentration of PRK ablation zone after excimer laser surgery for myopia. J Cataract Ref Surg; 1996; 22: 299-303.
4. Deitz MR, Piebenga LW, Matta CS et al: Ablation zone centration after PRK and its effect on visual outcome. J Cataract Ref Surg 1996; 22: 696-701.
5. Doane JF, Cavanaugh TB, Durrie DS et al: Relation of visual symptoms to topographic ablation zone decentration after excimer laser PRK. Ophthalmology 1995; 102: 42-47.
6. Hersh PS, Schwartz-Goldstein BH: Corneal topography of phase III excimer laser PRK: optical zone centration analysis. Ophthalmology 1995; 102: 951-962.

7. Braunstein RE, Jain S, McCally RL et al: Objective measurement of corneal light scattering after excimer laser PRK. Ophthalmology 1996; 103: 439-443.
8. Gartry DS, Kerr-Muir MG, Marshall J: PRK with an argon fluoride excimer laser: a clinical study. J Ref Corn Surg 1991; 7: 420-435.
9. Lim-Bon-Siong R, Williams JM et al: Retreatment of decentred excimer PRK ablations. Am J Ophthalmol 1997; 123: 122-124.
10. Talamo JH, Wagoner MD, Lee SY: Management of ablation decentration following excimer PRK. Arch Ophthalmol 1995; 113: 706-707.
11. Mulhern mg, Foley-Nolan A, O'Keefe M et al: Topographic analysis of ablation centration after excimer laser PRK and LASIK for high myopia. J Cataract Ref Surg 1997: 23 (4): 488-494.
11a. Vinciguerra P, Camesasca FI: Decentration after refractive surgery. J Refract Surg 2001; 17(2 Suppl): S190-191.
12. McCarty CA, Garrett SK, Alfred G: Assessment of subjective pain following photorefractive keratectomy. Melbourne Excimer Laser Group. J Ref Surg 1996; 12: 365-369.
13. Gimbel HV, DeBrof BM, Beldavs RA: Comparison of laser and manual removal of epithelium for PRK. J Ref Surg 1995; 11 (1): 36-41.
13a. Breil P, Frisch L, Dick HB: Diagnosis and therapy of LASIK-induced neurotrophic epitheliopathy. Ophthalmologe 2002 Jan; 99(1): 53-57.
14. Sher NA, Krueger RR, Teal p et al: Role of topical corticosteroids and NSAID in the etiology of stromal infiltrates after excimer laser PRK. J Ref Corneal Surg 1994; 10: 587-8.
15. Teal P, Berlin C, Arsbinoff S et al: Corneal sub-epithelial infiltrates following excimer laser PRK. J Cataract Ref Surg 1995; 21: 516-18.
16. Teichmann KD, Cameron J, Human A et al: Wessely-type immune ring following PTK. J Cataract Ref Surg 1996; 22: 142-146.
17. Seiler T, Mc Donnell PJ: Excimer laser PRK. Survey Ophthalmology 1995; 40: 89-118.
18. Faschinger C, Faulborn J, Ganser K: Infectious corneal ulcer–once with endophthalmitis- after PRK with disposable lens. Klin Monatsbl Augenheilkd 1995; 206: 96-102.
19. al-Rajhi AA, Wagoner MD, et al: Bacterial keratitis following photorefractive keratectomy: J Ref Cata Surg 1996; 12: 123- 1.27.
20. Gallo JP, Raizman MD: PTK for superficial corneal disorders. Int Ophthal Clin 1997; 37: 155-170.
21. Kim HM, Song JK, Han HS, Jung HR: Streptococcal keratitis after myopic LASIK. Korean J Ophthalmol 1998; 12: 108-111.
22. Webber SK, Lawless MA, Sutton GL, Rogers CM: Staphylococcal infection under a LASIK flap. Cornea 1999; 18(3): 361-365.
23. Perez-Santonja JJ, Sakla HF, Abad JL et al: Nocardial keratitis after LASIK. J Ref Surg 1997; 13:314-317.
24. Haw WW, Manche EE: Sterile peripheral keratitis following LASIK. J Ref Surg 1999; 15: 61-63.
25. Aras C, Ozdamar A, Bahcecioglu H, Bozkurt S: Corneal interface abscess after excimer LASIK. J Ref Surg 1998; 14: 156-157.
26. Peng Q, Mike PH, Peter HK et al: Interface fungal infection after LASIK presenting as diffuse lamellar keratitis. J Cat Ref Surg 2002; 28: 1400-1408.
27. Roger MK, John ES: Acanthamoeba keratitis after PRK. Cat Ref Surg 2002; 28: 364-368.
28. Fulcher SF, Fader RC, Rosa Jr RH, Holmes GP: Delayed-onset mycobacterial keratitis after LASIK. Cornea 2002 Aug; 21(6): 546-54.
29. Pushker N, Dada T, Sony P, Ray M, Agarwal T, Vajpayee RB: Microbial keratitis after laser in situ keratomileusis. J Refract Surg 2002 May-Jun; 18(3): 280-6.
30. Perry HD, Doshi SJ, Donnenfeld ED, Levinson DH, Cameron CD: Herpes simplex reactivation following laser in situ keratomileusis and subsequent corneal perforation. CLAO J 2002 Apr; 28(2): 69-71
31. Davidorf JM: Herpes simplex keratitis after LASIK. Letter to the editor. J Ref Surg 1998; 14: 667.
32. Maloney RK, Thompson V, Ghiselli G et al: A prospective multi-center trial of phototherapeutic keratectomy for corneal vision loss. Am J Ophthalmol 1996; 60: 149-160.
33. McGhee CNJ, Weed KH, Bryce IG: Minor and major complications of excimer laser PRK and PARK. Proc Int Soc Refract Surg: midsummer symposium 1995: 93-94.
34. Caubert E: Cause of sub-epithelial corneal haze over 18 months after photorefractive keratectomy for myopia. Refract Corneal Surg 1993; 9 (Suppl): S65-S70.
35. Corbett MC, Prydall JI, Verma S et al: An in vivo investigation of the structures responsible for corneal haze after PRK and their effect on visual functions. Ophthalmology 1996. 103: 1366-1380.
36. Moller-Pedersen T, Vogel M, Li HF et al: Quantification of stromal thinning, epithelial thickness and corneal haze after PRK using in vivo confocal microscopy. Ophthalmology 1997. 104: 362-368.
37. Taylor HR, McCarty CA, Aldred GF: Predictability of excimer laser treatment of myopia. Arch Ophthalmol 1996; 114: 248-251.
38. Seiler T, Holcshbach A, Derse M et al: Complications of myopic PRK with the excimer laser. Ophthalmology 1994; 101: 153-160.
39. Meyer JC, Stulting RD, Thompson KP, Durrie DS: Late onset of corneal scar after excimer laser PRK. Am J Ophthalmol 1996; 121: 529-539.

40. Lipshitz I, Loewenstein A, Varssano D et al: late onset corneal haze after PRK for moderate and high myopia. Ophthalmology 1997. 104: 369-374.
41. Siganos DS, Kasanevaki VJ, Pallikaris IJ: Correlation of subepithelial haze and refractive regression I month PRK for myopia. J Ref Surg 1999; 15: 338-342.
42. Nagy ZZ, Hiscott P, Seitz B et al: ultraviolet-B enhances corneal stromal response to 193 nm excimer laser treatment. Ophthalmology 1997; 104: 375-380.
43. Fagerholm P, Hamberg-Nystrom H, Tengroth B et al: Effect of postoperative steroids on the refractive outcome of PRK for myopia with the Summit excimer laser. J Cata Ref Surg 1994; 20 (Suppl): 212-215.
44. Carones F, Brancato R, Venturi E et al: Efficacy of corticosteroids in reversing regression after myopic PRK. J Ref Corn Surg 1993; 9(Suppl): S52-S56.
45. Carr JD, Patel R, Hersh ES: Management of late corneal haze following PRK. J Ref Surg 1995; 11(Suppl): S309-S313.
46. Loewenstein A, Lipshitz I, Lazar M: Scrapping of epithelium for treatment of undercorrection and haze after PRK. J Ref Corn Surg 1994; 10(Suppl): S274-S276.
47. Kang F, Tao J, Li Q et al: Mechanism of regression and haze after PRK. Hua Yen Ko Tsa Chih 2002; 38 (7): 433-437.
48. Pallikaris IG, Siganos DS: Excimer laser in situ keratomileusis and PRK for correction of high myopia. J Cataract Ref Surg 1994; 10: 498-510.
49. El-Maghraby A, Salah T, Warring GO III et al: Randomized bilateral comparison of excimer laser in situ keratomileusis and PRK for 1.2 to 8.0 diopter of myopia. Ophthalmology 1999; 106: 447-457.
50. Wang Z, Chen J, Yang B: Comparison of LASIK and PRK to correct myopia from −1.25 to −6.0 diopters. J Ref Surg 1997; 13: 528-534.
51. Snibson GR, McCarty CA, Aldred GF et al: Retreatment after excimer laser PRK; the Melbourne Excimer Laser Group. Am J Ophthalmol 1996; 121: 250-157.
52. Iskander NG, Peters NT, Anderson Penno EE, Gimbel HV: Postoperative complications in LASIK. Current Opinion In Ophthalmology. 2000; 11(4): 273-279.
53. Taylor HR, Guest CS, Kelly P et al: Comparison of excimer laser treatment of myopia and astigmatism. Arch Ophthalmol 1993; 111: 1621-1626.
54. Snibson GR, Carson CA, Aldred GF, Taylor HR: One-year evaluation of excimer laser PRK for myopia and myopic astigmatism. Arch Ophthalmol 1995: 113: 994-1000.
55. Tailey AR, Hardten DR, Sher NA et al: Results one year after using the 193 nm excimer laser for PRK in mild to moderate myopia. Am J Ophthalmol 1994; 101: 1548-1557.
56. Kim JH, Sah WJ, Hahn TW, Lee YC: Some problems after PRK. Refractive Corn Surg 1994; 10: S226-S230.
57. Seiler T, Wollensak J: Myopic PRK with the excimer laser. One-year follow-up. Ophthalmology 1991; 98:1156-1163.
58. Gartry D, KerrMuir M, Marshall J: Excimer laser PTK: 18 months follow up. Ophthalmology 1992; 99: 1209-1219.
59. Ehlers N, Bramsen T, Sperling S: Applanation tonometry and central corneal thickness. Arch Ophthalmol 1975; 53: 34-43.
60. Nomura H, Ando F, Niino N, Shimokata H, Miyake Y: The relationship between age and intraocular pressure in a Japanese population: The influence of central corneal thickness. Curr Eye Res 2002 Feb; 24 (2): 81-5.
61. Mark HH: Corneal curvature in applanation tonometry. Am J Ophthalmology 1973; 76: 223-224.
62. Agudelo LM, Molina CA, Alvarez DL: Changes in intraocular pressure after laser in situ keratomileusis for myopia, hyperopia, and astigmatism. J Refract Surg 2002 Jul-Aug; 18(4): 472-4.
63. Najman-Vainer J, Smith RJ, Maloney RK: Interface fluid after LASIK: misleading tonometry can lead to end stage glaucoma (letter). J Cataract Ref Surg 2000; 26: 471-472.
64. Lyle WA, Jin GJC: Interface fluid associated with diffuse lamellar keratitis and epithelial ingrowth after LASIK. J Cataract Ref Surg 1999; 25: 1009-1112.
65. Rehany U, Bersudsky V, Rumelt S: Paradoxical hypotony after LASIK. J Cataract Ref Surg 2000; 26: 1823-1826.
66. Portellinha W, Kuchenbuk M, Nakano K, Oliveira M: Interface fluid and diffuse corneal edema after LASIK. J Ref Surg 2001; 17: S192-S195.
67. Wang X, Shen J, McCulley JP, Bowman RW, Petroll WM, Cavanagh HD: Intraocular pressure measurement after hyperopic LASIK. CLAO J 2002 Jul; 28(3): 136-9.
68. Lee DH, Seo S, Shin SC, Chung EH, Turner TT: Accuracy and predictability of the compensatory function of Orbscan II in intraocular pressure measurements after laser in situ keratomileusis. J Cataract Refract Surg 2002 Feb; 28(2): 259-64.
69. Gartry DS, Kerr-Muir MG. Marshal J: The effect of topical corticosteroids on refraction and corneal haze following excimer laser treatment of myopia: an update. A prospective, randomized, double-masked study. Eye 1993; 7: 584-590.
70. Trabuchi G, Brancato R, Verdi M et at: Corneal nerve damage and regeneration after excimer laser photorefractive keratectomy in rabbit eyes. Invest Ophthalmol Vis Sci 1994; 35: 229-235.

71. Tervo K, Latwala TM, Tervo MT: Recovery of innervations following PRK. Arch Ophthalmol 1994; 112; 1466-1470.
72. Campos M, Hertzog L, Grabus JJ et al: Corneal sensitivity after photorefractive keratectomy. Am J Ophthalmol 1992; 14: 51-54.
73. Ishikawa T, Park SB, Cox C et al: Corneal sensation following excimer laser PRK in humans. J Ref Cat Surg. 1994; 10: 414- 422.
73a. Matsui H, Kumano Y, Zushi I, Yamada T, Matsui T, Nishida T: Corneal sensation after correction of myopia by photorefractive keratectomy and laser in situ keratomileusis. J Cataract Refract Surg 2001 Mar; 27(3): 370-3.
74. Sutton G, Kalski RS, lawless MA, Rogers CM: Excimer laser retreatment for scarring and regression after PRK for myopia. Br J Ophthalmol 1995; 79: 756-759.
75. Pepose JS, Laycock KA, Miller JK et al: Reactivation of latent herpes simplex virus by excimer laser photokeratectomy. Am J Ophthalmol 1992; 114: 45-50.
76. Fagerholm P, Fitzsimmons TD, Orndhal M et al: Phototherapeutic keratectomy: long term results in 166 eyes. J Ref Cata Surg 1993; 9: S76-S81.
77. Campos M, Nielsen S, Szerenyi K et al: Clinical follow-up of phototherapeutic keratectomy for treatment of corneal opacities. Am J Ophthalmol 1993; 115: 443-440.
78. Hersh PS, Spinak A, Carrana R, Mayer M: Phototherapeutic keratectomy: strategies and results in 12 eyes. Refract Corneal. Surg (1993) 9: S90-S95.
79. Talamo JH, Steinert RF, Puliafito CA: Clinical strategies for excimer laser therapeutic keratectomy. Refractive Corneal Surg 1992; 8: 319-324.
80. Chamon W, Azar DT, Stark JW et at: Phototherapeutic keratectomy. Ophthalmol Clin North Am 1993; 6: 399-413.
81. Sher NA, Barak M, Daya S, et al: Excimer laser photorefractive keratectomy. Arch Ophthalmol 1993; 111: 1022.
82. Rapuano CJ, Laibson PR: Excimer laser phototherapeutic keratectomy for anterior corneal pathology. CLAO Journal 1994; 20: 253-7.
83. Rene Din, Christopher J, Rapuano CJ et al: Recurrence of corneal dystrophies after phototherapeutic keratectomy. Ophthalmology 1999; 106 (8): 1490-1497.
84. Rapuano CJ, Labison PR: Excimer laser phototherapeutic keratectomy. CLAO Journal 1993; 19: 235- 240.
85. Campos M, Hertzog I Grabus J et al: PTK for severe post keratoplasty astigmatism. Am J Ophthalmol 1992; 114: 429- 436.
86. Christine RE, McGhee CNJ: Phototherapeutic keratectomy: Clinical studied. In "Excimer Lasers In Ophthalmology: Principles and Practice ". Eds McGhee CNJ, Martin Dunitz Ltd 1977; 372.
87. Loewenstein A, Lipshitz I, Levanon D et al: Influence of patient age on PRK for myopia. J Ref Surg 1997; 13 23-26.
88. Condon PI, Mulhern M, Fulcher T et al: LASIK for myopia and myopic astigmatism. Br J Ophthalmol 1997; 81 (3); 199-206.
89. Wilson SE: LASIK complications. Cornea 1998; 17 (5): 459-467.
90. Durrie DS, Lesher MP, Hunkeler JD: Treatment of overcorrection after myopic PRK. J Refract Corneal Surg 1994; 10 (Suppl): S295.
91. Hersh PS, Schwartz-Goldstein BH: Corneal topography of phase III excimer laser PRK. Ophthalmology 1995; 102: 963-978.
92. Salz JJ, Maguen E, Nesburn AB, et al: A two-year experience with excimer laser photorefractive keratectomy for myopia. Ophthalmology 1993; 100: 873-882.
93. Lin DTC: Corneal topographic analysis after excimer laser PRK. Ophthalmology 1994; 101: 1432-1439.
94. Levin S, Carson C, Garret SK et al: Prevalence of central islands after excimer laser refractive surgery. J Cataract Ref Surg 1995; 21: 21-26.
95. Parker PJ, Klyce SO, Ryan SL et al: Central topographic islands following photorefractive keratectomy. Invest Ophthalmol Vis Sci 1993; 34 (Suppl): 803.
96. Bor ZS, Hopp B, Bacz B et at: Plume emission, shock wave and surface wave formation during excimer laser ablation of the cornea. Refract Corneal Surg 1993; 9 (suppl): S111-S115.
97. Campos M, Cuevas K, Garbus J et al: Corneal wound healing after excimer laser ablation: effects of nitrogen gas blower. Ophthalmology 1992; 99: 893-897.
98. Colin J, Cochener C, Gallinaro C: Central steep islands immediately following excimer laser PRK for myopia. Refract Corneal Surg 1993; 9: 395-396.
99. Slade SG: Abnormal induced topography; Central islands. In: Machat JJ, ed. "Excimer Laser Refractive Surgery: Practice and Principles". Thorofare NJ: SLACK Incorporated; 1996:399.
100. McGhee CNJ, Bryce IG: The natural history of central steep islands following excimer laser PRK. J Cataract Ref Surg 1996; 22: 1151-1158.
101. Krueger RR, Saedy NF, McDonnell PJ: Clinical analysis of steep central islands after excimer laser photorefractive keratectomy. Arch Ophthalmol 1966; 114: 377-381.
102. Warring GO, O'Connell MA: PRK for myopia for using a 4.5 mm ablation zone. J Ref Surg 1995; 11: 170-180.
103. Shimizu K, Amano S, Tanaka S: PRK for myopia: one-year follow-up in 97 eyes. Ref Corneal Surg 1994; 10: S178-S187.
104. Ambrosio G, Gennamo G, De Marco R et al: Visual function before and after PRK for myopia. J Refractive Corneal Surg 10: 129-136.

105. Esente S, Passarelli N, Falco L et al: Contrast sensitivity under photopic conditions in PRK: a preliminary report. Ref Corneal Surg 1993; 9: S70-S72.
106. Stevens J, Giubilei M, Ficker L, Rosen P: Prospective study of photorefractive keratectomy for myopia using the VISX StarS2 excimer laser system. J Refract Surg 2002 Sep-Oct; 18(5): 502-8.
107. Stevens JD, Ficker LA: Results of photorefractive keratectomy for hyperopia using the VISX star excimer laser system. J Refract Surg 2002 Jan-Feb; 18(1): 30-6.
108. Perez-Santonja JJ, Sakla HF, Alio JL: Contrast sensitivity after LASIK. J Cataract Ref Surg 1998; 24: 183-189.
109. Mutyala S, McDonald MB, Scheinblum KA et al: Contrast sensitivity evaluation after LASIK. Ophthalmology 2000; 107: 1864-1867.
110. Chan WWJ, Edwards MH, George CW et al: Contrast sensitivity after LASIK. J Cataract Ref Surg 2002; 28: 1774-1779.
111. Nakamura K, Bissen-Miyajima H, Toda I, Hori Y, Tsubota K: Effect of laser in situ keratomileusis correction on contrast visual acuity. J Cataract Refract Surg 2001 Mar; 27(3): 357-61.
112. Chen J, Wang Z, Yang B, et Al: Laser in situ keratomileusis for correction of myopia. Chung Hua Yen Ko Tsa Chih 1998 Mar; 34(2): 141-5.
113. O'Brart DPS, Lohman CP, Fitze FW et al: Disturbances in night vision after excimer laser PRK. Eye 1994; 8: 46-51.
114. Brancato R, Tavola A, Caronas F et al: Excimer laser PRK for myopia in 1165 eyes. Refract Corneal Surg 1993; 9: 95-104.
115. Seiler T, Reckman W, Maloney RK: Effective spherical aberrations of the cornea as a quantitative descriptor in corneal topography. J Cataract Ref Surg 1993; 19 (Suppl): 155-165.
116. O'Brart D, Gartry DS, Lohman CP et al: Excimer laser PRK for myopia: comparison of 4.0 mm and 5.0 mm ablations zones. J Ref Corneal Surg 1994; 10 (2): 87-94.
117. O'Brart D, Corbett MC, Lohman CP: The effect of ablation zone diameter on the outcome of excimer laser PRK: A prospective randomized, double blind study. Arch Ophthalmology 1995; 113: 438-443.
118. Corbett MC, Verma S, O'Brart D et al: Effect of ablation profile on the wound healing and visual performance one year after excimer laser PRK. Br J Ophthalmol 1996; 80: 224-234.
119. Lohman CP, Fitzke F et al: Halos-a problem for all myopes? Ref Corneal Surg 1993; 9 (2): S72-S75
120. O'Brart D, Lohman CP Fitzke F et al: Night vision after PRK: haze and halos. Eur J Ophthalmol 1994; 4: 43-51.
121. O'Brart D, Lohman CP Fitzke F et al: Disturbances in night vision after excimer PRK. Eye 1994; 8: 46-51.
122. Epstein D, Fagerholm P, Hamberg-Nystrom H: Twenty-four month follow-up of myopic PRK. Ophthalmology 1994; 101: 1558-1563.
123. Kim JH, Sah WJ, Kim MS et al: Three-year results of PRK for myopia. J Ref Surg 1995; 11 (Suppl): S248-S252.
124. Stevens JD: One-year wait urged for PRK retreatment. Ocular Surgery News 1995; 13(15): 24.
125. Williams DK: Excimer laser PRK for extreme myopia. J Cataract Ref Surg 1996; 22: 910-914.
126. Pang G, Zhan S, Li Y, et Al: Myopic regression after photorefractive keratectomy. Chung Hua Yen Ko Tsa Chih 1998 Nov; 34(6): 451-3.
127. Ditzen K, Anschutz T, Schroder E: PRK to treat low, medium and high myopia: a multicenter study. J Cataract Ref Surg 1994; 20 (Suppl): 234-238.
128. Dausch D, Klein R, Schroder E et al: Excimer laser PRK with tapered transition zone for high myopia. A preliminary report of 6 cases. J Cataract Ref Surg 1993; 19 (5): 590-594.
129. Gimbel HV, Levy SG: Indications, results and complications of LASIK. Current Opinion in Ophthalmology 1998; 9: IV; 3-8.
130. Salah T, Warring GO, El Maghraby A et al: Excimer laser in situ keratomileusis under corneal flap for myopia of 2 to 20 diopters. Am J Ophthalmol 1996; 121: 143-155.
131. Zadok D, Maskaleris G, Garcia V et al: Outcomes of retreatment after LASIK. Ophthalmology 1991; 106: 2391-2394.
132. Perez-Santonja JJ, Bellot J, Claramonte P et al: LASIK to correct high myopia. J Cataract Ref Surg 1997; 23: 372-385.
133. O'Brart D, Corbett MC, Lohman CP: The effect of ablation zone diameter on the outcome of excimer laser PRK: A prospective randomized, double blind study. Arch Ophthalmology 1995; 113: 438-443.
134. Corbett MC, O'Brart DP, Warburton FG et al: Biological and environmental risk factors for regression after PRK. Ophthalmology 1996; 103: 1381-1389.
135. Snibson GR: Regression and retreatment, in "Excimer Lasers In Ophthalmology: Principles and Practice". Eds McGhee CNJ, Martin Dunitz Ltd 1997: 404-405.
136. Miyata K, Kaimiya K, Takashahi T et al: Time course of change in corneal forward shifting after excimer laser PRK. Arch Ophthalmol 2002; 120(7): 896-900.
137. Chayet AS, Assil KK, Montes M, Espinosa-Lagana M, Castellanos A, Tsioulias G: Regression and its mechanisms after laser in situ keratomileusis in moderate and high myopia. Ophthalmology 1998 Jul; 105(7): 1194-9.
138. Pop M, Aras M: PRK treatment for regression. One-year follow-up. Ophthalmology 1996; 103: 1979-1984.
139. Comaish IF, Domniz YY, Lawless MB et al: LASIK for residual myopia after PRK. J Cataract Ref Surg 2002; 28: 775-781.

140. McGhee CNJ, Ellerton CR: Complications of excimer laser PRK, in "Excimer Lasers In Ophthalmology: Principles and Practice". Eds McGhee CNJ, Martin Dunitz Ltd 1997: 39-395.
141. Hovanesian JA, Shah SS, Maloney RK: Symptoms of dry eye and recurrent erosion syndrome after refractive surgery. Cataract Refract Surg 2001 Apr; 27(4): 577-84.
142. Ti SE, Tan DT: Recurrent corneal erosion after laser in situ keratomileusis. Cornea 2001 Mar; 20(2): 156-8.
143. Pallikaris IG, Kymionis GD, Panagopoulou SI et al: Induced optical aberrations following formation of LASIK flap. J Cataract Ref Surg 2002; 28: 1737-1741.
144. Holladay JT, Janes JA: Topographic changes in corneal asphericity and effective optical zone after LASIK. J Cataract Ref Surg 2002; 28: (6): 942-947.
145. Gimbel HV, Penno EEA, Westenbrugge JAV et al: Incidence and management of intraoperative and early postoperative complications in 1000 cases of consecutive LASIK. Ophthalmology 1998; 105: 1839-1847.
146. Gimbel HV, Penno EE et al: In 'LASIK Complications: Prevention and Management, second edition, Slack Incorporated publications, 2001.
147. Gimbel HV, Iskander NG, Peters NT, Anderson Penno EE: Prevention and management of microkeratome-related LASIK complications. J Cataract Ref Surg 2000; 16(2): 226-229.
148. Jacobs JM, Taravella MJ: Incidence of intraoperative flap complications in laser in situ keratomileusis. J Cataract Ref Surg 2002; 28: 23-28.
149. Knorz MC: Flap and interface complications in LASIK. Curr Opin Ophthalmol 2002 Aug; 13(4): 242-5.
150. Lin RT, Maloney RK: Flap complications associated with lamellar refractive surgery. Am J Ophthalmol 1999; 127: 129-136.
151. Ambrosio R Jr, Wilson SE: Complications of laser in situ keratomileusis: etiology, prevention and treatment. J Ref Surg 2001; 17: 350-379.
152. Holland SP, Srivannaboon S, Reinstein DZ: Avoiding serious corneal complications of laser assisted in situ keratomileusis and photorefractive keratectomy. Ophthalmology 2000; 107: 640-652.
153. Leung ATS, Rao SK, Cheng ACK et al: Pathogenesis and management of LASIK flap button-hole. J Cataract Ref Surg 2000; 26: 358-362.
154. Pulaski JP: Etiology of buttonhole flaps. (Letter). J Cataract Ref Surg 2000; 26: 1270-1271.
155. Jain VK, Abell TG, Bond WI, Stevens G Jr: Immediate transepithelial photorefractive keratectomy for treatment of laser in situ keratomileusis flap complications. J Refract Surg 2002 Mar-Apr; 18(2): 109-12.
156. Wong VW, Zhu CC, Rao SK, Lam DSC: Corneal perforation during laser in situ keratomileusis. (Letter). J Cat Ref Surg 2000; 26: 1103-1104.
157. Hori Y, Watanabe H, Maeda N et al: Medical treatment of operated corneal perforation caused by LASIK. Arch Ophthalmol 1999; 117: 1422-1423.
158. Von Kulazta P, Stark WJ, O'Brien TP: Management of flap striae. Int Ophthalmol Clin 2000; 40 (3): 87-92. 23 in article by Shahinian
159. Melki SA, Talamo JH, Demetriades AM: Late traumatic dislocation of LASIK corneal flaps. Ophthalmology 2000; 107: 2136-2139
160. Aldave AJ, Hollander DA, Abbott RL: Late-onset traumatic flap dislocation and diffuse lamellar inflammation after laser in situ keratomileusis. Cornea 2002 Aug; 21(6): 604-7.
161. Dastgheib KA, Clinch TE, Manche EE et al: Sloughing of corneal epithelium and wound healing complications associated with LASIK in patients with epithelial basement membrane dystrophy. Am J Ophthalmol 2000; 130: 297-303.
162. Quiros PA, Chuck RS, Smith RE et al: Infectious ulcerative keratitis after LASIK. Arch Ophthalmol 1999; 117: 1423-1427.
163. Garf P, Bansal AK, Sharma S, Vemuganti GK: Bilateral infectious keratitis after LASIK; a case report and review of the literature. Ophthalmology 2001; 108: 121-125.
164. Fraenkel GE, Cohen PR, Sutton GL, et al: Central focal interface opacity after LASIK. J Ref Surg 1998; 14: 571-576.
165. Smith RJ, Maloney RK: Diffuse lamellar keratitis; a new syndrome in lamellar refractive surgery. Ophthalmology 1998; 105: 1721-1726.
166. Kaufman SC, Maitchauk DY, Chiou AGY, Beuerman RW: Interface inflammation after LASIK; sands of the Sahara Syndrome. J Cat Ref Surg 1999; 24: 1589-1593.
167. Maddox R, Hatsis A: Shifting Sands of Sahara: interface inflammation following LASIK. IN: Gimbel HV, Anderson Penno EE. Eds. LASIK Complications, Prevention and Management. Thorofare, NJ: SLACK Incorporated; 1999: 30-36.
168. Wilson SE, Ambrosio Jr R: Sporadic Diffuse Lamellar Keratitis (DLK) After LASIK. Cornea 2002 Aug; 21(6): 560-3.
169. Samuel MA, Kaufman SC, Ahee JA et al: diffuse lamellar keratitis associated with 1% carboxymethyl sodium after LASIK. J Cat Ref Surg 2002; 28: 1409-1411.
170. Haw WW, Manche EE: Late onset diffuse lamellar keratitis associated with an epithelial defect in 6 eyes. J Ref Surg 2000; 16: 744-748.
171. Shah MN, Misra M, Wilhelmus KR et al: diffuse lamellar keratitis associated with epithelial defects after LASIK. J Cat Ref Surg 2000; 26: 1312-1318.
172. Weisenthal RW: Diffuse lamellar keratitis induced by trauma 6 months after LASIK. J Ref Surg 2000; 16: 749-751.

173. Linebarger EJ, Harden DR, Lindstrom RI: Diffuse lamellar keratitis: diagnosis and management. J Cat Ref Surg 2000; 26: 1072-1077.
174. Johnson JD, Harissi-Dagher M, Pineda R, Yoo S, Azar DT: Diffuse lamellar keratitis: incidence, associations, outcomes, and a new classification system. J Cataract Refract Surg 2001 Oct; 27(10): 1560-6.
175. Buhren J, Baumeister M, Chicocki M et al: Confocal microscopic characteristics of stage 1 to 4 diffuse lamellar keratitis after LASIK. J cataract Ref Surg 2002; 28: 1390-1399.
176. Leu G, Hersh PS: PTK for the treatment of diffuse lamellar keratitis. J Cat Ref Surg 2002; 28: 1471-1474.
177. Walker MB, Wilson SE: Incidence and prevention of epithelial growth within the interface after LASIK. Cornea 2000; 19: 170-173.
178. Warring GO III: Epithelial ingrowth after LASIK. Am J Ophthalmol 200; 131: 402-403.
179. Perez-Santonja JJ, Bellot MJ, Sakala HF et al: Retreatment after LASIK. Ophthalmology 1998; 106: 21-28.
180. Lyle WA, Jin GJC: Retreatment after initial LASIK. J cataract Ref Surg 2000; 26: 650-659.
181. Stulting RD, Carr JD, Thompson KP et al: Complications of LASIK for the correction of myopia. Ophthalmology 1999; 106: 13-20.
182. Casker S, Er H, Kahvecioglu AR et al: Laser in situ keratomileusis to correct hyperopia from +4.25 D to +8.0 D. J Ref Surg 1998; 14: (1): 26-30.
183. Castillo A, Diaz-Valle D, Guttierrez AR et al: Peripheral melt of flap after LASIK. J Ref Surg 1998; 14: 61-63.
184. Helena MC, Meisler D, Wilson SE: Epithelial ingrowth within the lamellar interface after LASIK. Cornea 1997; 16(3): 300-305.
185. Cameron BD, Saffra NA, Strominger MB: LASIK-induced optic neuropathy. Ophthalmology 2001; 108: 660-665.
186. Lee AG, Kohnen T, Ebner R et al: Optic neuropathy associated with laser in situ keratomileusis. J Cat Ref Surg 2000; 26: 1581-1584.
187. LASIK induced optic neuropathy: Letters to the editor. Ophthalmology 2002; 109 (5); 817-820.
188. Luna JD, Artal MN, Pelizzari MF et al: Posterior pole complications after LASIK for the past 4 years. Pre-American Acadamy of Ophthalmollogy Meeting. San Francisco. CA 1997.
189. Luna JD, Artal MN, Pelizzari MF et al: Effects of suction ring on the posterior pole during LASIK: An animal model. ARVO (Abstract) 2000; 41: S349.
190. Bushley DM, Parmley VC, Paglen P: Visual field defects associated with LASIK. Am J Ophthalmol 2000; 129: 668-671.
191. Weiss HS, Rubinfeld RS, Anderschat JF: LASIK associated visual field loss in a glaucoma suspect. Arch Ophthalmol 2001; 119: 774-775.
192. Cubbit CL, Lausch RN, Okes JE: difference in interleukin 6 gene expression between cultured human corneal epithelial cells and keratocytes. Invest Ophthalmol Vis Sci 1995; 36(2): 330-336.
193. Seiler T, Koufala K, Richter G: Iatrogenic keratoconus after LASIK. J Ref Surg 1998; 14: 312-317.
194. Geggel HS, Talley AR: Delayed onset corneal ectasia following LASIK. J Cataract Ref Surg 1999; 25: 582-586.
195. Leung ATS, Rao KS, Lam DSC: Delayed onset corneal ectasia following LASIK. Letter to the editor. J Cataract Ref Surg 1999; 25: 1036-1037.
196. Seiler T, Quurke AW: Iatrogenic Keratectasia after LASIK in case of forme fruste keratoconus. J Cataract Ref Surg 1998; 24: 1007-1009.
197. Wang Z, Chen J, Yang B: Posterior corneal surface topographic changes after Lasik are related to residual corneal bed thickness. Ophthalmology 1999; 106(2): 409-410.
198. Baek T, Lee K, Kagaya F et al: Factors affecting forward shift of posterior corneal surface after Lasik. Ophthalmology 2001; 108 (2): 317-320. Comments in Ophthalmology 2002; 108 (3): 407-410.
199. Seitz B, Torres F, Langenbucher A et al: Posterior corneal curvature changes after myopic Lasik. Ophthalmology 2001; 108 (4): 666-673.
200. Rao SN, Epstein RJ: Early onset ectasia following Lasik: case report and literature review. J Ref Surg 2002; 18(2): 177-184.
201. Pallikaris IG, Kymionis GD et al: Corneal ectasia induced by Lasik. J Ref Cataract Surg 2001; 27 (11): 1796-1802.
202. Argento C, Cosentino MJ, Tytiun A et al: Corneal ectasia after laser in situ keratomileusis. J Cataract Ref Surg 2001; 27 (9): 1440- 1498.
203. Rao SK, Padmanabhan P: Posterior keratoconus: An expanded classification scheme based on corneal topography. Ophthalmology; 1998; 105: 1206-1212.
204. Vinciguerra P, Camesaska FI: Prevention of corneal ectasia after Lasik. J Ref Surg 2001; 17 (3 suppl): S 187- 189.
205. Schmitt-Bernard CF, Lesage C, Arnaud B: Keractesia induced by Lasik in keratoconus. J Ref Surg 2000; 16 (3): 368- 370.
206. Speicher L, Gottinger W: Progressive corneal ectasia after Lasik. Klin Monatsbl Augenheilkd 1998; 213 (4) 247-151.
207. Genth U, Mrochen M, Walti R et al: Optical low coherence reflectometry for noncontact measurement of flap thickness during laser on situ keratomileusis. Ophthalmology 2002; 109: 973-978.
208. Chakrabarty HS, Craig JP, Brahma A, Malik TY et al: Comparison of corneal thickness using ultrasound and

Orbscan slit-scanning topography in normal and post-LASIK eyes. J Cat Ref Surg 2001; 27:1823-1828.
209. Francesco B, Maria G, Giovanni A, Carlo S: Accuracy of Orbscan optical pachymetry in corneas wit haze. J Cataract Ref Surg 2002; 18: 253-258.
210. Mohamed A F, Alberto A, Jose IB et al: Comparison of corneal pachymetry using ultrasound and Orbscan II. J Cat Ref Surg 2001; 28: 248-252.
211. Vinciguerra P, Torres I, Camesasca FI: Application of confocal microscopy in refractive surgery. J Ref Surg 2002; 18 (3 Suppl): S378-81.
212. Durairaj BD, Balentine J, Kouyoumdjian G et al: The predictability of corneal flap thickness and tissue laser ablation in laser in situ keratomileusis. Ophthalmology 2000; 107: 2140-2143.
213. Siganos CS, Kymionis GD, Astyrakakis N, Pallikaris IG: Management of corneal ectasia after LASIK with INTACS. J Ref Surg 2002; 18(1): 43-46.
214. Rumelt S, Cohen I, Skandarni P et al: Ultrastructure of the lamellar corneal wound after Lasik in human eye. J Cataract Ref Surg 2001; 27(8) 1323- 1327.

Chapter 27

Management of Refractive Complications: Conservative and Reoperations

Many refractive and visually disturbing complications following photorefractive procedures require attention at some stage to provide better quality of vision to the patient. These complications are:

1. Primary undercorrection/overcorrection
2. Regression
3. Corneal haze
4. Central steep islands
5. Decentered ablation
6. Asymmetrical healing
7. Halos and glare

Some of these complications like haze, regression, steep islands and asymmetrical healing are more of a problem after PRK. They are less common after LASIK. The initial management of these complications is conservative, as mentioned in Chapter 26 under the respective heads.

MEDICAL MANAGEMENT

Corneal Haze, Regression and Asymmetrical Healing

Corneal haze and regression are found in association in most of the cases after PRK. Low potency topical steroids are the mainstay for treatment of corneal haze, regression and asymmetrical healing following PRK. They have been used for even up to 9-12 months after this refractive surgery in some cases. Other pharmacological agents have also been tried to modulate the stromal healing response in case of these problems. This aspect has already been discussed in Chapter 5 and 16.

Low potency topical steroids are also useful for management of occasional cases of corneal haze after LASIK, though haze is infrequent following LASIK. *But their role in management of regression following LASIK is limited, as regression after this procedure is associated with different etiological mechanisms than after PRK (Chapter 26).* Treatment of regression following LASIK needs a definitive enhancement procedure after stability of refraction (usually about 3 months).

Overcorrections

Overcorrections may be treated by abrupt withdrawal of the postoperative steroid therapy after PRK. This is supposed to stimulate wound-healing response and induce regression. *Medical management is not expected to help in case of overcorrections (consecutive hyperopia) following LASIK,* since such a healing response does not occur after this procedure. Overcorrections following LASIK need to be dealt with retreatment.

Halos and Glare

These problems are likely to occur in patients with large pupil size in dim illumination and with smaller ablation zone diameter. However, modern algorithms use an ablation zone of 6 mm or more, particularly in patients with larger preoperative pupils. Other causes that may result in glare and halos, their prevention and management with anti-glare glasses, diluted (0.5%) pilocarpine and topical steroids (if halos and glare are associated with significant haze) have been discussed in Chapter 26.

OTHER MODALITIES

Contact lenses

Many patients with primary over- and undercorrection and regression without haze would benefit with use of contact lenses. Those patients, who are unwilling to undergo retreatment or are unsuitable for a repeat procedure as well as cases where refraction has not yet stabilized, are also candidates for contact lens fitting[1]. *Rigid contact lenses* are not useful for residual corrections because of vaulting over the central corneal flattening, which necessitates prescription of power almost equal to the preoperative refraction. Soft contact lenses would generally conform to the new surface curvature. *Specifically designed contact lenses* are now available, which cause less stagnation of tear-fluid over the apex of flat ablation zone and minimum trapping of air bubbles. They are useful alternatives for treating under- and overcorrection.

Hard contact lenses are used for management of central steep islands, while waiting for their natural resolution.

Epithelial Debridement

Scrapping of epithelium to treat *regression* following PRK had been advocated because epithelial hyperplasia might be a major contributory factor for this complication[3]. Durrie et al[2] recommended epithelial debridement for treating *overcorrections*. It was thought to stimulate a stronger healing response and induce regression in cases of persisting overcorrection.

But one must be cautious because this procedure may result in increased haze/subepithelial opacity. Fagerholm et al[4] reported that this procedure was not sufficient to correct significant primary undercorrection or regression.

Epithelial debridement has not been advocated for post-LASIK residual refractive errors and regression. This is because epithelial hyperplasia and corneal haze are not primary factors contributing to these problems. Moreover, epithelial debridement may result in increased risk for epithelial ingrowth following LASIK.

REOPERATIONS

Reoperations becomes necessary in above case if conservative management fails; and in cases of decentered ablation, and persistent central steep islands.

Repeat excimer laser surgeries *(reoperations)* for refractive complications of photorefractive procedures can be divided into the following types, depending upon the primary and secondary procedures used[6].

Simple Reoperations

For simple reoperations same procedure is used for the secondary surgery as was used for the primary procedure, e.g. secondary PRK in case of primary PRK and re-LASIK following primary LASIK.

Mixed Reoperations

The reoperation is termed 'mixed' if the secondary procedure is different from the primary one. For example LASIK after PRK and PTK for irregular astigmatism due to flap wrinkling following LASIK.

Reoperations are again divided into the following two groups, depending upon the indications.

Enhancements

If the reoperation is performed for primary undercorrection or regression, it is termed enhancement procedure.

Retreatments

Retreatments are repeat surgeries performed for treatment of other complications like decentered zone, steep islands, subepithelial scarring; enlargement of ablation zone in case of glare and halos, etc.

Planning Reoperations

When planning retreatment, certain crucial factors need consideration before retreatment in a given case. This is an essential step to achieve the best possible results after retreatment.

Retreatment: Preoperative Considerations

1. Refractive stability.
2. Postoperative refraction
3. Analysis of corneal topography.
4. Unaided visual acuity less than 20/40 or unacceptable to the patient.
5. No improvement with pharmacological agents.
6. Visually significant decentration.
7. No natural improvement in central islands after 6 months.
8. Adequate residual bed thickness.
9. Reconsideration of treatment algorithms.
10. Choice of refractive procedure.
11. Intraoperative technical variables.

Refractive Stability

Refractive stability is the most important criteria before retreatment. This is more applicable to PRK, where refraction remains unstable for 6 months or longer due to continued stromal remodeling, keratocytic activity and development of corneal haze (see Chapters 5, 16 and 24). LASIK induces minimal healing response and refraction stabilizes as early as 3 months following this procedure.

Stability of refraction and determination of accurate refraction should be done following the principles and methods already described in chapter 19. Additional points to be followed for determination of refraction in cases of retreatment are:

1. The topical steroids, which are being given for management of regression and/or haze, should be withdrawn for 3 months.
2. Refraction is evaluated on 3 consecutive, one monthly intervals. The difference should not be >0.5 D spherical equivalent.
3. This preoperative refraction before retreatment would decide the exact treatment protocol and the treatment strategy to be followed in an individual case.

Postoperative Refraction

Refractive ablation is contraindicated in cases of emmetropia and overcorrection. A plano-PTK approach should be followed if retreatment is needed for decentered ablation, central islands or for enlargement of the optical zone in case of troublesome glare and halos; and if the patient is emmetropic or overcorrected.

Failure of Medical Management

Retreatment would be indicated if the pharmacological agents given for modulating corneal haze and/or reverting regression have not worked after a sufficient trial. These agents are given for about 6 months for treating regression following PRK. In case significant corneal haze is also present, then they may be tried for up to one year.

Decentered Ablation

Treatment for decentered ablation is indicated if it is visually significant, i.e. it causes decrease in UCVA of < 20/40, uniocular diplopia, halos or glare disability.

Corneal Topography and Slit-Lamp Examination

The importance of computerized videokeratography (CVK) in planning retreatment has already been discussed earlier in Chapter 19. Serial topography and subtraction/difference maps are crucial in differentiating decentered ablation zone from asymmetrical healing and focal regression. They are also useful in following resolution of central islands.

Slit-lamp examination combined with CVK analysis helps in differentiating an *apparently* decentered ablation, detected during late postoperative period, from focal regression due to asymmetric healing. Slit-lamp examination in the latter case would document substantial haze in the area of increased corneal power.

Central Steep Islands

Usually a waiting for about 12 months is advised before taking a case of central steep island for retreatment. This is because most of the central islands show a natural tendency to subside by 6 months and all by 12 months. However, the timing of repeat surgery for central islands should also be considered against the severity of visual disability suffered by the patient, which may necessitate an earlier retreatment.

Residual Bed Thickness

The RBT must be adequate for considering a case for retreatment for undercorrection and regression. *A mandatory RBT of > 325 microns after retreatment is advised to avoid corneal ectasia.* Apart from the available corneal tissue, estimation of the probable RBT that would be left after re-surgery is based on the required corrections and the treatment algorithm employed by a particular laser system. Calculation of RBT after re-LASIK is not complicated by the flap thickness factor, unlike in case of primary LASIK. This is because variability of the cut is not a concern, as a flap of previously known thickness is relifted. *However, measurement of the stromal bed after relifting the flap should be done as a precautionary measure even for re-LASIK.*

When measuring the CCT, *the epithelial factor should be taken into account in case of repeat PRK.* This is because there may be variable degree of epithelial hyperplasia varying from 15-20 microns more than the normal epithelial thickness. Now confocal microscopy (Confoscan) can actually measure the epithelial thickness. If this facility is not available, the epithelium is assumed to be approximately 55 microns thick. The maximum permissible ablation is calculated as follows:

For PRK

Permissible
Ablation depth = CCT − epithelial thickness − 325 μ

For re-LASIK

Permissible
Ablation depth = CCT − flap thickness − 325 μ or, Stromal bed thickness − 325 μ

Treatment Algorithms

The results after retreatment are greatly modified by the treatment algorithms. New improved treatment algorithms, which are known to give better results, are to be employed to improve accuracy of results after re-operations. The treatment algorithms are dependent on the laser system employed. The laser system should be the one, which is known for more accuracy and predictability. *Older laser systems using broad beam laser or scanning systems used for the primary procedure should preferably be avoided.* A smaller error of algorithm of the laser system that was used previously is expected to reproduce the same results.

Intraoperative Factors

All efforts must be made to maintain strict adherence to appropriate conditions of tissue hydration and atmospheric conditions of the operating room like humidity and temperature. These factors are known to alter the ablation rate of the stroma and result in undesired refractive outcome.

Choice of Surgical Procedure

The excimer laser procedure employed for reoperations depends on a number of factors. These are:

Primary Refractive Procedure

PRK

For **enhancements** after PRK, either secondary PRK or LASIK may be chosen. Generally, surgeons preferred to perform PRK for enhancements after pervious PRK. The preference has now shifted towards LASIK as the secondary procedure due to better results after this procedure, particularly in cases of regression (vide infra). However, **retreatment** for central islands, topographical abnormalities (asymmetrical healing, focal regression) and decentered ablation would require repeat PRK, as these are surface based problems, which can be corrected with surface ablation only (PRK, alone or combined with PTK).

LASIK

For **enhancements** following LASIK, the secondary procedure has to be re-LASIK or wavefront-guided LASIK (if wavefront-sensing is possible). *PRK is not recommended as the secondary procedure after LASIK* because of presence of corneal flap, which would be damaged by surface ablation. If the residual stroma does not permit re-LASIK in case of residual refractive errors, the patient is to be rehabilitated with contact lens or spectacle correction.

However, **retreatment** for central islands and decentered ablation can be performed using the minimum possible ablation. PTK may be performed to smoothen the surface irregularities due to late detected flap wrinkles. Occasionally, in selected cases of thin flaps or buttonholes, a PRK approach may be used[5,6], but recutting of a deeper flap at a later date may be beneficial because of increased risk of haze following PRK[6] in these cases. PRK may also be indicated in case of previously failed attempts in applying suction ring or failure of flap cutting due to loss of suction[2].

The Results and Safety of the Procedure

LASIK procedures are known to be more predictable and associated with better visual results, less regression and corneal haze than PRK. However the risk of flap complications and corneal ectasia associated with LASIK is avoided with PRK. LASEK avoids drawbacks of both these procedures.

Available Corneal Thickness

Low residual thickness of cornea after the primary surgery may not allow LASIK as the secondary procedure.

Degree of Refractive Error

For enhancement procedures, if the correction to be made is unlikely to leave a safe residual bed thickness, LASIK would not be advisable. One may utilize the conventional correction with lenses or resort to LASEK (Chapter 24).

REOPERATIONS FOLLOWING PRK

For enhancements in case of regression and residual refractive errors, LASIK is to be preferred to repeat PRK. The reason are:

1. The factors which have led to regression following primary PRK would operate in a similar manner after repeat PRK[7].
2. Similarly repeat PRK following primary undercorrections is likely to produce more healing response in the form of stromal remodeling, haze and epithelial hyperplasia because the healing response is more with deeper ablation (Chapter 5 and 26). These factors, then, would result in regression.
3. Less chances of steroid induced increase in intraocular pressure because their requirement is minimized following LASIK as compared to PRK.
4. Regression is an infrequent problem after LASIK than after PRK[8].
5. The reported success rate of retreatments by PRK is even lower than the primary procedure[7,9].
6. Results of LASIK enhancement procedures in cases of residual myopia and regression after PRK are encouraging[10-13].

Enhancement Strategies For Secondary PRK

1. Regression is frequently associated with significant subepithelial haze. Corneal haze results in an irregularity of anterior stroma, forming ridges and valleys.
2. PRK enhancement procedures after epithelial debridement must be accompanied with an initial minimal PTK for anterior stromal smoothening.
3. A transepithelial approach has been found to give good results, where the epithelium acts as a smoothening agent.
4. Laser ablation is preferably performed using an advanced scanning laser system, as discussed previously. Extra laser pulse are delivered to smoothen peripheral ablation edge, in view of the different ablation rate of epithelium and the presumed epithelial hyperplasia, if using transepithelial approach.
5. A slight under-treatment is advocated because of a heightened healing response and activation of the same mechanisms that had resulted in regression previously.
6. A larger ablation zone, with multizone approach is to be employed in cases of larger corrections and if ablation zone diameter was small previously.

REOPERATIONS FOLLOWING LASIK

As mentioned earlier, every care should be taken to obtain an accurate refraction in cases of reoperations, more so for enhancements. Refraction must be stable for at least one month following LASIK. Refractive corrections can be performed as early as 3–6 months after LASIK. Three months is the earliest period, when refraction can be stable in case of LASIK.

Lifting of the Flap

The flap can be easily relifted from the stromal bed for up to one year after LASIK. There are reports of relifting the flap as late as 2–3 years[6,14,15]. Relifting of the flap may be difficult sometimes. This can occur due to increased adherence of the flap due to previous inflammation, irregular cut and uneven ablation resulting in fibrosis. A flap that has its edge near the limbus (e.g. in case of hyperopic LASIK) may also be difficult to relift. Such cases are managed by recutting a new flap after about 12 months, when the previous flap is reasonably secure to its bed. The following steps are followed for relifting of the flap.

1. The hinge of the flap is located carefully at the slit-lamp. The flap margins are marked gently with a fine instrument or with a dye such as gential violet or a fine tipped marker pen.
2. Adhesions at the flap edge are broken with a Sinsky hook..
3. The flap is gently 'peeled off' from the stromal bed with the help of forceps. The flap must be handled carefully throughout all these maneuvers.

4. If one meets with resistance in lifting the flap, it is best to leave it in place and plan for a recut at a later date.

Recutting of the Flap

1. A new flap can be recut after about 3 months in case of buttonhole or partial flap. A new blade and deeper than the previous depth plate setting (20–60 micron) should be used in this case.
2. But this option is postponed for about 12 months in case of an adherent flap as mentioned earlier. In this case, the same depth plate setting must be used to avoid slivers of the stromal tissue.

Laser Ablation and Flap Repositioning

1. Same steps and all the precautions are followed regarding laser ablation and care of the flap during ablation, as described for the primary procedure (Chapter 23).
2. Special care is taken to avoid ablation of the edge of stromal bed and the flap hinge, particularly in case of hyperopic enhancements, where ablation has to be extended towards the periphery. This is essential to avoid risk of epithelial ingrowth.
3. In case of re-LASIK, extra care is required for removal of any interface debris, epithelial tags and for smoothening of the flap wrinkles after repositioning of the flap.

Special Complications after Re-LASIK

1. Corneal haze is more common problem after re-LASIK in patients who had PRK as the primary procedure[10, 11]. However, Comaish et al[13] did not find significant haze after LASIK in 32 eyes treated for PRK enhancements.
2. Epithelial ingrowth rate is found to be higher (up to 31%) in case of re-LASIK. This because the flap edge becomes irregular after relifting and provides channel for epithelial ingrowth[16, 17]. Rojas et al[18] did not find higher incidence of epithelial ingrowth in 36 eyes treated for myopic overcorrection with re-LASIK.
3. Higher incidence of other complications like flap striae (5.5–5.6%), flap melting (10.9%) and decentered ablation (1.8%) has been reported after re-LASIK[16, 17].

RETREATMENT OF CENTRAL STEEP ISLANDS

1. Central steep islands spontaneously resolve within 6 months in majority of cases after PRK. Retreatment for persistent central islands, not amenable to rigid contact lens treatment, is generally indicated after this period following PRK[19, 20]. The tendency of the steep islands to resolve following LASIK is less[21, 22].
2. Early retreatment would be indicated in cases of central steep islands following LASIK and in cases associated with intolerable visual symptoms not relieved with hard contact lenses.
3. it is very difficult to ascertain refraction in presence of central islands. Therefore, treatment is mostly based on CVK data, which shows the diopteric power of the steep island and its size.
4. Due to lack of accurate postoperative refraction, retreatment is performed in PTK-mode, confined to the central steep island. This is facilitated by use of a suitable masking agent, which protects the surrounding cornea. A conservative approach during ablation is recommended to avoid hyperopic shift.
5. Use of a spot scanning laser system is mandatory for retreatment because broad beam laser is associated with increased risk of central steep islands[22] (Chapter 26).
6. In cases, where refraction is possible and it shows undercorrection, refractive ablation after a minimum possible PTK smoothening can be performed.
7. Treatment of central islands following PRK is performed after epithelial debridement because transepithelial approach has been found to increase the incidence of this topographical abnormality.
8. Treatment of central islands following LASIK is performed after relifting the flap.

RETREATMENT OF CORNEAL HAZE

1. Corneal haze following LASIK is minimal and no case of retreatment for corneal haze following LASIK has been reported.
2. Significant corneal haze after PRK is generally associated with regression. Retreatment for regression may address to this problem also. In this situation, first a minimal PTK treatment is given to clear subepithelial haze, followed by refractive ablation, as mentioned previously.

3. Isolated corneal haze is managed medically for about 1–2 years, because the natural history of corneal haze is one of complete resolution. Retreatment is indicated for persistent haze causing subepithelial opacity/scarring without significant refractive error. A conservative PTK ablation is utilized after epithelial debridement.

RETREATMENT FOR DECENTRATION

Retreatment is indicated for significant decentered ablation zone (several millimeters), associated with loss of BCVA and/or troublesome visual symptoms.

Results of retreatment for decentered ablation zone have significantly improved with newer technologies like CVK analysis (difference maps), scanning laser systems and topography linked ablation (TopoLink, Chapter 19).

1. Retreatment for decentered ablation zone can be performed using 3–4 mm ablation zone. For retreatment, ablation zone is decentered in an opposite direction to the original one, thus ablating the edge of the pervious ablation zone. This approach enlarges the optical zone and brings the edge of the previous ablation zone out of the papillary axis.

2. The depth of ablation of this secondary small zone ablation is equal to the previous preoperative correction.

3. This treatment is likely to produce hyperopic shift because of tissue removal from the central cornea as well. Protecting the already ablated area with a suitable masking agent may help in avoiding the hyperopic shift. This treatment strategy, similar to the one used for treating focal areas of regression/topographical abnormalities, has been discussed in Chapter 19, under role of CVK in postoperative management.

4. Corneal ablation assisted by topography (Topo Link) or customized ablation are better modalities for retreatment of decentered ablation, so as in case of other postoperative topographical abnormalities (asymmetrical healing, focal regression, central steep islands).

SPECIAL PROBLEMS FOR RETREATMENT OF DECENTERED ABLATION FOLLOWING LASIK

Retreatment of decentered ablation zone with conventional methods of ablation is difficult. It is limited by the diameter of corneal flap and the size of the stromal bed. The edge of stromal bed may inadvertently get ablated. This would increase the risk of epithelial ingrowth. Topography linked ablation might minimize the chances of ablation of the edge of stromal bed but may not be able to completely avoid this problem.

Gimbel et al[23] have suggested an "Epithelial template technique" in desperate cases of decentered ablation following LASIK. The essential steps of this technique are:

1. First, epithelial ablation is performed using the epithelium as a template. Here caution must be exercised not to ablate through epithelium and reach the anterior stroma.
2. If the immediate postoperative topography is satisfactory and the ablation pattern is centered within the flap diameter, same treatment can be performed on the stromal bed after relifting the flap.
3. This secondary procedure is performed after allowing sufficient time for the healing of ablated epithelial.

Suggested readings

1. Schipper I, Businger V, Pfarrer R: Fitting contact lenses after excimer laser photorefractive keratectomy for myopia. CLAO J 1995; 21: 281-284.
2. Durrie DS, Lesher MP, Hunkeler JD: Treatment of overcorrection after myopic PRK. J Refract Corneal Surg 1994; 10 (Suppl): S295.
3. Loewenstein A, Lipshitz I, Lazar M: Scrapping of epithelium for treatment of undercorrection and haze after PRK. J Ref Corn Surg 1994; 10(Suppl): S274-S276.
4. Fagerholm PP, Epstein D, Tengroth BM et al: Refractive outcome following epithelial abrasion in eyes with regression after PRK for myopia. Invest Ophthalmol Vis Sci 1994; 35 (Suppl): 1724 (abst).
5. Jain VK, Abell TG, Bond WI, Stevens G Jr: Immediate transepithelial photorefractive keratectomy for treatment of laser in situ keratomileusis flap complications. J Refract Surg 2002 Mar-Apr; 18(2): 109-12.
6. Gimbel HV, Penno EE et al: LASIK enhancement and retreatment concerns, in 'LASIK Complications: Prevention and Management', second edition, Slack Incorporated publications, 2001.

7. Snibson GR, McCarty CA, Aldred GF et al: Retreatment after excimer laser PRK; the Melbourne Excimer Laser Group. Am J Ophthalmol 1996; 121: 250-157.
8. Pallikaris IG, Siganos DS: Excimer laser in situ keratomileusis and PRK for correction of high myopia. J Cataract Ref Surg 1994; 10: 498-510.
9. Gartry DS, Larkin DFP, Hill AR et al: Retreatment for significant regression after excimer laser photorefractive keratectomy: a prospective, randomized, masked trial. Ophthalmology 1998; 105: 131-141.
10. Alio JL, Artola A, Attia WH et al: LASIK for retreatment of residual myopia after PRK. Am J Ophthalmol 2001; 132: 196-203.
11. Lazaro C, Castillo A, Hernandez-Matamoros JL et al: LASIK enhancement after PRK. Ophthalmology 2001; 108: 1423-1429; discussions by SN Rao. PA Mazumdar, 1429.
12. Agarwal A. Agarwal T et al: LASIK for residual myopia after radial keratotomy and PRK. J Cataract Ref Surg 2001; 27: 901-906.
13. Comaish IF, Domniz YY, Lawless MB et al: Laser in-situ keratomileusis for residual myopia after PRK. J Cataract Ref Surg 2002; 28: 775-781.
14. Iskander NG, Peters NT, Anderson Penno EE, Gimbel HV: Postoperative complications in LASIK. Current Opinion In Ophthalmology. 2000; 11(4): 273-279.
15. Salah T: Reoperations following LASIK. In: Pallikaris IG, Siganos D, eds. LASIK. Thorofare, NJ; SLACK Incorporated; 1998: 307.
16. Zadok D, Maskaleris G, Garcia V et al: Outcomes of retreatment after LASIK. Ophthalmology 1991; 106: 2391-2394.
17. Lyle WA, Jin GJC: Retreatment after initial LASIK. J cataract Ref Surg 2000; 26: 650-659.
18. Rojas MC, Haw WW, Manche EE: LASIK enhancement for consecutive hyperopia after myopic overcorrection. J Cataract Ref Surg 2002; 28: 37-43.
19. Lin DTC: Corneal topographic analysis after excimer laser PRK. Ophthalmology 1994; 101: 1432-1439.
20. McGhee CNJ, Bryce IG: The natural history of central steep islands following excimer laser PRK. J Cataract Ref Surg 1996; 22: 1151-1158.
21. Wilson SE: LASIK complications. Cornea 1998; 17 (5): 459-467.
22. Slade SG: Abnormal induced topography; Central islands. In: Machat JJ, ed. "Excimer Laser Refractive Surgery: Practice and Principles". Thorofare NJ: SLACK Incorporated; 1996:399.
23. Gimbel HV, Penno EE et al: In 'LASIK Complications: Prevention and Management, second edition, Slack Incorporated publications, 2001.

Index

A

Aberrometers 2, 19
Ablatable mask 176, 191
Ablation depth 30
Ablation, excimer laser
   large area 47, 124
   paracentral 130
   scanning 14, 50
Ablation rate 30
Ablation threshold 30
Ablation zone
   decentration 177
   diameter 177
Ablative photodecomposition 20, 28
Absorption coefficient of lasers 37
Acoustic shock waves 42
Acyclovir, and excimer laser surgeries 107
Adherence of epithelium 33
Alignment system 46
Ammetropia 81
Amplification, laser 8
Apical zone diameter 56
Arc lamp 10
Arcus juveniles 63
Arcus senile 63
Argon fluoride laser 1, 28
Argon laser 10, 17
Astigmatic keratotomy 96
Astigmatism, corneal 55
Automated lamellar keratoplasty, (ALK) 87
Axial length 81

B

Bacterial keratitis, following
   contact lenses 156
   excimer laser surgeries 232
Band keratopathy
   rough 65
   smooth 65
   treatment 65
Bandage contact lens 72, 133
Basement membrane 56
Basement membrane ablation 125
Basement membrane dystrophy 70
Bare sclera surgery, for pterygium 110
Barrier function of
   endothelium 60
   epithelium 56
Bettie's dystrophy 73
Biber-Hab-Dimer dystrophy (lattice dystrophy) 72
Biomask 125
Bleachable dye 11
Bread crumb dystrophy (Granular dystrophy, Groenouw-I dystrophy) 71
Boltzmann's energy distribution 7
Bowman's layer 29, 33, 55
Bowman's layer dyasrophy 70
Buttonholes 248

C

Calibration of laser energy 47
Carbon-dioxide laser 10, 19
Cataractogenesis 37
Cavitation, after photodisruption 19
Central corneal thickness (CCT) 40
Central steep islands 42, 240
Centration of ablation zone during laser ablation 129
Chromophores 16
Clear lens extraction 99
Chiron-Technolas Keracor excimer laser system 51
Climatic droplet keratopathy (spheroidal degeneration) 66
Cogan's epithelial dystrophy, (microcystic epithelial dystrophy, epithelial basement membrane dystrophy, map-dot-fingerprint dystrophy) 70
Coherent waves 8
Cold-spots, in laser beam 49
Collateral damage 20
Collateral damage due to laser ablation 20, 32
Complications of excimer laser surgeries 266
Computerized videokeratography (CVK) 60
Contact lens, and management of refractive complications 266
Continuous wave mode 11
Contrast visual acuity 242
Cornea farinata 64
Corneal blindness 1
Corneal clarity following PTK 145
Corneal degenerations 62
Corneal dimensions 55
Corneal dystrophies 69
Corneal ectasia 38
Corneal edema 256
Corneal flap
   diameter 188
   orientation 188
   thickness 39, 188
Coupling fluids 256
Corneal haze 33, 145, 233
Corneal hypoesthesia 35, 235
Corneal hypoxia 59, 155
Corneal neovascularization 155
Corneal perforation, following LASIK 249
Corneal sensitivity 35, 113, 171
Corneal surgical procedures 82
Corneal topography 165
Corneal transparency 60
Crocodile shagreen of Vogt 64
Cryotherapy/laser photocoagulation, before myopic ablation 41, 170
Customized LASIK or C-LASIK 2, 190

D

Decentred ablation zone 277
Degenerations, corneal
   age-related 63
   lipid degeneration 66
   hyaline degeneration 67
   pigmentary degeneration 67
   pellucid marginal 68
   Terrien's marginal degeneration 69
   spheroidal degeneration 66
Delayed epithelial healing 235

Derby-shaped beam 49
Descemet's membrane response 34
Difference maps 167
Diffraction of light 189
Diclofenac sodium after excimer
　laser ablation 132
DNA, and excimer laser ablation 42
Diffuse lamellar keratitis 251
Displaced flap 250
Divergence of laser waves 8
Drug hypersensitivity 227
Drug toxicity 227
Dye lasers 10, 17
Dystrophies, corneal
　Bowman's layer 70
　endothelial 73
　epithelial 70
　epithelial-endothelial (Fuchs') 74
　stromal 71

E

Electronically controlled devices
　and laser pulse shortening 11
Elevation maps 108
Elliptical method 180
Enantiomorphism 169
End point of PTK ablation 128
Endothelial cell count 58, 171
Endothelial dystrophies 73
Endothelial pump 59
Endothelial response to excimer laser
　ablation 33
Entrance pupil 129
Epikeratophakia 88
　after corneal ectasia 255
Epithelial functions 56
Epithelial hyperplasia 31
Epithelial debridement,
　during surface ablation 119, 120
Epithelial healing after surface
　ablation 131
Epithelial ingrowth, following
　LASIK 253
Erbium: YAG laser 10, 19
Erodible mask 176, 191
Excimer lasers 10, 27, 37
　ablation threshold 30
　beam smoothening 49
　clinical applications 2
　energy calibration 47
　large (wide) beam 47
　　advantages 49, 107
　　disadvantages 40, 49, 107
　output failure 225
　　intraoperative 225
　　cause 225
　　management 225

solid state 14
scanning beam 50
Excimer laser delivery,
　broad beam/wide beam 45
　scanning 50
Excimer laser delivery systems
　Chiron-Technolas Keracor-116 51
　Chiron-Technolas Keracor-117 and
　　217 C 51
　Coherent-Schwind Keratome 51
　Kera Technology ISO beam 51
　Meditek MEL 60 51
　Nidek EC-500 51
　Nidek MK 2000 51
　Summit apex plus laser system
　Visx 2015 51
　Visx 2020 51
Excimer lasers interaction with ocular
　tissues 30
Excimer laser intrastromal
　keratomileusis 2
Excited state, of atoms 7
Eye-tracker 46

F

Failure to remove the epithelium
　adequately 229
FDA approval for PRK 174
FDA approval for PTK 111
FDA studies 111
Ferry line 67
Flap edema 250
Flap folds 250
Flap shrinkage 250
Flap wrinkling 250
Flash lamp 10
Fleck dystrophy 73
Fleisher ring 67
Fluorometholone, after excimer laser
　surgery reduction of haze 132, 234
Fluence 29
Fluorescence, and
　spontaneous emissions 7
　secondary 35
Focal smoothening 125
Forward shift of corneal curvature 38, 245
Free caps 249
Frequency conversion 13
　second harmonic (doubling) 14
　third harmonic (tripling) 14
　fourth harmonic (quadrupling) 14
　fifth harmonic (quintupling) 14
Free radicals, and excimer
　laser surgery 41
Fuchs' dystrophy 74
Fundus evaluation, before excimer laser
　surgeries 170

G

Gas medium 10
Giant papillary conjunctivitis (GPC) 156
Glare 243
Glare visual acuity 242
Gold vapor laser 11
Granular dystrophy
　(bread-crumb dystrophy,
　Groenouw-I dystrophy) 71
Groenouw-II dystrophy
　(macular dystrophy) 72
Graft failure, after PTK 236
Ground state, of atoms 7
Guttae, corneal, see
　corneal guttata

H

Halos and ghost images, after
　excimer laser refractive surgeries 243
Hansatome 127
Hassal-Henle bodies 64
Healing response of the stroma 33
Herpes simplex keratitis scars 109
Hexagonal keratotomy 98
Higher-order aberrations 191
Holmium: YAG 10, 83, 96
Homogenization of laser beam 49
Hot-spots in laser beam 49
Hydrogen fluoride laser 10
Hydrokeratomes 188
Hyperopic PRK 180
Hyperopic shift after PTK 129, 143, 236

I

Inadequate exposure 246
Inadequate suction 247
Inappropriate ablation 239
Incomplete flap 247
Induced astigmatism, after
　PTK 129, 143, 236
　excimer laser refractive surgeries 239
Interface debris 251
Interferon-alpha-2b 134
Intracorneal lenses 89
Intraocular lenses 100
Intraocular surgical procedures 99
Intrastromal refractive keratectomy 2, 12
Intrastromal ring segment 90
Irradiance, of excimer lasers 29
Irregular astigmatism 56
Isopropyl alcohol, and
　epithelial removal 119

K

Keratoconus 108
Keratomileusis 86

mechanical 86
  manual 87
  automated
    escimer laser 184
Keratophakia 88
Krypton chloride excimer laser 28
Krypton fluoride excimer laser 28
Krypton laser 10, 17

L

Large area photoablation 47, 175
Large beam laser systems 51
Laser assisted in-situ keratomileusis:
  LASIK 184
Laser-assisted subepithelial keratectomy:
  LASEK 205
Laser beam smoothening 49
Laser beam
  derby-shaped 49
  flat top/hat-shaped 49
  gaussian 49
  truncated gaussian 49
Laser cavity 9, 45
Laser delivery
  continuous mode 11
  fundamental mode 12
  monomode 12
  multimode 12
  pulse mode 11
Laser failure of ablation 227
Laser mechanical failure 227
Laser microkeratomes 189
Laser pump 9, 45
Laser scalpel 2
Laser system 9
Laser thermokeratoplasty 17, 83
Laser waves
  in phase 14
  out of phase 14
Lasing media 10
Lattice dystro 72
Lid edema and blepharoptosis 229
Liquid medium 10
Loss of BCVA 241
Lost flap 249
Lower-order optical aberrations 190

M

Manual superficial keratectomy 125
Masking agents 127, 130
Mechanical damage to flap 247
Mechanical microkeratomes,
  maintenance 186
Methods of measuring the optical
  aberrations 191
Microkeratome 185
Microkeratome blade 186
Microkeratome
  automated 186
    electromechanical 188
    turbine operated 188
  hydro-jet 188
  laser 189
  manual 186
Mitomycin- C, and stromal healing
  modulation 134
Mode locking 11
Modified taper technique 124
Monochromatic rays 8
Mucus plaques or tags 229
Multipass ablation 177
Multizone ablation 48
Multizone multipass 178
Multizone technique 177
Mutagenesis 42
Myopic regression 239

N

Nd: YLF 10
Near vision, and refractive surgeries 161
Non-ablatable mask 191
Non-linear crystals 14
Normalized maps 167
NSAIDs, topical and postoperative
  management 131-134

O

Optical breakdown 18
Optical mixing 13
Orbscan I 40
Orbscan II 257
Overcorrection 238
Overlapping zones ablation 124
Oxygen free-radical and excimer laser
  ablation 41

P

Pachymetry 40
Pancorneal photoablation 124
Para-central ablation 130
Partial ablation 130
Pellucid marginal degeneration 68
Penetrating keratoplasty 1, 77
Phakic intraocular lens 100
Phase matching and frequency
  conversion 13
Photochemical effect 19, 28
Photocoagulation 16
Photodisruption 18
Photodynamic effect 22
Photodynamic therapy 20
Photokeratitis 42
Photon 7
Photorefractive keratectomy for
  astigmatism: PARK 179
Photorefractive keratectomy: PRK 2
Photosensitizing agents 20
Phototherapeutic keratectomy: PTK 2, 108
Photothermal effect 16
Photothermal tissue shrinkage 17
Phototoxicity 37
Photovaporization 19
Pigmentary degenerations 67
Plasma formation, and
  photodistruption 18
Plasminogen-inhibitors 133
Point and shoot technique 124
Polishing technique 125
Population inversion 9
Posterior corneal topography 40
Postoperative pain 230
Preoperative evaluation
  for PTK 112
  for refractive surgeries 158
Pretreatment of corneal surface 118
Prophylaxis, against bacterial
  keratitis after laser surgery 232
Pseudomembrane after excimer laser
  ablation 32
Pseudopterygium 68
Pterygium 67
Pulsed mode delivery of lasers 11

Q

Q -switching 11

R

Radial keratotomy 91
Reactivation of herpes simplex keratitis
  after excimer ablation 235
Recurrent corneal erosion
  syndrome 75, 108
Recurrent corneal microerosions 246
Refractive changes after
  PTK 129, 143, 236
Regression 235
Relaxing incisions 97
Reoperations 266
Repetition rate 29
Residual stromal bed thickness
  (RBT) 39, 256, 270
Results of excimer laser surgeries 212
Retinal detachments 41
Ruby laser 10

S

Salzmann's nodular degeneration 66
Scanning laser systems 50, 14
Secondary fluorescence 38
Shock wave generation 19
Single zone ablation 176
Single-pass multizone ablation 177

Single-ring technique 84
Slit scanning 51, 176
Smoothening technique 127
Solid medium 10
Solid state excimer lasers 14
Specular microscopy 58
Spheroidal degeneration 66
Spontaneous emission 7
Spot scanning 50
Standard taper technique 124
Stem cells 57
Sterile corneal infiltrates/sterile stromal infiltrates 231
Steroid induced elevation of IOP 237
Stimulated emission 8
Stokes law 8
Stromal dystrophies 71
Stromal melts 256
Subtraction maps 167
Suction ring 189
Surface heating 42
Surface waves 42

T

Tangential maps 168
Tapered transition zone ablation 179
Tear-film changes after PTK 146
Terrien's marginal degeneration 69
Thermal effect of lasers 16, 83
Thermokeratoplasty 83
Thickness plate 187
Thin flaps 248
Thyraton 10
Top hat-shaped ablation 49
Topical anaesthetics 133
Topical medication 131–134
TopoLink 168, 171
Traccomatous scarring 1, 109
Transition zone ablation 48
Transpupillary thermotherapy (TTT) 20
Traumatic rupture 38
Two-ring technique 84

U

Undercorrection 238

V

Viability of epithelial cells after LASEK 210
Vision-2020 program 1
Vogt's limbal girdle 63

W

Water-jet microkeratomes 188
Wavefront-guided LASIK 190
Wedge-resection 97
Wetting agents 127
Wrinkled flap 250

X

Xenon chloride excimer laser 28
Xenon fluoride excimer laser 28